Children and Exercise X

Children and Exercise XXVIII presents the latest scientific research into paediatric exercise physiology, endocrinology, kinanthropometry, growth and maturation, and youth sport. Including contributions from a wide-range of leading international experts, the book is arranged into eight sections :

- The Josef Rutenfranz lecture
- Keynote lectures
- Physiology
- Neuromuscular issues
- Cardiovascular and cardiorespiratory fitness
- Physical fitness and health
- Physical activity and sedentary behaviour
- Sport participation and the young athlete

Offering critical reviews of current topics and reports of current and on-going research in paediatric health and exercise science, this is a key text for all researchers, teachers, health professionals and students with an interest in paediatric sport and exercise science, sports medicine and physical education.

Manuel Coelho e Silva is Associate Professor of Auxology and Kinanthropometry, and coordinator of the Research Center for the Study of Sport and Physical Activity in the University of Coimbra, Portugal.

Amândio Cupido-dos-Santos is Assistant Professor of Exercise Physiology and Assessment of Elite Athletes in the University of Coimbra, Portugal.

António J Figueiredo is Assistant Professor of Training Methods and Youth Sports, and Dean in the Faculty of Sport Science and Physical Education in the University of Coimbra, Portugal.

José P Ferreira is Associate Professor, coordinator of the master program in Exercise and Health for Special Groups, and coordinator of the Sport Psychology Laboratory in the University of Coimbra, Portugal.

Neil Armstrong is Professor of Paediatric Physiology, Vice-President and Senior Deputy Vice-Chancellor of the University of Exeter, UK.

First published 2014
by Routledge
2 Park Square, Milton Park, Abingdon, Oxfordshire OX14 4RN

Simultaneously published in the USA and Canada
by Routledge
711 Third Avenue, New York, NY 10017

First issued in paperback 2014

Routledge is an imprint of the Taylor and Francis Group, an informa business

British Library Cataloguing in Publication Data
A catalogue record for this book is available from the British Library

Library of Congress Cataloging in Publication Data

ISBN 978-0-415-82972-4 (hbk)
ISBN 978-1-138-91694-4 (pbk)
ISBN 978-0-203-40458-4 (ebk)

Typeset in Times New Roman
by MJCS

Children and Exercise XXVIII

The Proceedings of the 28th Pediatric Work Physiology Meeting

Edited by Manuel J Coelho-e-Silva, Amândio Cupido-dos-Santos, António J Figueiredo, José P Ferreira and Neil Armstrong

London and New York

Contents

PREFACE

Children and Exercise XXVIII contains the Proceedings of the 2013 Symposium of the European Group of Pediatric Work Physiology held in Curia, Anadia, PORTUGAL. This symposium was hosted by the Research Centre for the Study of Sport and Physical Activity, University of Coimbra.

1968	Dortmund, Germany	J. Rutenfranz
1969	Liblice, Czechoslovakia	V.S. Seliger
1970	Stockholm, Sweden	C. Thoren
1972	Netanya, Israel	O. Bar-Or
1973	De Haan, Belgium	M. Hebblinck
1974	Sec, Czechoslovakia	M. Macek
1975	Trois Rivieires, Canada	R.J. Shephard
1976	Bisham Abbey, UK	C.T.M. Davies
1978	Marstand, Sweden	B.O. Eriksson
1981	Jousta, Finland	J. Ilmarinen
1983	Papendahl, Netherlands	R.A. Binkhorst
1985	Hardenhausen, Germany	J Rutenfranz
1987	Hurdal, Norway	S. Oseid
1989	Leuven, Belgium	G Beunen
1989	Seregelyes, Hungary	R. Frenkl
1991	St. Sauves, France	J Coudert, E. Van Praagh
1993	Hamilton, Canada (*)	O. Bar-Or
1995	Odense, Denmark	K. Froberg
1997	Exeter, UK	N. Armstrong
1999	Rome, Italy	A Calzolari
2001	Corsedonk, Belgium	D. Matthys
2003	Porto, Portugal	J. Maia
2005	Gwatt, Switzerland	S. Kriemler, N Farpour-Lambert
2007	Tallinn, Estonia	T. Jurimae
2009	Le Touquet, France	G. Baquet, S. Berthoin
2010	Niagara, Canada (*)	B. Timmons
2011	Mawgan Porth, UK	C. Williams
2013	Anadia, Portugal	M. Coelho-e-Silva

(*) Joint meetings with NASPEM (North American Society of Pediatric Exercise Medicine.

The 2013 International Symposium followed PWP tradition with an emphasis on discussion of issues and research relating exercise, physical activity and sport in children and youth. This volume reflects the formal programme and contains the Josef Rutenfranz Lecture, keynote presentations and 45 "peer-reviewed" communications.

ACKNOWLEDGMENTS AND WORKING GROUPS

Chair
Manuel J Coelho-e-Silva
University of Coimbra, PORTUGAL

Co-chairs
Amândio Cupido dos Santos, António J. Figueiredo, José P. Ferreira
[University of Coimbra, PORTUGAL]

Committee of Honor
Emídio Guerreiro [XIX Government of Portuguese Republic, State Secretary]. *Litério Marques* [Anadia Municipality]. *João Gabriel Silva* [Rector of the University of Coimbra]. *Augusto Baganha* [Portuguese Institute of Sport and Youth]. *Miguel Seabra* [Fundação para a Ciência e a Tecnologia]. *José Manuel Constantino* [President of the Portuguese Olympic Committee]. *Pedro Machado* [Regional Tourism Office]. *Marcos Onofre* [Portuguese Society of Physical Education] *António Guerra* [Portuguese Society of Pediatrics]. *Jorge Laíns* [Portuguese Society of Physical Medicine and Rehabilitation]. *J Fonseca Esteves* [Portuguese Society of Sports Medicine]. *Davide Carvalho* [Portuguese Society for the Study of Obesity]

International Scientific Committee
Adam Baxter-Jones [University of Saskatchewan, CANADA]. *Alon Eliakim* [Tel-Aviv University, ISRAEL]. *Christons Kotzamanidis* [Aristotl University Thessaloniki, GREECE]. *Craig Williams* [University of Exeter, UK]. *Daniel Courteix* [Blaise Pascal University of Clermont-Ferrand, FRANCE]. *Emmanuel Van Praagh* [Blaise Pascal University of Clermont-Ferrand, FRANCE]. *Gareth Stratton* [University of Swansea, UK]. *Georges Baquet* [University of Lille 2, FRANCE]. *Geraldine Naughton* [Australian Catholic University, AUSTRALIA]. *Han CG Kemper* [Vrije University of Amsterdam, NETHERLANDS]. *Helge Hebestreit* [University of Würzburg, GERMANY]. *Joey C. Eisenmann* [Michigan State University, USA]. *Jorge Mota* [University of Porto, PORTUGAL]. *José Maia* [University of Porto, PORTUGAL]. *Lars Bo Andersen* [University of Southern Denmark, DENMARK]. *Manuel J Coelho-e-Silva* [University of Coimbra, PORTUGAL]. *Mark Tremblay* [University of Ottawa, CANADA]. *Nathalie Farpour-Lambert* [Geneve University Hospital, SWITZERLAND]. *Neil Armstrong* [University of Exeter, UK]. *Philippe Obert* [University of Avignon, FRANCE]. *Robert Malina* [University of Texas, USA]. *Susi Kriemler* [Universit of Zurich, SWITZERLAND]. *Thomas Rowland* [Baystate Medical Center, USA]. *Tim Takken* [University Medical Center Utrecht, NETHERLANDS].

Local Scientific Committee
Ana Teixeira [University of Coimbra, PORTUGAL]. *Carlos Fontes Ribeiro* [University of Coimbra, PORTUGAL]. *Isabel Fragoso* [Technical University of Lisbon, PORTUGAL]. *João Páscoa Pinheiro* [Medical School, PORTUGAL]. *Luís Bettencourt Sardinha* [Technical University of Lisbon, PORTUGAL]. *Luís Rama* [University of Coimbra, PORTUGAL]. *Paula Tavares* [University of Coimbra, PORTUGAL]. *Raul Martins* [University of Coimbra, PORTUGAL]. *Rui Gomes* [University of Coimbra, PORTUGAL]

International Organizing Committee
Albrecht Claessens [Catholic University of Leuven, BELGIUM]. *António Prista* [Pedagogical University of Maputo, MOZAMBIQUE]. *Chris Visscher* [University Medical Center Groningen, NETHERLANDS]. *Edilson Cyrino* [Londrina State University, BRAZIL]. *Kevin Finn* [University of Northern Iowa, USA]. *Laura Capranica* [University di Roma Foro Italico, ITALY]. *Lauren Sherar* [Loughborough University, UK]. *Luíz dos Anjos* [Federal University Fluminense, BRAZIL]. *Maria Eugenia Peña Reyes* [Escuela Nacional de Antropologia e Historia, MEXICO]. *Marije Elferink-Gemser* [University Medical Center Groningen, NETHERLANDS]. *Ning ZiHeng* [Politechnic Institute of Macau, CHINA]. *Renaat Philippaerts* [University of Ghent, BELGIUM]. *Richard Fisher* [St Mary's University College, UK]. *Roel Vaeyens* [University of Ghent, BELGIUM]. *Sean P Cumming* [University of Bath, UK].

Local Organizing Committee
Alain Massart. Aristides Machado-Rodrigues. Artur Santos. Beatriz Gomes. Carlos E. Gonçalves. Elsa Silva. Ivo Rego. João Valente-dos-Santos. Maria João Campos. Miguel Fachada. Miguel Oliveira. Paulo Nobre. Pedro Gaspar. Vasco Vaz.

Committee of the Oral Comunication Award
Karin Pfeiffer [Michigan State University]. *Marije T. Elferink-Gemser* [University of Groningen; HAN University of Applied Sciences]. *José Pedro Ferreira* [University of Coimbra]

Committee of the Poster Presentation Award
Lauren Sherar [University of Loughborough]. *Edilson Cyrino* [Londrina State University]. *Maria Eugenia Peña Reyes* [Escuela Nacional de Antropologia e Historia, MEXICO]. *Amândio Cupido-dos-Santos* [University of Coimbra]

Committee of the Hans Stoboy Award
Han C. G. Kemper [Amsterdam]. *Shannon R Siegel* [California State University, San Bernardino]. *António J Figueiredo* [University of Coimbra]

Accreditation of Medical Education

Carlos Fontes Ribeiro [Medical School, *University of Coimbra*]. *Luís Horta* [Portuguese Agency for Doping Prevention]

Delegates of Coimbra Network

Rosane Rosendo da Silva [Federal University of Santa Catarina, BRAZIL]. *Betty M. Pérez* [Universidad Central de Venezuela]. *Dalmo Machado* [University of São Paulo, Ribeirão Preto, BRAZIL]. *Dartagnan Pinto Guedes* [Northern Parana University, BRAZIL]. *Edilson Cyrino* [Londrina State University, BRAZIL]. *Enio Ronque* [State University of Londrina, BRAZIL]. *Hugo Tourinho Filho* [São Paulo University - USP, BRAZIL]. *Joice Stefanello* [Federal University of Paraná, BRAZIL]. *Luís Gobbo* [University of São Paulo, BRAZIL]. *Luíz dos Anjos* [Federal University Fluminense, BRAZIL]. *Beatriz Rocha-Ferreira* [Federal University of Grande Dourados, BRAZIL]. *Neiva Leite* [Federal University of Paraná, BRAZIL]. *Rômulo Fernandes* [UNESP - University of São Paulo State, BRAZIL]. *Vanildo Pereira* [State University of Maringá, BRAZIL]

Part I

The Josef Rutenfranz Lecture

THE JOSEF RUTENFRANZ LECTURE

Professor Dr Josef Rutenfranz was the leader of the group of eight scientists who conceived PWP in a café in Berlin in 1967, and organized the first PWP symposium in Dortmund in 1968. Josef Rutenfranz chaired the first meeting and remained the unofficial "Chairman of the Board" until his untimely death at the age of 60, on 28th February 1989. At PWP 1989, in Hungary, later that year it was decided that subsequent PWP symposia should begin with the Josef Rutenfranz Lecture.

1991	Per-Olaf Astrand	Children and Adolescents: Performance Measurements, Education
1993	Dan M. Cooper	New Horizons in Paediatric Exercise Research
1995	Oded Bar-Or	Safe Exercise for the Child with a Chronic Disease
1997	Han C. G. Kemper	A Scientific Voyage through Research in Children's Health – From Heart via Muscle to Bone
1999	Frank Galioto	The Challenges of the Future: Are We Ready?
2001	Anna Farkas	What About Girls?
2003	Gaston Beunen	Physical Growth, Maturation and Performance: Back to the Future
2005	Beat Villiger	News on Exercise-Induced Asthma
2007	Willem Van Mechelen	A Behavioural and Ecological Perspective to Energy-Balance-Related Behaviours in Children
2009	Emmanuel Van Praagh	The Child as a Source of Mechanical Power
2010	Viswanath Unnithan	Preventive Efficacy of Team Sports: Cardiovascular and Cardio-Respiratory Insights for Health and Performance
2011	Neil Armstrong	From Playground to Podium
2013	Robert M Malina	Youth, Sport, and Physical Activity

YOUTH, SPORT, AND PHYSICAL ACTIVITY

Robert M. Malina

University of Texas at Austin and Tarleton State University, USA

Several key topics in the long history of paediatric work physiology research are highlighted in the title. Youth are the children and adolescents who are the focus of research. Sport is perhaps the most popular and visible context of physical activity (PA) among youth. PA is a topic of heightened public health interest. Organized youth sports are a major feature of the lives of children and adolescents in many parts of the world, and are driven largely by adults – administrators, coaches and parents.

Paediatric work physiology has evolved from a largely physiological focus into a variety of disciplines highlighting interactions of biology and behaviour in the context of physical activity and sport from laboratory to the playing field to the clinic. This overview evaluates (1) trends in PA, physical fitness (PF) and associated factors among youth in the past 50 years or so, and (2) trends and issues in organized youth sport, and then attempts to relate the two. Primary focus is on data for the U.S., though data from other countries are cited where appropriate.

1.1 TRENDS IN PHYSICAL ACTIVITY

Productivity statistics for agriculture and manufacturing suggest a decline in physically demanding work in the U.S. Estimated hours of work required to produce 100 bushels of corn or wheat declined by about 75% between 1900 and 1950, and then by 91% for corn and 70% for wheat between 1950 and 1980. Weekly hours in manufacturing work declined by 30% between 1900 and 1950, but did not change between 1950 and 2000 (Floud *et al.*, 2011). Improvements in agricultural and industrial technologies contributed to more efficient production and reduced physical activity demands.

The shift to less physically demanding occupations was more apparent over the past two generations. Moderate intensity occupations (≥ 3 METS) in U.S. adults decreased from about 48% in 1960 to 20% in 2008 while light intensity (2.0-2.9 METS) and sedentary (<2 METS) occupations increased over this interval from 37% to 55% and from 15% to ~25%, respectively. Mean occupation-related energy expenditure also decreased by about 100 calories per day (Church *et al.*, 2011). Estimated weekly time in occupational and home/domestic work, work-related travel and active leisure among U.S. adults declined from 235 to 160 MET hours/week (32%) between 1965 and 2009, while time sedentary increased, ~25 to 37 hours/week. Estimates for U.K adults between 1961 and 2005 indicated a, decline in physical activity from 216 to 173 MET hours/week (20%) and an increase in time sedentary from 27 to 42 hours/week (Ng and Popkin, 2012).

Corresponding estimates for earlier samples of youth are not available. Many youth were engaged in agricultural and manufacturing work early in the twentieth century, while boys in "street" occupations (errands/delivery, newspapers, shoeshine) were quite active. Lower heart rates, for example, were noted in boys with a newspaper route; their "efficiency" was attributed to regular activity: the boys covered 3 to 9 miles daily delivering papers (McCurdy, 1913).

Estimates of daily energy expenditure (EE) among students at a boarding school in the U.K. in 1919–1921 provide early insights (Bedale, 1922–1923). The Douglas bag technique was used; BMR was measured in bed. Energy costs of school and non-school activities (walking, sports, outdoor work, gardening, haymaking, etc.) were derived and total daily EE on "typical school days" was estimated. Estimated costs of some activities in younger students were based on observation. Results are summarized in Table 1.1.

EE (total, per unit mass) based on heart rate (HR, some with calorimetry) and doubly labeled water (DLW) in contemporary youth are included for comparison. HR estimates date to the 1980s and DLW to the 1990s. Allowing for age and methodological variation, EE is lower in all samples compared to the estimates from ~1920 (except boys 14-18 years, DLW). EE is related to body size; trends must be viewed in context of secular gains in body mass compared to youth of 3–4 generations ago. Estimated absolute and relative EE (HR) declined between ~1920 and the 1980s; HR estimates also suggested a continued decline in relative EE from the 1990s to the present in boys and girls <14 years of age. DLW estimates suggested a decline in relative EE between ~1920 and the 1990s, but no subsequent changes.

The most variable component of EE is PA (AEE). The prevalence of Canadian youth 12–14 and 15–19 years with leisure time AEE ≥ 3 and ≥ 6 kcal/kg/day (questionnaire) increased between 1981 and 1988 in only boys, but did not change appreciably between 1988 and 1998 in both sexes (Eisenmann *et al.*, 2004). About 20% of boys in both age groups and girls 12–14 years and 10% of girls 15–19 years exceeded the AEE recommendation for youth (≥ 6 kcal/kg/day) in 1998.

In contrast to EE, PA is a behaviour and contexts of PA are variable. Estimates of PA based on questionnaires and diaries are subjective. Accelerometry is objective, but there is a need to relate accelerometry to specific contexts of PA. Both subjective and objective estimates of PA show a decline in PA from late childhood through adolescence, although there is variation among studies, contexts and scales. Boys are more active than girls, on average; the sex difference is attenuated during adolescence if data are expressed relative to maturation rather than chronological age (Thompson *et al.*, 2003). Current emphasis is largely focused on levels of PA associated with health benefits; the current

6

recommendation for school age youth is ≥60 minutes of moderate-to-vigorous PA (MVPA) daily (Strong *et al.*, 2005).

Table 1.1 Estimated energy expenditure (EE) in youth: 1920–2011.

Sex	n	Age, yrs	EE, kcal/day	kg/day
Boys, 6–13 years				
Bedale, 1919–1921*	12	9.6	2401	84.5
HR, 1980–1989	979	9.8	2217	70.8
1990–1999	59	11.1	2247	61.9
2000–present	111	11.2	2515	50.2
DLW, 1990–1999	197	8.2	1822	58.8
2000–present	551	8.3	2028	60.5
Girls, 6–13 years				
Bedale, 1919–1921	27	11.5	2500	67.3
HR, 1980–1989	896	10.0	2002	62.6
1990–1999	40	10.6	1948	57.6
2000–present	101	12.2	2111	49.0
DLW, 1990–1999	264	8.8	1848	55.4
2000–present	875	8.9	1848	56.7
Boys, 14–18 years				
Bedale, 1919–1921	25	15.5	3270	62.6
HR, 1980–1989	304	15.1	2812	50.5
1990–1999	12	15.1	2791	51.8
2000–present	131	15.1	2934	50.4
DLW, 1990–1999	50	15.4	3267	55.0
2000–present	73	16.4	3307	50.1
Girls, 14–18 years				
Bedale, 1919–1921	27	15.8	2866	53.8
HR, 1980–1989	393	15.1	2439	45.2
1990–1999	21	14.7	2322	45.0
2000–present	104	15.2	2597	41.6
DLW, 1990–1999	48	15.3	2487	43.4
2000–present	122	15.8	2686	44.8

*Data for 1919–1921 are calculated from Bedale (1922–1923); others are means weighted for sample sizes of individual studies (Malina, unpublished); HR=heart rate, includes calorimetry; DLW=doubly labeled water. Studies are grouped by year of publication.

It is often assumed that levels of habitual PA of children and adolescents have declined over time. Data addressing this issue, however, are limited in time depth. Self-reported PA and variable criteria for levels of PA have also been used and data are limited to adolescents. The Youth Risk Behavior Survey (YRBS) is a major source of data for American high school youth. A slight decline was noted in physically active boys ("exercise and sports activities that make you sweat and breathe hard for 20 minutes or more on three or more days in the past week") between 1993 and 2003, 75% to 70%, but not in girls, 56% to 55% (Adams, 2006). In contrast, no change was noted in percentages of boys and girls reporting moderate PA (did not make students sweat or breathe hard) and vigorous PA (made students sweat or breathe hard) between 1993 and 2005 (Li *et al.*, 2010). Moderate PA did not appreciably differ between boys (29%) and girls (24%), while vigorous PA was higher in boys (72%–75%) than girls (56%). Guidelines in the U.S. have since been modified to include both aerobic ($\geq$60 minutes per day, 7 days per week) and muscle strengthening ($\geq$3 days per week) activities (US Department of Health and Human Services, 2010). In the 2010 National Youth Physical Activity and Nutrition Study, small percentages of boys (22%) and girls (8%) met the aerobic criteria ("increased your heart rate and made you breathe hard for some of the time"), while more youth (boys 65%, girls 37%) met the muscle strengthening criteria ("such as push-ups, sit-ups, or weight lifting"). Only 19% of boys and 26% of girls met the criteria for both. Results for muscle strengthening were similar to the 2003 YRBS while those for aerobic activities were consistent with the 2009 YRBS (Centers for Disease Control and Prevention, 2011).

Similar trends over time were apparent in European youth. Percentages of Finnish boys and girls participating in leisure time MVPA did not vary appreciably between 1977 and 2005, and more boys than girls participated in MVPA (Telama and Laakso, 2009). Vigorous PA at least four times a week did not change between 1986 and 2002 in nationally representative samples of 11–15 year old boys and girls in six of seven European countries; Finnish youth showed a slight increase over time (Samdal *et al.*, 2007). Surveys of Iceland youth 14–15 years indicated a 7%–8% increase in vigorous PA between 1992 and 1997, but negligible changes between 1997 and 2006 (Eiðsdóttir *et al.*, 2008). In contrast, sports participation scores of Flemish parents and offspring both observed as adolescents did not differ between 1969–74 and 2002–04 in males, and 1979–80 and 2002–04 in females (Matton *et al.*, 2007).

In contrast to U.S. and European youth, higher percentages of South Australian youth of both sexes reported vigorous PA (that makes "you huff and puff and lasts at least 30 minutes" in most weeks) in 2004 compared to 1985. Boys, especially the most active, also increased in total leisure time PA in the previous week, while girls did not (Lewis *et al.*, 2007). Percentages of Australian youth 12–15 years in New South Wales also reported increased PA (60 minutes MVPA per day) and time in MVPA between 1985 and 2004 (Okely *et al.*, 2008). The interval from 1997 to 2004 showed larger increases in MVPA during the summer in contrast to the winter school terms (Hardy *et al.*, 2008).

Allowing for variation among studies, methodology and criteria, evidence for largely adolescent samples does not indicate a decline in PA among youth for the past 25 years or so. On the other hand, many youth do not meet recommended levels of MVPA. Data for younger children are limited. Accelerometry data indicated no changes in habitual PA in Danish children 8–10 years between 1998 and 2004 (Møller *et al.*, 2009), but an increase in overall and weekend PA (counts/minute) but not in overall MVPA and VPA in Norwegian children 9 years of age between 1999 and 2005 (Kolle *et al.*, 2009).

1.2 TRENDS IN PHYSICAL FITNESS

Physical fitness (PF) is a correlate of PA, though definitions of PF have changed from a performance to a health-related focus. Earlier surveys generally included more extensive test batteries, but more recent data tend to focus on aerobic and strength-related items in addition to the BMI. Reduced levels of PF are often attributed to declines in physically active and/or increases in physically inactive behaviours.

Data for grip strength date to the 1830s. Changes across time must be tempered as instruments change; motivation for maximal effort is also a factor. Nevertheless, secular gains in grip strength in Belgian (1830s–1971), American (1899–1964) and Japanese (1923–1969) youth were proportional to changes in body size (Malina, 1978). More recently, muscular strength declined in Danish youth since the 1950s (Heebøll-Nielsen, 1982) and in Russian youth since the 1960s (Godina, 1998). Arm pull strength of Flemish adolescents also declined between 1969–74 and 2002–04 in males, and 1979–80 and 2002–04 in females (Matton *et al.*, 2007). Changes in other fitness items across these intervals were not consistent in the Flemish youth. Comparisons of four national surveys of U.S. youth between 1958 and 1985 indicated major improvements in PF between 1958 and 1965, but little change from 1965 to 1985. The early improvement (1958–1965) reflected in part national emphasis on PF testing in schools in the 1960s. One mile run (1600 m) also did not change between 1979 and 1986 (Malina, 2007).

Strength and endurance of youth in southwestern Poland declined in decennial surveys from 1965 to 1995, especially after 12–14 years (Raczek, 2002), while EUROFIT scores of national samples of Polish youth 7–19 years improved between 1979 and 1989, but deteriorated between 1989 and 1999 (Przewęda and Dobosz, 2003). The decline in fitness marked in power of the upper and lower extremities and endurance. Swedish youth 16 years of age declined in the bench press, sit-ups and endurance run but improved in the two-hand lift between 1974 and 1995 (Westerstahl *et al.*, 2003). Increases in the BMI explained variable portions of the variance in the fitness, suggesting a significant role for decreased PA. Comparisons of South Australian youth 10–11 years in 1985 and 1997 indicated a decline in aerobic fitness (1.6 km run-walk time) and running speed (50 m dash), but no differences in power (standing long jump) (Dollman, 2003).

Trends for PF in Japanese youth 12–17 years between 1964 and 1997 showed a different pattern. PF scores improved from 1964 to 1974, were variable between 1975 and 1985, and declined from 1986 through 1997. The early changes may be related to increases in height from 1964 to 1984, while subsequent declines may be related to changing patterns of PA (Nishijima *et al.*, 2003a, 2003b). Improvements in PF (1964–1974) were also attributed to national emphasis on practice and fitness testing, while the variable results (1975–1985) were attributed to increased television viewing and subsequent declines (1986–1997) to emphasis on scholarship and PA for pleasure and increased video game time (Shingo and Takeo, 2002). Composite data for the 20m multistage shuttle run (cardiorespiratory endurance) in youth 6–19 years from 33 countries worldwide indicated a systematic decline between 1960 and 2003. The estimated decline was -0.46% per year since 1970 (Tomkinson and Olds, 2007). Similar analyses for tests of power and speed (anaerobic fitness) indicated more variable patterns. Both items improved somewhat through the mid-1980s; power then declined to 2003, while speed showed no change to about 2000 (Tomkinson, 2007).

Data for maximal aerobic power ($\dot{V}O_2$ peak) for American youth date to the late 1930s in boys and 1960s in girls. The data were based on relatively small samples combined across several ages and included both treadmill and cycle protocols; $\dot{V}O_2$ peak for the cycle was multiplied by 1.075 (Eisenmann and Malina, 2002). It is also likely that overweight/obese youth were not included. Regression lines indicated fairly stable levels for relative $\dot{V}O_2$ peak (ml/kg/min) from the 1930s through the 1990s in boys 6–12 and 13–18 years. Regression lines were stable from the 1970s in girls 6–11 years and from the 1960s in girls 12–14 years of age, but were curvilinear in girls 15–18 years. The latter suggested an increase from the 1960s through the 1970s and a decline into the late 1990s. Trend lines should be interpreted with care, since the number of data points in most age groups was limited. Examination of individual data points for absolute $\dot{V}O_2$ peak in boys indicated highest values in the late 1960s and 1970s, while subsequent values were somewhat lower. From this perspective, the general trend may be consistent with the decline in aerobic capacity assessed with the 20 m shuttle run (Tomkinson and Olds, 2007, see above). On the other hand, estimated $\dot{V}O_2$ peak did not differ in three cohorts of Danish adolescents of both sexes between 1983 and 2003 (Andersen *et al.*, 2010).

1.3 TRENDS IN PHYSICAL INACTIVITY

Physically inactive behaviours or behaviours with potential for inactivity are often cited in discussions of PA and PF. Physically inactive behaviours have been and are a fact of life – school, study, leisure reading, sitting and talking, etc. Technological advances have added to the potential for physically inactive behaviours, and the pace of introducing technology accelerated over time. Dates of ownership of technological innovations by 25% of the U.S. population provide an estimate of the rapidity with which advances reached society at large: telephone 1911, radio 1928, automobile 1941, television 1952, personal computers 1991, cell phones 1996, and internet 1998 (Ross, 2003). More recently, emphasis on extra-curricular classes for music, art, tutoring, among others offers high potential for physical inactivity (U.S. Department of Education, 2006).

Surveys of youth have used television viewing (TV) and more recently computer use as indicators of inactivity. TV ≥3hrs/day among American youth in the YRBS declined linearly from 1999 to 2009 with no change to 2011, while computer use (other than homework) ≥3 hrs/day was ~22% in 2003 and 2005, increased to 25% in 2007 and 2009, and to 31% in 2011 (Centers for Disease Control and Prevention, 2012). Boys consistently spent more time using computers than girls. Among European youth in seven countries, percentages of youth 11–15 years who watched at least 4 hours TV per day did not change between 1986 and 1998. Boys watched more TV than girls. Of interest, vigorous PA and TV behaviours were not correlated over this interval (Samdal *et al.*, 2007). Similar trends were suggested for U.K. and Australian youth (Dollman *et al.*, 2005).

A comprehensive survey of "media" use highlights more recent changes in opportunities for physical inactivity associated with technology (Rideout *et al.*, 2010). After adjusting for multitasking, American youth 8–18 years devoted 7:38 hours:minutes daily to media in 2009: TV, music/audio, computer, video games, print and movies. Estimates for 1999 and 2004 were, respectively, 6:21and 6:19. Talking on cell phones (0:33 per day) was not included; listening to music or watching videos and playing games on cell phones were included with the respective media types. Ownership of cell phones in 2009 increased with age: 8–10 years, 31%; 11–14 years, 69%; 15–18 years, 85%. Youth in 7–12th grades spent 1:35 per day sending-receiving text messages in 2009. Consistent with other observations, media use was not associated with PA: heavy users 1:59, moderate users 1:43, light users 1:44. Age-group specific estimates of media use time are summarized in Table 1.2. Overall, boys spent more time with media than girls; time spent with video games accounted for most of the sex difference.

Table 1.2 Age variation in daily time (hours: minutes) spent with media in 2009*.

Media	Age Group, yrs		
	8–10	11–14	15–18
TV content	3:41	5:03	4:22
Music	1:08	2:22	3:03
Computers	0:46	1:46	1:39
Video games	1:01	1:25	1:08
Print	0:46	0:37	0:33
Movies	0:28	0:26	0:20
Total media exposure	7:51	11:53	11:23
% multitasking	30%	27%	30%
Total media use	5:29	8:40	7:58

*Adapted from Rideout *et al.* (2010).

1.4 TRENDS IN TIME USE

Interest in the use of free time by children and adolescents has deep historical roots. Early studies of American youth have enumerated activities in which they participated, specifically play interests and preferences, beginning in the 1890s (e.g., Croswell, 1899; McGhee, 1900; Terman, 1926; Foster, 1930; Schwendener, 1932). Although surveys varied in detail and scope, play preferences included a variety of physically active games (e.g., tag, chase) and sports. Preferences of boys included more sports than girls. Rope jumping and skates/roller skating were among the top preferences among girls. Time devoted to the activities was not considered.

One of the earliest studies of time use was based on interviews in the form of a time-activity schedule to identify the most common and most popular play interests and activities of 200 adolescent boys 12–14 years. Boys were followed for

2 years, so that mixed-longitudinal trends from 12 to 16 years of age were estimated (Dimock, 1937). Play activities before school, during recess and other free time at school, and after school were noted. The mean number of hours per week as a participant in "physical play" declined with age from about 11 hours at 12 years to 7 hours at 16 years. In contrast to "physical play," time spent as a spectator of "physical play" increased from <1 hour at 12 to 2 hours at 16 years. The decline in physical play was accompanied by an increase in time devoted to work from ~3 hours at 12–13 years to 5 hours at 16 years. Delivering or selling newspapers was the most common work activity. Work time was complemented by time traveling to school, amusements, work and other activities, which increased, on average, with age by ~3 hours per week, from 10 hours at 12 years to 13 hours at 16 years. Walking to school was the common means of transport at 12 years, whereas bicycling was more common at 16 years, i.e., greater distance to high school (Dimock, 1937). A major difference between boys in the 1930s and at present would appear to be PA associated with work after school and transport.

Systematic studies of time use by children conducted in 1981, 1997 and 2003 provide information relevant to play and sport and by inference PA (Hofferth, 2009; Hofferth and Sandberg, 2001a, 2001b). The initial survey was motivated by interest in the influence of family circumstances on children's activities. The 1997 survey was motivated by increases in level of education of the population and number of women in the work force and decreases in two-parent households and family size. The 2003 survey was motivated by a political shift to conservatism, legislation establishing academic landmarks in schools, change in welfare provisions and events of September 11, 2001. The last mentioned contributed to heightened concern for child safety. The current scene includes continued political conservatism, safety as reflected in gun violence and child abuse (clergy, coaches), and increasing numbers of immigrant children in schools.

Time use diaries documented daily activities in the three surveys, although age groups considered varied somewhat (Juster et al., 2004). Time can be viewed as non-discretionary and discretionary (Hofferth, 2009). The former is reasonably set: time for sleeping, personal care and eating, and time in day care and school. Discretionary time is selective and optional: chores, shopping, study, church attendance, youth groups, play, outdoor activities, sports, hobbies, art, television, reading, passive leisure; more recently video, computers and cell phones.

Percentages of children 6–12 years of age participating in selected activities in the three surveys are summarized in Table 1.3. Almost all children spent time watching television and playing. The next most reported activity was sports; children participating in sport increased from 1981 to 1997 but declined from 1997 to 2003.

Time spent in specific activities by children 6–12 years in the three surveys is given in Table 1.4. Three activities dominated weekly time: school, television and play. Time in school increased from 1981 to 1997 but changed negligibly from 1997 to 2003. Time studying increased across surveys, with variation between children 6–8 and 9–12 years. Younger children spent more time playing than older children. Play time decreased in younger and increased in older children between 1981 and 1997, but did not change appreciably between 1997 and 2003. Somewhat surprisingly, television time declined from 1981 to 1997 in both age groups; it also decreased among children 6–8 years from 1997 to 2003, but increased in children 9–12 years.

Table 1.3 Percentages of children 6–12 years involved in selected activities: 1981, 1997, 2003*.

Activity	6–8 yrs				9–12 yrs			
	1981	1997	1997	2003	1981	1997	1997	2003
Sports	69	75	74	57	65	76	77	62
Outdoors	13	14	15	13	21	17	16	8
Playing	93	91	93	94	90	88	88	84
Youth groups	33	25	26	33	42	27	27	34
Television	97	96	96	97	97	94	94	97
Reading	37	43	42	54	32	34	35	43
Art activities	20	24	26	35	17	21	22	21
Other passive leisure	53	45	46	38	73	51	52	44

*Adapted from Hofferth and Sandberg (2001) and Hofferth (2009).

Table 1.4 Weekly time (hours:minutes) in selected activities of children 6–12 years: 1981, 1997, 2003*.

Activity	6–8 yrs				9–12 yrs			
	1981	1997	1997	2003	1981	1997	1997	2003
School	27:52	32:46	31:39	33:05	29:02	34:03	33:35	33:22
Daycare	0:12	1:33	1:35	1:22	0:18	0:24	0:32	0.44
Studying	0:52	2:08	1:58	2:36	3:22	3:41	3:36	4:20
Sports	6:01	5:13	5:03	2:46	4:51	6:33	6:31	4:31
Outdoors	0:28	0:30	0:31	0:34	0:46	0:36	0:39	0:18
Playing	14:58	11:10	12:09	11:36	7:24	8:54	9:00	8:43
Youth groups	0:41	0:42	0:37	0:50	0:56	0:49	0:49	1:09
Television	15:55	12:54	12:40	11:36	20:01	13:36	13:32	14:54
Reading	0:59	1:09	1:09	1:31	1:03	1:14	1:13	1:38
Art activities	0:21	0:45	0:51	1:05	0:22	0:54	0:56	0:54
Other passive leisure	1:58	1:33	1:35	1:18	3:24	2:19	2:18	1:57

*Adapted from Hofferth and Sandberg (2001) and Hofferth (2009).

Time in sports decreased across surveys in children 6–8 years; the decrease in sport time between 1997 and 2003 was >2 hours. Time in sports increased by about 2 hours between 1981 and 1997 in children 9–12 years, but decreased by the same amount between 1997 and 2003. Of relevance to the present discussion, the percentage of children involved in sport and time devoted to sport declined between 1997 and 2003. Time outdoors was limited, but decreased by more than one-half between 1981 and 2003 in children 9–12 years.

As noted earlier, widespread availability of computers is relatively recent. Weekly time (hours:minutes) devoted to computer activities in 2003 increased with age: 6–8 years (0:57), 9–11 (1:27), 12–14 (3:23), 15–17 (5:08). Television time increased from 6–8 (12:57) to 9–11 (15:01) years, but was stable at about 15 hours at the older ages (Juster *et al.*, 2004).

Although time in school has not appreciably changed, legislation establishing academic landmarks influence physical activity during the school day. Between 2000–2001 (*No Child Left Behind* legislation) and 2006–2007, 44% of school districts increased instructional time in English, Language Arts and Math, while 20% of districts decreased time in recess, i.e., free play time outdoors. Time for recess was reduced, on average, from 184 to 144 minutes per week (Center for Public Education, 2008).

Time use by children 3–5 years is limited to the 1981 and 1997 surveys (Hofferth and Sandberg, 2001a). Weekly time (hours:minutes) in school decreased (-2:25) while time in daycare increased (+7:20). Weekly time playing decreased (-8:29). In addition to more time in day care, play time was replaced by school work (+0:11), art activities (+0:44), reading or being read to (+0:55) and sports (+2:37). The percentage of preschool children involved in sports increased from 41% to 74% between 1981 and 1997. The trend for sports probably reflected the downward extension of organized sports to 4–5 years of age, e.g., t-ball, soccer, gymnastics, swimming and perhaps others. About 20% of children reported outdoor activities in both years, but weekly time outdoors, though limited, increased (0:13 to 0.37). More recently, children enrolled in Head Start spent 63 minutes per day outdoors (Tandon *et al.*, 2013), while only 58% of children not enrolled in day care went outdoors daily (Tandon *et al.*, 2012). And, children who spend more time outdoors tend to be more physically active (Mackett and Paskins, 2008).

1.5 THE OBESITY EPIDEMIC

The preceding trends in PA, PF, physical inactivity and time use among American youth are often discussed in the context of the obesity epidemic which had its antecedents in the 1980s as its prevalence doubled between national surveys of 1976–1980 and 1988–1994, and continued to increase through 2007–2008 (Table 1.5). Childhood obesity begins early; 10% of American children 2–5 years of age were already obese in 1999–2000; the prevalence increased to 14% among boys but remained stable in girls through 2009–2010 (Ogden *et al.*, 2012).

The epidemic is usually viewed as an imbalance of energy intake and expenditure. There is a need to decompose the equation into more specific correlates, e.g., increases in food supply and decreases in food prices likely altered demand for food and feeding practices (i.e., the food industry). Estimated PA declined over time in adults, but estimates for youth are inconclusive or suggest otherwise. There is a need for critical evaluation of correlates of food intake, PA and inactivity, and related behaviours as well as their interactions among youth.

Table 1.5 Emergence of obesity in American youth*.

Survey Years	6–11 Years		12–17 Years	
	Boys	Girls	Boys	Girls
'63–70	4.0	4.5	4.5	4.7
'71–74	4.3	3.6	6.1	6.2
'76–80	6.6	6.4	4.8	5.3
'88–94	11.6	11.0	11.3	9.7
'99–00	15.7	14.3	14.8	14.8
'03–04	19.9	17.6	18.3	16.4
'07–08	21.2	18.0	19.3	16.8
'09–10	20.1	15.7	19.6	17.1

*Adapted from Odgen *et al.* (2002, 2006, 2008, 2010, 2012), BMI ≥ P95, age, sex-specific.

1.6 YOUTH SPORT

Youth sports programmes vary among and within countries in structure and operation (De Knop *et al.*, 1995; Heinemann, 1999). They also vary in accessibility, participant selectivity and degree of specialization. Programmes include national sport federations which are top-down in operation; sport clubs ranging from local to professional (many with academies for the elite); school sport teams or clubs; community centers and youth service organizations; and commercial clubs. Given programme diversity and related factors, it is difficult to compare countries.

Youth sports in the U.S. are largely agency-sponsored and school-based. The former is the major level of youth participation, e.g., Little League baseball, Pop Warner Football, United States Youth Soccer, among others. Agency-sponsored sports involve seasonal fees which vary considerably among programmes. High school sport is the primary school-based entity, although interschool sport at lower grade levels is also popular. Public and private schools have extensive interscholastic sport programmes, which are funded by local tax revenues and parental resources, respectively. Corporate involvement is increasing, especially in football (American) and basketball. Selectivity of high school sport is more marked than at younger ages. Clubs sports are largely commercial and often highly selective – gymnastics, swimming and diving, figure skating, tennis and increasingly soccer.

1.7 ANTECEDENTS OF ORGANIZED YOUTH SPORTS IN THE U.S.

Organized sports for youth in the U.S had their roots in concerns for the welfare of children and adolescents in the late nineteenth and early twentieth centuries, specifically in the context of rapidly growing cities and associated living conditions and child labour (White House Conference on Child Health and Protection, 1931). Concern for delinquency was a primary force in the origin of public and philanthropic programmes, collectively known as Boys' Work (Stone, 1931), aimed at play, recreation and character development of boys <18 years in the 1890s. Many had religious interests, and largely involved volunteers from education, hygiene, recreation, social work and religion. Many programmes attempted to divert delinquent to more socially acceptable activities with sport an integral part of "gang busting" efforts (Thrasher, 1927). More than 100 different clubs based on interests of boys were listed in 1902, including the Young Men's Christian Association and Boys' Clubs, among others, and were significant in the origin of community-based youth sports programmes.

The Play Movement developed at the same time as Boy's Work (Curtis, 1917). Reduction in child labour and school attendance contributed to a perceived need for play, which was viewed as important in overall physical, motor and psychosocial development, including character building (North, 1931). Many playgrounds were established in cities early in the twentieth century; some also established "play streets" closed to traffic for specific periods (Curtis, 1917; North, 1931). The Play Movement emphasized space for organized games, including volleyball and basketball for children <14 years, and supervised sports – baseball, football and tennis for youth ≥14 years (North, 1931). In contrast, the Playground Association of America (1913) developed athletic badge tests of "physical efficiency" in part as a reaction to specialized athletics. Competitions were held to determine the awarding of the badges.

1.7.1 Community-Based Sport

Sport activities of Boys' Work and the Play Movement were aimed at youth of elementary school age (grades 1–8, 6 to ~14–15 years). Although there were some earlier efforts, competitive sport programmes were organized by in many communities in the 1920s–1930s (Berryman, 1975). For example, baseball tournaments were organized for boys <13 years of age in Cincinnati in 1913. A tackle football programme was organized for boys <12 years in Denver in 1927, while Pop Warner Football for boys ≥15 years began with four teams in Philadelphia in 1929. The latter was begun at the request of building owners in an effort to prevent the breaking of factory windows by teenagers throwing stones (Pop Warner Little Scholars, 2013). Church-based groups also influenced community sports, primarily in cities. The Catholic Youth Organization (CYO) was founded in Chicago in 1930 (Gems, 2005), and spread to other cities. Many offered a variety of organized sport programmes; inter-church sport leagues were in place in the 1930s and 1940s. Although these early efforts were important, the founding of Little League Baseball in 1939 by Carl Stotz (Little Baseball and Softball Media Guide, 2012) is often viewed as a singularly important event in the spread of community-based sports in the U.S. as suburbs developed and expanded with economic prosperity after World War II.

1.7.2 Scholastic Sport

School sports developed simultaneously with but independently of Boys' Work and the Play Movement. There were two major forces, the school programme and students. Within the school programme, Luther Gulick established the New York

Public Schools Athletic League (PSAL) in 1903; similar leagues were organized in 177 cities by 1915 (Rice, 1939). The PSAL initially conducted "class athletics" in elementary school (grades 5 to 8) at specific times each year, and not interschool athletics as we know them. "Class athletics" included standard tests in the schools: Fall, standing long jump; Winter, chinning the bar; Spring, sprint runs. Test results from each school were sent to the PSAL, which declared the winner based on comparisons of results (Reilly, 1917). The PSAL also emphasized swimming, baseball, football and basketball, and several minor games (Rice, 1939). An interschool programme for grades 5–8, labeled "Rational Athletics" was also proposed (Reilly, 1917). The competitions would involve a field day of neighbouring schools in which 80% of the boys from each school would perform a specified set of events. The school winning the majority of events would be declared the winner. Additional events for boys and events for girls were also proposed.

A downward drift of intercollegiate sports, especially football, baseball and track and field in the 1880s influenced interscholastic sport. High school sport originated with student organizations and not with school authorities (Gutowski, 1988), and were reasonably well established early in the twentieth century. Activities of high school sports clubs attracted the attention of faculty and administrators concerned with time and energy devoted to sports and their effects on the schools. Concerns included the small number of boys involved, quality of coaching (clubs often hired their own coaches), use of "ringers" (professionalism), out of town travel, length of schedule, unsportsmanlike conduct, interference with school work, lack of carry-over value, injury (especially football), emphasis on winning, among others. In addition to the welfare of athletes, faculty and administrators were concerned for the reputation of the schools and saw a need for adult control (Mirel, 1982; Gutowski, 1988). These factors contributed to the formation of state high school athletic associations, 1895 in Michigan (Mirel, 1982) and 1903 in Indiana (Rice, 1939). State associations in Illinois, Indiana, Iowa, Michigan and Wisconsin formed the Midwest Federation of State High School Athletic Associations in 1921, which became the National Federation of State High School Athletic Associations in 1923. It became the National Federation of State High School Associations in the 1970s when the fine arts were established as a programme area (National Federation of State High School Associations, 1999–2000).

1.7.3 Sports for Girls

It should be apparent that little or no attention was devoted to sports for girls. This reflected views on societal roles and expectations for girls and physiological sex differences, and the organizations offering youth sports. Nevertheless, play preferences of girls in early studies included a number of sports – baseball, volleyball, tennis, and "ball", while interscholastic sport events were available for boys and girls in 95% and 70% of city schools, respectively, in the early 1920s (Rice, 1939). Interestingly, no sports were listed among the top 25 game preferences of girls in northwestern Ohio in 1959 (Sutton-Smith and Rosenberg, 1961). However, sport opportunities for girls and women would change dramatically with Title IX legislation (see below).

1.8 PARTICIPATION IN ORGANIZED SPORT

Community-based and interscholastic sports increased from the 1930s through the 1950s (with the exception of World War II), a time when medical and physical education communities raised concerns or were opposed to competitive sports for children of elementary and junior high school age (e.g., Journal of Health and Physical Education, 1932; Lowman, 1947; AAHPER, 1952; American Academy of Pediatrics, 1956; Reichert, 1958). Organized programmes for youth flourished and spread to younger ages, and the attitude of the public, especially parents, was generally favorable (Scott, 1953). Expansion of suburbs after WW II necessitated more schools with a corresponding increase in interschool competitions and scholastic leagues.

Title IX of the Education Amendments in 1972 was the important milestone in sport participation for girls. Accordingly, "No person in the United States shall, on the basis of sex, be excluded from participation in, be denied the benefits of, or be subjected to discrimination under any education program or activity receiving Federal financial assistance" (Pieronek, 1994). Regulations implementing Title IX were put into effect in 1975 and influenced participation of girls in sport at all levels.

Historical statistics for organized youth sport participants are limited. Data for two specific sport organizations highlight the increase in the second half of the twentieth century (Table 1.6). Little League baseball began before WW II and flourished after the war. Soccer did not emerge on the U.S. youth sports scene until the mid-1970s. Participants in both sports increased steadily to 2000. Subsequently, participants in baseball/softball declined while numbers in soccer were rather stable through 2010.

Table 1.6 Estimated numbers of participants in two youth sports organizations.

Year	Little League Baseball*		U.S. Youth Soccer**
	Baseball	Softball	
1950	18,300		
1960	825,000		
1970	1,371,200		
1974	1,640,000	29,696	103,432
1980	1,736,600	141,696	810,793
1990	2,107,590	259,080	1,615,041
2000	2,467,110	378,315	3,020,442
2010	2,168,850	344,910	3,036,438

* http://www.littleleague.org/
**http://www.usyouthsoccer.org/

Children 4–12 years comprised the majority of participants in U.S. Youth Soccer (~72% in 2012) and Little League Baseball/Softball (87%/80% in 2010). Based on data from sport organizations and sporting goods manufacturers (Hainline, 2012), participants 6–11 years as a percentage of all participants 6–18 years varied among sports: volleyball (65%), soccer (62%), baseball (57%), basketball (42%) and football (23%); basketball was equally popular among youth 12–14 (29%) and 15–18 (28%) years, while football was most popular among youth (mostly boys) 15–18 years (46%).

The National Council of Youth Sports (2008) is an advocacy group for youth sport; participation statistics are provided by officers of member organizations. Estimated participants ≤ 6 through18 years increased from ~17 million in 1987 to ~33 million in 1997 and to ~44 million in 2008, which approximated 37%, 71% and 80% of the pre-kindergarten through 12th grade school enrollment in the respective years (author calculations). More boys participated in sport (63%, 66%) than girls (37%, 34%) in 1997 and 2008, respectively.

Numbers of high school (grades 9–12) sport participants though variable in the 1970s and early1980s, increased steadily since the mid-1980s (Table 1.7). The numbers are overestimates, to some extent, as many youth participated in multiple sports. The number of girls approximated 8% of that for boys in 1971–1972 (school year) and 40% in 1975–1976, and then gradually increased to 71% in 2000–2001 with no change to 2010–2011. Male athletes approximated ~25% of estimated total enrollments in grades 9–12 from the 1970s through 2010; percentages of female athletes increased from ~10% in the mid-1970s to about 20% in 2010 (author calculations). The high school statistics include >45 sports-activities, but five sports have historically accounted for the majority of participants: football, basketball, outdoor track and field, baseball and soccer in boys; outdoor track and field, basketball, volleyball, softball (fast pitch) and soccer in girls. These sports accounted for 65% of athletes in each sex in 2010–2011 (http://www.nfhs.org, accessed March 24, 2012).

Table 1.7 Estimated numbers of participants in high school sports.

School Year	Boys	Girls	Girls as % of Boys
'71–72	3,666,917	294,015	8.0
'75–76	4,109,021	1,645,039	40.0
'80–81	3,503,124	1,853,789	52.9
'85–86	3,344,275	1,807,121	54.0
'90–91	3,406,355	1,892,316	55.6
'95–96	3,634,052	2,367,936	65.2
'00–01	3,921,069	2,784,154	71.0
'05–06	4,206,549	2,953,355	70.0
'10–11	4,494,406	3,173,549	70.6

*http://www.nfhs.org

Other U.S. data suggested more variable recent participation trends for school athletics ("all students who have participated to any degree in school athletics teams" during the school year) between 1991 and 2010 (Child Trends Data Bank, 2012). Male participants declined across grade levels: 8th, 73% to 67%; 10th, 69%

to 64%; 12th, 65% to 61%, while female participants declined only in the 8th grade, 65% to 61%, but increased slightly in the 10th (52% to 55%) and 12th (47% to 51%) grades. The declines across grade levels probably reflected differential drop-out and persistence in sport and also the selectivity of sport.

As noted, the structure of sport programmes vary among countries; age groups also vary in the comparative data. Several examples illustrate trends over time. Canadian youth 5–14 years of age "regularly" participating in organized sports declined from 1992 to 2005, more so in boys than in girls: 5–10 years, boys 60% to 52%, girls 45% to 43%; 11–14 years, boys 74% to 62%, girls 54% to 48% (Clark, 2008). The decline in regular sport participation was also apparent among Canadian youth 15–18 years (sexes combined), 77%, 68% and 59% in 1992, 1998 and 2005, respectively. In 2005, the late adolescents participated more in structured compared to unstructured sport, males 51% vs 30% and females 42% vs 19% (Ifedi, 2008).

The percentage of Australian children playing sport, especially more than one sport, declined from 1985 to 2000 (Norton et al., 2001). The decline occurred primarily in organized sports and especially "mainstream" team sports. In contrast, participation in organized sport (club and school) among South Australian youth did not differ between 1985 and 2004 (Lewis et al., 2007). More recently, participation in organized sport among Australian youth 5–15 years has increased from 2000 to 2009, 65% to 71% (Government of South Australia, 2011).

Data for sport participation trends in European youth are less extensive. Participation in sport clubs by Icelandic youth 14–15 years of age increased from 1992 to 2006, 21% to 36% among boys and 13% to 27% among girls (Eiôsdóttir et al., 2008). Percentages of Italian youth "practicing sport" also increased from 1995 to 2000, but there was some variation by age group: 6–10 years, boys 55% to 62%, girls 49% in both years; 11–14 years, boys 71% to 73%, girls 50% to 55%; 15–19 years, boys 62% to 70%, girls 37% to 46% (Istituto Nazionale di Statistica, 2005). Largest relative gains occurred among girls 11–19 years and boys 6–10 and 15–19 years.

1.9 IMPLICATIONS

It is reasonable to evaluate sport, specifically organized youth sports, in the context of the trends in PA, PF, physical inactivity, time use and obesity. Potential interactions among trends merit critical evaluation. For example, what is the influence of participation in organized sports on informal play and sport, and in turn PA? What is the contrast in PA or EE in informal and formal sport activities? In the context of concern for obesity, organized youth sport as currently structured is, with few exceptions, not conducive to participation by the overweight/obese.

1.9.1 Sport and PA

Children and adolescents involved in sport had higher levels of MVPA, estimated daily EE and AEE (Katzmarzyk and Malina, 1998; Wickel and Eisenmann, 2007; Ribeyre et al., 2007; Machado Rodrigues et al., 2012), and self-reported more PA than non-participants (Trost et al., 1997; Pfeiffer et al., 2006; Aarnio et al., 2002).

Participation in sports during adolescence tended to track at higher levels than other indicators of PA (Malina, 2001), while frequency of sport participation (Tammelin et al., 2003), membership in sport clubs (Telama et al., 1994, 1997; (Barnekow-Bergkvist et al., 2001), and sport club training and competition during adolescence (Telama et al., 2006) were significant predictors of PA in the mid-20s and early-30s.The preceding were derived from Scandinavian countries. In the Michigan Study of Adolescent Life Transitions, childhood (time spent on sports) and adolescent (time in sports, kinds of after school activities) sport participation was a significant predictor of sport and PF activities in young adulthood (Perkins et al., 2004).

Given the strong association between adolescent participation in sport and adult PA, more attention should be given to this context of PA among adolescents as sports participation declines and sport programmes become more selective. Sport offerings for youth with less skill or less interest in elite competition are limited and probably not available in most communities in the U.S and perhaps other countries. There is need to modify sport programmes to accommodate youth with a wide range of skills and interests, and to study of the process through which sport participation during adolescence translates into an active lifestyle in adulthood.

1.9.2 Organized Vs. Informal Sport

Since contemporary youth in most parts of the world participate in organized in contrast to informal sport, it is reasonable to inquire about PA and skill acquisition in the respective sport settings. How do PA levels and skills compare between participants in organized and informal sport? Organized sport is adult-directed and structured while informal sport is youth-directed and unstructured. Data addressing these issues are limited. Estimated intensities of unstructured and structured ball games based on activity diaries and accelerometry were, for example, 3.4 and 2.5 calories per minute, respectively, among U.K. boys 12–13 years, and 3.2 and 2.6 calories per minute, respectively, in girls. Respective estimates were 2.0 vs 1.9 and 2.3 vs. 1.9 calories per minutes for 10–11 year old boys and girls (Mackett and Paskins, 2008).

Organized sport routinely involves specific instruction and practice of sport-specific skills and strategies. Systematic evaluations of the influence of instruction and practice on learning and refining sport-specific skills in the youth sports setting are lacking. Casual observation of youth participants indicates improvement. In contrast, informal sport (e.g., street games) involves frequent repetitions without supervision of an adult, trial and error, experimentation, variable settings, and exposure to different conditions, skills and rules. Sport-related skills are learned without awareness or explicit knowledge of the skills (Malina, 2013). Skills learned informally may be adaptable to a variety of sports and sport circumstances. Research on implicit learning in sport is in its infancy but is expanding (Masters et al., 2013).

There is a need to compare skill acquisition under organized and informal conditions. Improvement in sport skills is a major motivation for children and adolescents to participate in sport. Moreover, children who are more proficient in movement skills, not necessarily sport-specific skills, are more likely to be more physically active and fit in adolescence (Barnett *et al.*, 2008, 2009; Wrotniak *et al.*, 2006).

1.9.3 Limitations of Time

Time use data for youth 6–12 years suggested a decrease in discretionary time and in informal (unstructured) activities, and an increase in organized (structured) activities between 1981 and 1997 which persisted through 2003. The increase in play among youth 9–12 years was related to more time with video games. Time in media-related activities also increased from 2004 to 2009. Many organized and media-related activities have high potential for physical inactivity. Time outdoors decreased by more than one-half between 1981 and 2003 in children 9–12 years. This has implications for PA as children who spend more time in outdoor activities tend to be more physically active.

Time in sport over time varied with age. Among children 6–8 years, it declined by ~1 hour between 1981 and 1997 and by >2 hours more between 1997 and 2003. In contrast, among children 9-12 years, time in sport increased by ~2 hours between 1981 and 1997, and then decreased by 2 hours between 1997 and 2003 (Table 1.4).

Time is a limited indicator of intensity of PA and specifically sport. Although PA is a major part of sport participation, it involves more than PA. Although there is variation by sport, time involves clothing change, warm-up, instruction and practice (drills, repetitions), rest, scrimmages, games, among others. Team sports such as soccer, basketball, ice and field hockey involve reasonably continuous activity which varies in intensity during practice or a match, whereas baseball and American football involve intermittent activities among frequent periods of relative inactivity. Intermittent activities are also characteristic of gymnastics, diving, racket sports and some field events in athletics, while continuous activity is a more likely feature of swimming and running events. Estimated EE (METs) varies among sports and by intensity of effort (Ridley *et al.*, 2008; Ridley and Olds, 2008).

An observational study of youth sport participants 11–14 years in several organized sports indicated considerable variation in intensity of activity within and among sports (Katzmarzyk *et al.*, 2001). Selected data are summarized in Table 1.8. Variation in activities has implications for estimates of EE based on time devoted to sport.

At a more elite level, observations of male gymnasts 10.5±0.9 years highlight the intermittent nature of training activities (Daly *et al.*, 1998, 1999). About 63% of total time was devoted to rest or recovery. Work-rest ratios varied: strength and conditioning, 1:1.44, development of routines, 1:1.78; and pre-competition, 1:1.94. Mean heart rate was 127.5 bpm, which was ~60% to ~65% of maximal values, while peak rates were transient and varied with event: 158 to 184 bpm on the high bar and 171 to 184 bpm on the parallel bars.

22

Table 1.8 Mean percentages of time devoted to specific activities in several youth sports among boys 11–14 years*.

Activity	Basketball (9)	Soccer		Hockey	
		Indoor (18)	Outdoor (6)	Ice (13)	In-Line (12)
Sitting	18	<1	<1	26	28
Standing	21	40	17	30	19
Walking	30	23	16	26	39
Jogging	20	21	32	13	13
Sprinting	11	15	35	5	3

*Adapted from Katzmarzyk *et al.* (2001), ice and in-line hockey: walking = coasting with few strides, jogging = steady skating at moderate intensity, sprinting = vigorous effort at greater speeds.

Descriptions of time in sport and PA need to be complemented with information on specific activities during practice and games. Hours provide limited information about demands placed upon youth. Sport-related activities and training vary among individuals and with age, by level of sport and phase of season, and with coaches and coaching styles. Intra-individual variation is probably considerable and merits attention.

1.9.4 Sport for the Overweight/Obese

Organized sport is increasingly indicated as a potentially important context of PA to combat the epidemic of obesity among youth. As presently organized and practiced, however, it is unlikely that overweight/obese youth will have equal opportunities with few exceptions, e.g., offensive line in American football, some throwing events in athletics. Obese youth tend to be less proficient in movement skills and components of PF. Excess body mass and fatness have a negative influence on most motor and fitness tests, specifically those requiring movement/projection of the body. In contrast, isometric and isokinetic strength are greater in obese compared to non-obese youth, reflecting the absolute size advantage of the obese (Malina *et al.*, 2004).

PA intervention programmes with overweight/obese youth have generally incorporated a variety of aerobic and resistance activities in an effort to accommodate individual differences in body mass and activity interests of the youth (Strong *et al.*, 2005), but generally did not address youth interests in sports per se and team games. On the other hand, there is increasing interest in using team sport activities as PA interventions for overweight/obese youth (Weintraub *et al.*, 2008; Faude *et al.*, 2010; Seabra *et al.*, under review).

1.10 REFERENCES

AAHPER, 1952, *Desirable Athletic Competition for Children: Joint Committee Report.* (Washington, DC: American Association for Health, Physical Education, and Recreation).

Aarnio, M., Winter, T., Peltonen, J., Kujala, U.M. and Kaprio J., 2002, Stability of leisure-time physical activity during adolescence-a longitudinal study among 16-, 17- and 18-year-old Finnish youth. *Scandinavian Journal of Medicine and Science in Sports,* **12**, pp. 179–185.

Adams, J., 2006, Trends in physical activity and inactivity amongst US 14-18 year olds by gender, school grade and race, 1993-2003: Evidence from the Youth Risk Behavior Survey. *BMC Public Health,* **6**, pp. 57 (1–7).

American Academy of Pediatrics, 1956, Report, committee on school health, competitive athletics. *Pediatrics,* **18**, 672–676.

Andersen, L.B., Froberg, K., Kristensen, P.L., Moller, N.C., Resaland, G.K. and Anderssen, S.A., 2010, Secular trends in physical fitness in Danish adolescents. *Scandinavian Journal of Medicine and Science in Sports,* **20**, pp. 757–763.

Barnekow-Bergkvist, M., Hedberg, G., Janlert, U. and Jansson, E., 2001, Adolescent determinants of cardiovascular risk factors in adult men and women. *Scandinavian Journal of Public Health,* **29**, pp. 208–217.

Barnett, L.M., van Beurden, E., Morgan, P.J., Brooks, L.O. and Beard, J.R., 2008, Does childhood motor skill proficiency predict adolescent fitness? *Medicine and Science in Sports and Exercise,* **40**, pp.2137–2144.

Barnett, L.M., van Beurden, E., Morgan, P.J., Brooks, L.O. and Beard, J.R., 2009, Childhood motor skill proficiency as a predictor of adolescent physical activity. *Journal of Adolescent Health,* **44**, pp. 252–259.

Bedale, E.M., 1922-1923, Energy expenditure and food requirements of children at school. *Proceedings of the Royal Society, London, Series B Biological Sciences,* **94B**, pp. 368–404.

Berryman, J.W., 1975, From the cradle to the playing field: America's emphasis on highly organized competitive sports for preadolescent boys. *Journal of Sport History,* **2**, pp. 112–131.

Center for Public Education, 2008, Time out: Is recess in danger? http://www.centerforpubliceducation.org/Main-Menu/Organizing-a-school/Time-out-Is-recess-in-danger accessed January 10, 2013.

Centers for Disease Control and Prevention, 2011, Physical activity levels of high school students – United States, 2010. *Morbidity and Mortality Weekly Report,* **60**, pp. 773–777.

Centers for Disease Control and Prevention, 2012, Youth risk behavior surveillance – United States, 2011. *Morbidity and Mortality Weekly Report,* **61**, pp. 1–162.

Child Trends Data Bank, 2012, Participation in school athletics. http://www.childtrendsdatabank.org accessed February 8, 2013.

Church, T.S., Thomas, D.M., Tudor-Locke, C., Katzmarzyk, P.T., Earnest, C.P., Rodarte, R.Q., Martin, C.K., Blair, S.N. and Bouchard, C., 2011, Trends over 5 decades in U.S. occupation-related physical activity and their associations with obesity. *PLoS One,* **6**, e19657.

Croswell, T.R., 1899, Amusements of Worcester school children. *Pedagogical Seminary,* **6**, pp. 314–371.

Curtis, H.S., 1917, *The Play Movement and Its Significance.* (Washington, D.C.: McGrath Publishing Company).

Daly, R.M., Rich, P.A. and Klein, R., 1998, Hormonal responses to physical training in high-level peripubertal male gymnasts. *European Journal of Applied Physiology*, **79**, pp. 74–81.

Daly, R.M., Rich, P.A., Klein, R. and Bass S., 1999, Effects of high-impact exercise on ultrasonic and biochemical indices of skeletal status: A prospective study in young male gymnasts. *Journal of Bone and Mineral Research*, **14**, pp. 1222–1230.

De Knop, P., Engstrom, L-M., Skirstad, E. and Weiss, M.R. (editors), 1996, *Worldwide Trends in Youth Sport*. (Champaign, IL: Human Kinetics).

Dimock, H.S., 1937, *Rediscovering the Adolescent: A Study of Personality Development in Adolescent Boys*. (New York: Association Press).

Dollman, J. 2003, *Trends and sociodemographic distribution of children's health-related fitness and behaviours*. Doctoral dissertation, University of South Australia, Mawson Lakes Campus.

Dollman, J., Norton, K. and Norton, L., 2005, Evidence for secular trends in children's physical activity behavior. *British Journal of Sports Medicine*, **39**, pp. 892–897.

Eiðsdóttir, S.P., Kristjánsson, A.L., Sigfúsdóttir, I.D. and Allegrante, J.P., 2008, Trends in physical activity and participation in sports clubs among Icelanding adolescents. *European Journal of Public Health*, **18**, pp. 289–293.

Eisenmann, J., Katzmarzyk, P.T. and Tremblay, M.S., 2004, Leisure-time physical activity levels among Canadian adolescents, 1981-1998. *Journal of Physical Activity and Health*, **1**, pp. 154–162.

Eisenmann, J.C. and Malina, R.M., 2002, Secular change in peak oxygen consumption among United States youth in the 20th century. *American Journal of Human Biology*, **14**, pp. 699–706.

Faude, O., Kerper, O. and Multhaupt, M., 2010, Football to tackle overweight in children. *Scandinavian Journal of Medicine and Science in Sports*, **20**, pp. 103–110.

Floud, R., Fogel, R.W., Harris, B. and Hong, S.C., 2011, *The Changing Body: Health, Nutrition, and Human Development in the Western World since 1700*. (Cambridge, UK: Cambridge University Press).

Foster, J.S., 1930, Play activities of children in the first six grades. *Child Development*, **1**, pp. 248–254.

Gems, G.R., 1993, Sport, religion, and Americanization: Bishop Sheil and the Catholic Youth Organization. *International Journal of the History of Sport*, **10**, pp. 233–241.

Godina, E.Z., 1998, Secular changes in Russia and the former Soviet Union. In *Secular Growth Changes in Europe*, edited by Bodzsar, E.B. and Susanne, C. (Budapest: Eotvos University Press), pp. 351–367.

Gutowski, T.W., 1988, Student initiative and the origins of high school extracurriculum: Chicago, 1980-1915. *History of Education Quarterly*, **28**, pp.49–72.

Hainline, B., 2012, *Positioning Youth Tennis for Success*. (White Plains, NY: United States Tennis Association).

Hardy, L.L., Okely, A.D., Dobbins, T.A. and Booth, M.L., 2008, Physical activity among adolescents in New South Wales (Australia): 1997 and 2004. *Medicine and Science in Sports and Exercise*, **40**, pp. 835–841.

Heebøll-Nielsen, K., 1982, Muscle strength of boys and girls, 1981 compared to 1956. *Scandinavian Journal of Sports Sciences,* **4**, pp. 37–43.

Hofferth, S.L., 2009, Changes in American children's time – 1997 to 2003. *International Journal of Time Use Research,* **6**, pp.26–47.

Hofferth, S.L. and Sandberg, J.F., 2001a, Changes in American children's time, 1981-1997. *Advances in Life Course Research,* **6**, pp. 193–229.

Hofferth, S.L. and Sandberg, J.F., 2001b, How American children spend their time. *Journal of Marriage and Family,* **63**, pp. 295–308.

Journal of Health and Physical Education, 1932, Trend of athletics in junior high schools (editorial). *Journal of Health and Physical Education,* **3**, p. 22.

Juster, F.T., Ono, H. and Stafford, F.P., 2004, Changing times of American youth: 1981–2003. *Child Development Supplement.* (Ann Arbor, MI: Institute for Social Research, University of Michigan).

Katzmarzyk, P.T. and Malina, R.M., 1998, Contributions of organized sports participation to estimated daily energy expenditure in youth. *Pediatric Exercise Science,* **10**, pp. 378–386.

Katzmarzyk, P.T., Walker, P. and Malina, R.M., 2001, A time-motion study of organized youth sports. *Journal of Human Movement Studies,* **40**, pp. 325–334.

Kolle, E., Steene-Johannessen, J., Klasson-Heggebø, K., Andersen, L.B. and Anderssen, S.A., 2009, A 5-yr change in Norwegian 9-yr-olds' objectively assessed physical activity level. *Medicine and Science in Sports and Exercise,* **41**, pp. 1368–1373.

Lewis, N., Dollman, J. and Dale, M., 2007, Trends in physical activity behaviours and attitudes among South Australian youth between 1985 and 2004. *Journal of Science and Medicine in Sport,* **10**, pp. 418–417.

Li, S., Treuth, M.S. and Wang, Y., 2010, How active are American adolescents and have they become less active? *Obesity Reviews,* **11**, pp. 847–862.

Lowman, C.L., 1947, The vulnerable age. *Journal of Health and Physical Education,* **18**, pp. 635–636.

Mackett, R.L. and Paskins, J., 2008, Children's physical activity: The contribution of playing and walking. *Child and Society,* **22**, pp. 345–357.

Malina, R.M., 1978, Secular changes in growth, maturation, and physical performance. *Exercise and Sport Sciences Reviews,* **6**, pp. 203–255.

Malina, R.M., 2007, Physical fitness of children and adolescents in the United States: status and secular change. *Medicine and Sports Science,* **50**, pp. 67–90.

Malina, R.M., 2013, Motor development and performance. In *Conditions of Children's Talent Development in Sport,* edited by Cote, J., Lidor, R. (Morgantown, WV: Fitness Information Technology), pp. 61–83.

Malina, R.M., Bouchard, C. and Bar-Or, O., 2004, *Growth, Maturation, and Physical Activity,* 2nd edition. (Champaign, IL: Human Kinetics).

Masters, R., van der Kamp, J. and Capio, C., 2013, Implicit motor learning by children. In *Conditions of Children's Talent Development in Sport,* edited by Cote, J. and Lidor, R. (Morgantown, WV: Fitness Information Technology), pp. 21–39.

Matton, L., Duvigneaud, N., Wijndaele, K., Philippaerts, R., Duquet, W., Beunen, G., Claessens, A.L., Thomis, M. and Lefevre, J., 2007, Secular trends in anthropometric characteristics, physical fitness, physical activity, and biological maturation in Flemish adolescents between 1969 and 2005. *American Journal of Human Biology,* **19**, pp. 345–357.

McCurdy, J.H., 1913, Physical efficiency tests during adolescence. *Transactions of the Fifteenth International Congress on Hygiene and Demography,* **3**, pp. 420–428.

McGhee, Z., 1900, A study of the play life of some South Carolina children. *Pedagogical Seminary,* 7, pp. 459–478.

Mirel, J., 1982, From student control to institutional control of high school athletics: Three Michigan cities, 1883–1905. *Journal of Social History,* **16**, pp. 83–100.

Møller, N.C., Kristensen, P.L., Wedderkopp, N., Andersen, L.B. and Froberg, K., 2009, Objectively measured habitual physical activity in 1977/1998 vs 2003/2004 in Danish children: The European Youth Heart Study. *Scandinavian Journal of Medicine and Science in Sports,* **19**, pp. 19–29.

National Federation of State High School Associations, 1999–2000, History and origins. In *NFHS Handbook.* (Indianapolis, IN: National Federation of State High School Associations).

Ng, S.W. and Popkin, B., 2012, Time use and physical activity: A shift away from movement across the globe. *Obesity Reviews,* **13**, pp. 659–680.

Nishijima, T., Kokudo, S. and Ohsawa, S., 2003a, Changes over the years in physical and motor ability in Japanese youth in 1964–97. *International Journal of Sport and Health Science,* **1**, 164–170.

Nishijima, T., Nakano, T., Takahashi, S., Suzuki, K., Yamada, H., Kokudo, S. and Obsawa, S., 2003b. Relationship between changes over the years in physical ability and exercise and sports activity in Japanese youth. *International Journal of Sport and Health Science,* **1**, pp. 110–118.

North, C.C., 1931, *The Community and Social Welfare: A Study of Community Organization.* (New York: McGraw-Hill Book Company).

Ogden, C.L., Carroll, M.D. and Flegal, K.M., 2008, High body mass index for age among US children and adolescents, 2003, 2006. *Journal of the American Medical Association,* **299**, pp. 2401–2405.

Ogden, C.L., Carroll, M.D., Curtin, L.R., McDowell, M.A., Tabak, C.J. and Flegal, K.M., 2006, Prevalence of overweight and obesity in the United States, 1999–2004. *Journal of the American Medical Association,* **295**, pp. 1549–1555.

Ogden, C.L., Carroll, M.D., Curtin, L.R., Lamb, M.M. and Flegal, K.M., 2010, Prevalence of high body mass index in US children and adolescents, 2007–2008. *Journal of the American Medical Association,* **303**, pp. 242–249.

Ogden, C.L., Carroll, M.D., Kit, B.K. and Flegal, K.M., 2012, Prevalence of obesity and trends in the body mass index among US children and adolescents, 1999–2010. *Journal of the American Medical Association,* **307**, pp. 483–490.

Ogden, C.L., Flegal, K.M., Carroll, M.D. and Johnson, C.L., 2002, Prevalence and trends in overweight among US children and adolescents. *Journal of the American Medical Association,* **288**, pp. 1728–1732.

Okely, A.D., Booth, M.L., Hardy, L., Dobbins, T. and Denney-Wilson, E., 2008, Changes in physical activity participation from 1985 to 2004 in a statewide survey of Australian adolescents. *Archives of Paediatric and Adolescent Medicine,* **162**, pp. 176–180.

Perkins, D.F., Jacobs, J.E., Barber, B.L. and Eccles, J.S., 2004, Childhood and adolescent sports participation as predictors of participation in sports and physical fitness activities during young adulthood. *Youth and Society,* **35**, pp. 495–520.

Pfeiffer, K.A., Dowda, M., Dishman, R.K., McIver, K.L., Sirard, J.R., Ward, D.S. and Pate, R.R., 2006, Sport participation and physical activity in adolescent females across a four year period. *Journal of Adolescent Health,* **39**, pp. 523–529.

Pieronek, C., 1994, A clash of titans: College football v. Title IX. *Journal of College and University Law,* **3**, pp. 351–381.

Playground Association of America, 1913, The athletic badge test for boys. *The Playground,* **7**, pp. 33–37, 57–60.

Pop Warner Little Scholars 2013, http://en.wikipedia.org/wiki/Pop_Warner_Little_Scholars, accessed April 1, 2013.

Przewęda, R. and Dobosz, J., 2003, Kondycja fizyczna Polskiej młodzieży. *Studia i Monografie, Akademia Wychowania Fizycznego Józefa Piłsudskiego w Warszawie,* no. 98.

Raczek, J., 2002, Entwicklungsveranderungen der motorischen Leistungsfahigkeit der Schuljugend in drei Jahrehnten (1965–1995). *Sportwissenschaft,* **32**, pp. 201–216.

Reichert, J.L., 1958, Competitive athletics for pre-teen-age children: A challenge to physicians. *Journal of the American Medical Association,* **166**, pp. 1701–1707.

Reilly, F.J., 1917, *New Rational Athletics for Boys and Girls.* (New York: D.C Heath and Company).

Ribeyre, J., Fellmann, N., Montaurier, C., Delaître, M., Vernet, J., Coudert, J. and Vermorel, M., 2000, Daily energy expenditure and its main components as measured by whole-body indirect calorimetry in athletic and non-athletic adolescents. *British Journal of Nutrition,* **83**, pp. 355–362,

Rice, E.A., 1939, *A Brief History of Physical Education.* (New York: A.S. Barnes and Company).

Rideout, V.J., Foehr, U.G. and Roberts, D.F., 2010, *Generation M2: Media in the Lives of 8- to 18-Year Olds.* (Menlo Park, CA: Henry J. Kaiser Family Foundation).

Ridley, K., Ainsworth, B.E. and Olds, S., 2008, Development of a compendium of energy expenditures for youth. *International Journal of Behavior, Nutrition and Physical Activity,* **5**, pp. 45–52.

Ridley, K. and Olds, T.S., 2008, Assigning energy costs to activities in children: A review and synthesis. *Medicine and Science in Sports and Exercise,* **40**, pp. 1439–1446.

Ross, K.L., 2003, Historical statistics and analysis on unemployment, poverty, urbanization, etc., in the United States. http://www.friesian.com/stats.htm, accessed 22 November 2010.

Samdal, O., Tynjäla, J., Roberts, C., Sallis, J.F., Villberg, J. and Wold, B., 2007, Trends in vigorous physical activity and TV watching of adolescents from 1986 to 2002 in seven European countries. *European Journal of Public Health,* **17**, pp. 242–248.

Schwendener, N., 1932, *Game preferences of 10,000 fourth grade children.* Doctoral dissertation, (New York, Columbia University).

Scott, P.M., 1953, Attitudes towards athletic competition in elementary schools. *Research Quarterly,* **24**, pp. 352–361.

Seabra, A.C., Seabra, A.F., Brito, J., et al. No date, Effects of a 6-month soccer intervention program on psychological well-being and body composition in overweight boys: A pilot study. Under review.

Shingo, N. and Takeo, M., 2002, The educational experiments of school health promotion for the youth of Japan: Analysis of the 'sport test' over the past 34 years. *Health Promotion International,* **17**, pp. 147–160.

Stone, W.L. 1931, *What Is Boys' Work.* (New York: Association Press).

Strong, W.B., Malina, R.M., Blimkie, C.J.R., Daniels, S.R., Dishman, R.K., Gutin, B., Hergenroeder, A.C., Must, A., Nixon, P.A., Pivarnik, J.M., Rowland, T., Trost, S. and Trudeau, F., 2005, Evidence-based physical activity for school youth. *Journal of Pediatrics,* **146**, pp. 732–737.

Sutton-Smith, B. and Rosenberg, B.G., 1961, Sixty years of historical change in the game preferences of American children. *Journal of American Folklore,* **74**, pp. 17–46.

Tammelin, T., Nayha, S., Hills, A.P. and Järvelin, M.R., 2003, Adolescent participation in sports and adult physical activity. *American Journal of Preventive Medicine,* **24**, pp. 22–28.

Tandon, P.S., Saelens, B.E., Zhou, C., Kerr, J. and Christakis, D.A., 2013, Indoor versus outdoor time in preschoolers at child care. *American Journal of Preventative Medicine,* **44**, pp. 85–88.

Tandon, P.S., Zhou, C. and Christakis, D.A., 2012, Frequency of parent-supervised outdoor play of US preschool-aged children. *Archives of Pediatric and Adolescent Medicine,* **166**, pp. 707–712.

Telama, R. and Laakso, L., 2009, Secular trends in youth physical activity and parents' socioeconomic status from 1977 to 2005. *Pediatric Exercise Science,* **21**, pp. 462–474.

Telama, R., Laakso, L. and Yang, X., 1994, Physical activity and participation in sports of young people in Finland. *Scandinavian Journal of Medicine and Science in Sports,* **4**, pp. 65–74.

Telama, R., Laakso, L., Yang, X. and Vikari, J., 1997, Physical activity in childhood and adolescents as predictor of physical activity in young adulthood. *American Journal of Preventive Medicine,* **13**, pp. 317–323.

Telama, R., Yang, X., Hirvensalo, M. and Raitakari, O., 2006, Participation in organized youth sport as a predictor of adult physical activity: A 21-year longitudinal study. *Pediatric Exercise Science,* **17**, pp.76–88.

Terman, L.M., 1926, *Genetic Studies of Genius. Volume I. Mental and Physical Traits of a Thousand Gifted Children,* 2nd edition (Stanford, CA: Stanford University Press).

Thompson, A., Baxter-Jones, A.D.G., Mirwald, R.L. and Bailey, D.A., 2003, Comparison of physical activity in male and female children: Does maturation matter? *Medicine and Science in Sports and Exercise,* **35**, pp. 1684–1690.

Thrasher, F.M., 1927. *The Gang: A Study of 1,313 Gangs in Chicago.* (Chicago: University of Chicago Press).

Tomkinson, G.R., 2006, Global changes in anaerobic fitness test performance of children and adolescents. *Scandinavian Journal of Medicine and Science in Sports,* **17**, pp. 497–507.

Tomkinson, G.R. and Olds, T.S., 2007, Secular changes in pediatric aerobic fitness test performance: The global picture. *Medicine and Sport Science,* **50**, pp. 46–66.

Trost, S.G., Pate, R.R., Saunders, R.P., Ward, D.S., Dowda, M. and Felton, G., 1997, A prospective study of the determinants of physical activity in rural fifth-grade children. *Preventive Medicine,* **26**, pp. 257–263.

U.S. Department of Education, National Center for Education Statistics, 2006, *The Condition of Education 2006.* (Washington, DC: U.S. Government Printing Office).

U.S. Department of Health and Human Services, 2010, Objectives PA-3.1, 3.2, 3.3. In *Health People 2020.* (Hyattsville, MD: U.S. Department of Health and Human Services). (Available at http://healthypeople.gov/2020/topicsobjectives2020).

Weintraub, D.L., Tirumalai, E.C., Haydel, K.F., Fujimoto, M., Fulton, J.E. and Robinson, T.N., 2008, Team sports for overweight children: the Stanford Sports to Prevent Obesity Randomized Trial (SPORT). *Archives of Pediatric and Adolescent Medicine,* **162**, pp. 232–237.

Westerstahl, M., Barnekow-Bergkvist, M., Hedberg, G. and Jansson, E., 2003, Secular trends in body dimensions and physical fitness among adolescents in Sweden from 1974 to 1995. *Scandinavian Journal of Medicine and Science in Sports,* **13**, pp. 128–137.

White House Conference on Child Health and Protection, 1931, *White House Conference 1930.* (New York: The Century Company).

Wickel, E.E. and Eisenmann, J.C., 2007, Contribution of youth sport to total daily physical activity among 6- to 12-yr-old boys. *Medicine and Science in Sports and Exercise,* **39**, pp.1493–1500.

Wrotniak, B.H., Epstein, L.H., Dorn, J.M., Jones, K.E. and Kondilis, V.A., 2006, The relationship between motor proficiency and physical activity in children. *Pediatrics,* **118**, pp. e1758–1765.

Part II

Keynote Lectures

PHYSICAL ACTIVITY FOR OBESE YOUTH: IMPLICATIONS FOR CHRONIC DISEASE RISK FACTORS

P. T. Katzmarzyk

Pennington Biomedical Research Center, Baton Rouge, LA

2.1 INTRODUCTION

Obesity and chronic diseases are becoming increasingly important health concerns among the world's youth. For example, in the United States it is estimated that approximately 32% of children are now overweight or obese (Ogden *et al.*, 2012). Data from the US National Health and Nutrition Examination Survey (NHANES) also indicates that the prevalence of prediabetes/diabetes increased from 9% to 23% between 1999–2000 and 2007/2008 among youth 12 to 19 years of age (May *et al.*, 2012).

In addition to the emergence of overt chronic conditions among children, there is a concern that risk factors for chronic diseases are also becoming more prevalent. The metabolic syndrome represents a clustering of chronic disease risk factors including abdominal obesity, dyslipidaemia, high blood pressure and hyperglycaemia (Alberti *et al.*, 2009). Approximately 50% of youth 12–19 years of age in the United States have at least one metabolic syndrome risk factor, while 8.6% have 3 or more risk factors (Johnson *et al.*, 2009). This does not portend well for future health, as there is evidence that the metabolic syndrome and its component risk factors demonstrate significant tracking from childhood to adulthood (Katzmarzyk *et al.*, 2001).

Among adults, physical activity is recommended for the primary prevention of chronic diseases such as cardiovascular disease, diabetes and cancer (Eyre *et al.*, 2004). The health benefits associated with physical activity in children and youth are also well recognized. Most current recommendations are that children and youth should accumulate at least 60 minutes of moderate-to-vigorous physical activity every day to obtain health benefits (Janssen and LeBlanc, 2010; Strong *et al.*, 2005).

Given the current high prevalence of obesity among youth, it is important to understand the health benefits associated with physical activity in this group. Although the focus of many physical activity interventions among obese youth has been on weight loss and the maintenance of weight loss (Atlantis *et al.*, 2006), there is also interest in understanding the other associated health benefits such as the reduction in cardiovascular risk factors. Thus, the purpose of this report is to briefly review the evidence for the effects of physical activity on chronic disease risk factors among obese youth.

2.2 PHYSICAL ACTIVITY AND WEIGHT LOSS IN YOUTH

Physical activity is a key component in the energy balance equation, and it is currently recommended as a strategy to invoke and maintain weight loss among adults (American Dietetic Association 2009; Donnelly *et al.*, 2009). Several studies have reported an inverse association between physical activity and adiposity in children and youth (Rauner *et al.*, 2013; Reichert *et al.*, 2009). Further, recent reviews have provided insights into the effects of physical activity interventions on adiposity in children and youth (Atlantis *et al.*, 2006; McGovern *et al.*, 2008; Reichert *et al.*, 2009).

Atlantis and colleagues (2006) conducted a meta-analysis of 14 randomized trials of physical activity for weight loss in overweight and obese children and adolescents. They found a significant effect of physical activity on percent body fat (standardized mean difference = -0.4%; 95% CI: -0.7, -0.1) but not on changes in weight (standardized mean difference = -0.27; 95% CI: -0.6, 0.1). It should be noted that nine of the 14 trials also included a dietary component in the intervention, whereas five studies used physical activity only. McGovern and colleagues (2008) also conducted a meta-analysis of 17 physical activity interventions among overweight youth. They found a significant moderate effect of physical activity on adiposity (effect size = -0.52; 95% CI: -0.71, -0.30) but no significant effect on BMI (effect size = -0.02; 95% CI: -0.21, 0.18).

The results of the available studies support the use of physical activity as an intervention to reduce adiposity in children and youth, and also highlight the limitations of using BMI or body weight as an outcome in physical activity interventions. BMI and body weight are composite measures of mass that include both fat and fat-free mass, and may not be sensitive enough measures to capture intervention effects. Despite the positive results, there is a lack of quality studies evaluating the effects of physical activity on adiposity or weight loss among youth. Further research is required to develop evidence-based recommendations for weight loss for obese children and youth (Reichert *et al.*, 2009).

2.3 PHYSICAL ACTIVITY AND CHRONIC DISEASE RISK FACTORS IN OBESE YOUTH

As described above, there are many benefits associated with physical activity in children and youth. The first line of evidence comes from cross-sectional studies, which have demonstrated robust associations between physical activity and cardiovascular disease risk factors in paediatric samples (Andersen *et al.*, 2006; Ekelund *et al.*, 2012; Katzmarzyk *et al.*, 1999). For example, we used a multivariate approach to examine the relationship between physical activity and cardiovascular disease risk factors in a sample of 610 boys and girls 9–18 years of age from the Quebec Family study. Using canonical correlation, we found that a set of physical activity variables (daily energy expenditure, moderate-to-vigorous physical activity, inactivity, and television viewing) explained between 5% and 20% of the variance in a group of risk factors (blood pressure, fasting glucose, triglycerides, LDL-cholesterol, and HDL-cholesterol) (Katzmarzyk *et al.*, 1999).

Two large cross-sectional studies provide compelling evidence for a link between physical activity and cardiovascular disease risk factors in children (Andersen *et al.*, 2006; Ekelund *et al.*, 2012). Andersen and colleagues (2006) conducted an analysis of accelerometry and cardiovascular risk factor data from 1732 9- and 15-year olds from the European Youth Heart Study. Their results demonstrate a significant inverse association between mean time spent in moderate-to-vigorous physical activity and a clustered cardiovascular disease risk score (systolic blood pressure, triglycerides, total cholesterol/HDL-cholesterol ratio, insulin resistance, sum of skinfolds, and aerobic fitness) (see Figure 2.1).

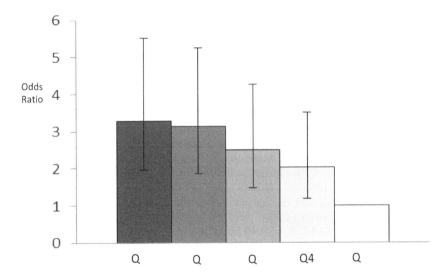

Figure 2.1 Odds ratios of clustered cardiovascular risk across quintiles of moderate-to-vigorous physical activity (>2000 counts per minute) among 1732 children from the European Youth Heart Study (Andersen *et al.*, 2006). Error bars indicate 95% confidence intervals.

Ekelund and colleagues (2012) recently analysed pooled accelerometry data from 14 studies comprising 20,871 children 4–18 years of age. Time spent in moderate-to-vigorous physical activity was significantly associated with systolic blood pressure, fasting triglycerides, HDL-cholesterol and insulin levels (Ekelund *et al.*, 2012). Higher levels of physical activity were associated with more favourable levels of the risk factors.

2.4 PHYSICAL ACTIVITY INTERVENTIONS AND CHRONIC DISEASE RISK FACTORS IN OBESE YOUTH

Several reviews have been published on the topic of physical activity interventions and chronic disease risk factors in children and adolescents. Rather than re-analysing data from primary research communications, the focus in this section will be on summarizing the results of these reviews. Despite a large evidence-base that indicates a positive association between physical activity and health, there are relatively few high quality randomized controlled trials that establish the efficacy of exercise training for the reduction of chronic disease risk factors in obese youth.

Two reviews published in 2005 came to somewhat different conclusions regarding the effects of physical activity on risk factors in children and adolescents (Strong *et al.*, 2005; Watts *et al.*, 2005). A narrative review by Watts and colleagues (2005) concluded that physical activity in children produced beneficial effects on body fat, lean mass and cardiorespiratory fitness; however, it had little effect on blood lipids or blood pressure. On the other hand, a systematic review published by a panel convened by the Divisions of Nutrition and Physical Activity and Adolescent and School Health of the U.S. Centers for Disease Control and Prevention indicated that there was "strong" evidence for physical activity having positive benefits for musculoskeletal health, several components of cardiovascular health, adiposity among overweight youth, and blood pressure among mildly hypertensive youth (Strong *et al.*, 2005). Further, the panel found that there was also "adequate" evidence for beneficial effects of physical activity on lipid and lipoprotein levels and adiposity in normal weight children and adolescents, blood pressure in normotensive youth, other cardiovascular variables, self-concept, anxiety, depressive symptom, and academic performance (Strong *et al.*, 2005).

A systematic synthesis of research conducted as part of a project to revise Canada's physical activity guidelines reiterated the level of evidence for a positive association between physical activity and health among children and youth (Janssen and LeBlanc, 2010). For aerobic physical activity interventions, the authors reported summary effect sizes of -3.03 (95% CI: -3.22, -2.84) for triglycerides, 0.26 (95% CI: 0.03, 0.49 for HDL-cholesterol), -1.39 (95% CI: -2.53, -0.24) for systolic blood pressure, 0.39 (95% CI: -1.72, 0.93) for diastolic blood pressure, and -0.60 (95% CI: -1.71, 0.5) for insulin. A recent narrative review has updated the evidence that contributed to the earlier systematic reviews (Andersen *et al.*, 2011). The conclusions of the authors were that physical activity was associated with lower blood pressure and a better lipid profile in children, and that the associations were generally stronger when using composite cardiovascular risk factor scores (Andersen *et al.*, 2011).

2.5 SUMMARY AND RECOMMENDATIONS FOR FUTURE RESEARCH

The available evidence suggests a strong association between physical activity and chronic disease risk factors in children and youth. Most studies were conducted among overweight and obese youth; however, the inclusion criteria varied from study to study. Further studies and systematic reviews among the obese paediatric population are required to determine if the effects of physical activity differ from normal weight adolescents. Given the paucity of data for some risk factors, it is difficult to determine dose-response associations, and further research is required to understand the optimal physical activity prescription.

The evidence for an effect of physical activity on chronic disease risk factors comes from a variety of sources, and studies were rarely designed specifically to address this question. For example, many risk factors are typically measured as outcome variables in studies that targeted weight loss as the primary outcome. Therefore, the subjects in many cases did not have elevated levels of the risk factors at baseline, and one would not expect physical activity to have significant effects given that values were already within the normal range. Future studies should be designed to test the efficacy and effectiveness of physical activity at lowering specific risk factors, using studies that were designed specifically for that risk factor (i.e. enrol hypertensive youth, dyslipidaemic youth, etc. at baseline). Another interesting area for future research is the disentanglement of the effects of physical activity *per se* from the effects of weight loss. In many studies the subjects lost weight as a consequence of the intervention, and it is difficult to determine if the changes observed in the risk factors are the result of the loss of body fat or if they arise from the physical activity itself. The role of physical activity in improving risk factors among obese youth is a fertile area for future research.

2.6 REFERENCES

Alberti, K.G., Eckel, R.H., Grundy, S.M., Zimmet, P.Z., Cleeman, J.I., Donato, K.A., Fruchart, J.C., James, W.P., Loria, C.M. and Smith, S.C., Jr., 2009, Harmonizing the Metabolic Syndrome. A Joint Interim Statement of the International Diabetes Federation Task Force on Epidemiology and Prevention; National Heart, Lung, and Blood Institute; American Heart Association; World Heart Federation; International Atherosclerosis Society; and International Association for the Study of Obesity. *Circulation,* **120**, pp. 1640–1645.

American Dietetic Association, 2009, Position of the American Dietetic Association: Weight Management. *Journal of the American Dietetic Association,* **109**, pp. 330–346.

Andersen, L.B., Harro, M., Sardinha, L.B., Froberg, K., Ekelund, U., Brage, S. and Anderssen, S.A., 2006, Physical activity and clustered cardiovascular risk in children: a cross-sectional study (The European Youth Heart Study). *Lancet,* **368**, pp. 299–304.

Andersen, L.B., Riddoch, C., Kriemler, S. and Hills, A., 2011, Physical activity and cardiovascular risk factors in children. *British Journal of Sports Medicine,* **45**, pp. 871–876.

Atlantis, E., Barnes, E.H. and Fiatarone Singh, M.A., 2006, Efficacy of exercise for treating overweight in children and adolescents: A systematic review. *International Journal of Obesity and Related Metabolic Disorders,* **30**, pp. 1027–1040.

Donnelly, J.E., Blair, S.N., Jakicic, J.M., Manore, M.M., Rankin, J.W. and Smith, B.K., 2009, American College of Sports Medicine Position Stand. Appropriate physical activity intervention strategies for weight loss and prevention of weight regain for adults. *Medicine and Science in Sports and Exercise,* **41**, pp. 459–471.

Ekelund, U., Luan, J., Sherar, L.B., Esliger, D.W., Griew, P. and Cooper, A., 2012, Moderate to vigorous physical activity and sedentary time and cardiometabolic risk factors in children and adolescents. *Journal of the American Medical Association,* **307**, pp. 704–712.

Eyre, H., Kahn, R., Robertson, R.M., Clark, N.G., Doyle, C., Hong, Y., Gansler, T., Glynn, T., Smith, R.A., Taubert, K. and Thun M.J., 2004, Preventing cancer, cardiovascular disease, and diabetes: a common agenda for the American Cancer Society, the American Diabetes Association, and the American Heart Association. *Stroke,* **35**, pp. 1999–2010.

Janssen, I. and LeBlanc, A.G., 2010, Systematic review of the health benefits of physical activity and fitness in school-aged children and youth. *International Journal of Behavioural Nutrition and Physical Activity,* 7, pp. 40.

Johnson, W.D., Kroon, J.J.M., Greenway, F.L., Bouchard, C., Ryan, D.H. and Katzmarzyk, P.T., 2009, Prevalence of risk factors for metabolic syndrome in adolescent: National Health and Nutrition Examination Survey (NHANES), 2001–2006. *Archives of Pediatrics and Adolescent Medicine,* **163**, pp. 371–377.

Katzmarzyk, P.T, Malina, R.M. and Bouchard, C., 1999, Physical activity, physical fitness, and coronary heart disease risk factors in youth: The Québec Family Study. *Preventive Medicine,* **29**, pp. 555–562.

Katzmarzyk, P.T., Perusse, L., Malina, R.M., Bergeron, J., Despres, J.P. and Bouchard, C., 2001, Stability of indicators of the metabolic syndrome from childhood and adolescence to young adulthood: the Quebec Family Study. *Journal of Clinical Epidemiology,* **54**, pp. 190–195.

May, A.L., Kuklina, E.V. and Yoon, P.W., 2012, Prevalence of cardiovascular disease risk factors among U.S. adolescents, 1999–2008. *Pediatrics,* **129**, pp. 1035–1041.

McGovern, L., Johnson, J.N., Paulo, R., Hettinger, A., Singhal, V., Kamath, C., Erwin, P.J. and Montori, V.M., 2008, Treatment of pediatric obesity: A systematic review and meta-analysis of randomized trials. *Journal of Clinical Endocrinology and Metabolism,* **93**, pp. 4600–4605.

Ogden, C.L., Carroll, M.D., Kit, B.K. and Flegal, K.M., 2012, Prevalence of obesity and trends in body mass index among US children and adolescents, 1999–2010. *Journal of the American Medical Association,* **307**, pp. 483–490.

Rauner, A., Mess, F. and Woll, A., 2013, The relationship between physical activity, physical fitness and overweight in adolescents: A systematic review of studies published in or after 2000. *BMC Pediatrics,* **13**, pp. 19.

Reichert, F.F., Menezes, A.M.B., Wells, J.C.K., Dumith, C. and Hallal, P.C., 2009, Physical activity as a predictor of adolescent body fatness: A systematic review. *Sports Medicine,* **39**, pp. 279–294.

Strong, W.B., Malina, R.M., Blimkie, C.J., Daniels, S.R., Dishman, R.K., Gutin, B., Hergenroeder, A.C., Must, A., Nixon, P.A., Pivarnik, J.M., Rowland, T., Trost S. and Trudeau F., 2005, Evidence based physical activity for school-age youth. *Journal of Pediatrics,* **146**, pp. 732–737.

Watts, K., Jones, T.W., Davis, E.A. and Green, D., 2005, Exercise training in obese children and adolescents: Current concepts. *Sports Medicine,* **35**, pp. 375–392.

CHILD HEALTH NEEDS OF YOUNG CHILDREN FROM FAMILIES LIVING IN SOCIAL AND ECONOMIC DISADVANTAGE

G. Naughton[1,2], K. Gibbons[1,2], and J. Myers[2]

[1] Australian Catholic University, Australia; [2] Murdoch Children's Research Institute, Australia

3.1 BACKGROUND

The 11% of children in Australia living in poverty, (UNICEF, 2012) have parents with low regular income, disconnection from services in employment, health and education, and feeling socially isolated from supportive networks. Refugees, newly arrived migrants and migrants from non-English speaking backgrounds are over-represented in areas of social disadvantage in Australia. Despite the availability of universal health services such as child health nurses, families from socially disadvantaged backgrounds are missing out on important support for the early years of childhood.

Living in social disadvantage places young children at risk of poor health outcomes (Power, 2005; Law *et al.*, 2012). The links between poor nutrition, inadequate physical activity, and socioeconomic disadvantage (e.g. low income, low educational attainment) are well established (Ebenegger *et al.*, 2011). For example, individuals from lower socioeconomic areas consumed less fruit and vegetables, and more fat than individuals living in higher socioeconomic areas in Australia (Williams *et al.*, 2011). Children from socially disadvantaged backgrounds are also over-represented in the prevalence of obesity from a young age (Shrewsbury and Wardle, 2008).

Child health practices in areas of social disadvantage in Australia are infrequently described. A Needs Assessment originally conducted in 1995 within more socially disadvantaged, outer western suburbs of Melbourne, (Australia) (Graham *et al.*, 2000; Gibbons *et al.*, 2000) was repeated in 2010. The overall purpose was to review family and child health practitioners' perceptions of child nutrition, physical activity and childhood obesity concerns in families from the same outer western suburbs of Melbourne as previously studied and a regional area with a matching socioeconomic demographic. A secondary purpose was to investigate differences between child health needs of families in regional and urban areas of similar socioeconomic disadvantage.

3.2 METHODS

The project received ethics approval from the Human Research and Ethics Committee, at the Royal Children's Hospital, Melbourne, and State Education and Early Childhood authorities. Replicating the methods from the Needs Assessment in 1997, 601 parents of children aged 2–8 years and 45 early child health practitioners were recruited from a random selection of early childhood settings appropriate for each age group: childcare for children aged 2–4 years, kindergartens for children aged 4–6 years and primary schools for children aged 6–8 years.

All parents aged 18 years and over, with children attending the setting on the day of the study, were invited to participate in a written parent survey. Families were assisted by researchers if needed and local interpreters were used as required. Primary school surveys were distributed to parents of children in their second year of schooling (aged 6–8 years). Surveys were made available in Vietnamese for schools, due to the high proportion of Vietnamese-speaking families.

The parents' survey comprised of questions about nutrition practices, active outdoor play and screen viewing time on the day prior to the survey. Responses were used to dichotomise outcomes into meeting or not meeting national or best practice guidelines for children's nutrition and physical activity. For example, parent reports of children's consumption of takeaway food, 'packaged' food (such as crisps, chocolates etc), greater than ½ cup sweet drinks and any tea / coffee each consumed on the day prior to the survey were used as cut-points for these practices. Similarly, estimated consumption of one or more 'serves' of fruit and vegetables per day were used as cut-points.

Parent reports of children's time spent in 'active outdoor play' were used to describe physical activity because the outdoor environment offers more opportunity for total body movement and outdoor play is more likely to be of a moderate to vigorous intensity than indoor play (Whittaker, 2003). The cut-points were >2 hours of active outdoor play for pre-school children and >1 hour for school-aged children. Similarly, hours of children's screen viewing time were reported by parents; with cut points of no more than 1 hour for pre-school children and 2 hours for school aged children. Parents were also asked to identify any concerns about their child's physical activity and nutrition in the preceding 6 months. Finally, parents were asked to list barriers to healthy behaviour in active play and nutrition as well as concerns about obesity-related issues.

Two sample tests of proportions were used to compare proportions between each group, and 95% confidence intervals for the estimated difference in proportions were constructed from the unpooled standard error of the difference. T-tests were used to compare continuous outcome measures. For qualitative data, taped interviews with practitioners were analysed using thematic analysis reviewed by two researchers. Data were managed using the EpiData programme (Odense M, Denmark, Version 3.1, 2006) and analysed using Stata 11 (StataCorp. 2009. Stata: Release 11. Statistical Software. College Station, TX: StataCorp LP).

3.3 RESULTS

With a response rate of 72%, we analysed parent reports from 395 pre-school children (52% boys) with a mean age of 3.8 (2.0 – 6.02) years and 206 school-aged children (54% boys) who had a mean age of 6.92 (6.92 (5.95 – 8.37). A language other than English was spoken in the homes of 39% of pre-school children's families and 43% of school-aged children. The proportion of children with mothers born overseas was also similar in pre-school (45%) and school-aged children (53%).

We found that 80% of pre-school-aged children were reported to exceed their recommended TV viewing time (1 hour per day for pre-school children) and 30% of school-aged children exceed their recommended time (2 hours per day for school-aged children) on week days ($p < 0.001$). However, at weekends, the number of school-aged children exceeding recommended TV viewing time doubled (62%) and computer time tripled (19%) ($p<0.001$).

The pre-determined physical activity criterion of 2 or more hours per day for children 2–5 years and 1 or more hours per day for children aged 5–12 years was more frequently not reached by pre-school children (76%) than school-aged children (41%) ($p < 0.001$).

Between the ages of 2–8 years (across three age groups) children living in the regional area (n = 298) were consistently reported to be more active than urban (n = 303) children. For example, among parents of children aged 6–8 years, the proportion of children having more than 1 hour of active outdoor play on the day prior to the survey was 72% in the regional area and 47% in the urban area. However, regional parents also reported their children aged 2–8 years viewed more television than their urban peers.

Concerns about high cost physical activities were expressed more from urban than regional parents. Higher parental concerns for neighbourhood safety were again more prevalent among parents from urban than regional areas.

Compared with parents in urban areas, parents of regional school-aged children were also less concerned about their child's fruit intake ($p<0.001$), overall growth ($p = 0.005$) and dental health ($p = 0.003$).

In both locations, despite practitioners reporting the availability of information, if mothers of preschool children were born overseas or spoke a language other than English at home, they reported greater difficulties accessing, using and practising key messages about child nutrition and physical activity.

Independent of age, parental concern about obesity risk in their child remained <5%, yet the estimated national prevalence even in pre-school children is approximately 25% (Vaska and Volkmer, 2004).

3.4 CONCLUSION

Across all age groups (2–8 years) screen time use for the majority of children exceeded national recommendations. Insufficient active outdoor play in young children also remains a concern, particularly in pre-school children. More urban than regional parents expressed concerns, and perceived proportionally greater barriers in child health issues. Resources in culturally-appropriate languages, with well-considered standards of literacy and sensitive images, placed-based experiences, and increased efforts in social connection may help meet the needs of families with young children from socially disadvantaged backgrounds.

3.5 REFERENCES

Ebenegger, V., Marques-Vidal, P-M,. Nydegger A., Laimbacher, J., Niederer I., Bürgi, F., Giusti, V., Bodenmann, P., Kriemler, S. and Pude, J.J., 2011, Independent contribution of parental migrant status and educational level to adiposity and eating habits in pre-school children. *European Journal of Clinical Nutrition,* **65**, pp. 210–218.

Gibbons, K., Graham, V., Marraffa, C. and Henry, L., 2000, 'Filling the Gap' - children aged between two and four years: sources of nutrition information used by families, and childcare staff. *Australian Journal of Nutrition and Dietetics*, **57**, pp. 208–14.

Graham, V., Gibbons, K., Marraffa, C. and Sultana, J., 2000, 'Filling the Gap' - children aged between six and eight years: sources of information used by families, school nurses and teachers. *Australian Journal of Nutrition and Dietetics,* **57**, pp. 90–94.

Law, C., Parkin, C. and Lewis, H., 2012, Policies to tackle inequalities in child health: why haven't they worked (better)? *Archives of Disease in Childhood,* **97**, pp. 301–303.

Power, E.M., 2005, Determinants of healthy eating among low-income Canadians. *Canadian Journal of Public Health,* **96**, pp. S37–42.

Shrewsbury, V. and Wardle, J., 2008, Socioeconomic Status and Adiposity in Childhood: A Systematic Review of Cross-sectional Studies 1990–2005. *Obesity,* **16**, pp. 275–284.

UNICEF Innocenti Research Centre, 2012, 'Measuring Child Poverty: New league tables of child poverty in the world's rich countries',Innocenti Report Card 10, UNICEF Innocenti Research Centre, Florence.

Vaska, V.L. and Volkmer, R., 2004, Increasing prevalence of obesity in South Australian 4-year-olds: 1995–2002. *Journal of Paediatrics and Child Health,* **40**, pp. 353–355.

Whittaker, R.C., 2003, Obesity prevention in pediatric primary care: four behaviours to target. *Archives Pediatric and Adolescent Medicine,* **157**, pp. 1050–1055.

Williams, L.K., Veitch, J. and Ball, K., 2011, What helps children eat well? A qualitative exploration of resilience among disadvantaged families. *Health Education Research,* **26**, pp. 296–307.

SCHOOL BASED PHYSICAL ACTIVITY INTERVENTIONS CAN WORK: HOW EFFECTIVE ARE THEY AND WHAT DOES IT TAKE TO GET THEM IMPLEMENTED?

L.B. Andersen[1,2], M. Ried-Larsen[1], T. Huang [1], G.K. Resaland[3], and A. Bugge[1]

[1]Institute of Sport Sciences and Clinical Biomechanics, University of Southern Denmark, Denmark; [2]Department of Sport Medicine, Norwegian School of Sport Sciences, Norway; [3]Faculty of Teacher Education and Sport, Sogn og Fjordane University College, Norway

4.1 INTRODUCTION

The world today is facing an increasing number of individuals with lifestyle related diseases such as cardiovascular diseases (CVD), type 2 diabetes and certain types of cancers (Lee *et al.*, 2012). This has tremendous consequences both at the individual and the societal level in terms of decreased quality of life, increased morbidity and mortality (Lee *et al.*, 2012). The economic burden on the health care system and lost productivity adds to the burden of the society. The reason for this increase is multifactorial but lack of physical activity, and excess body fat contribute (Grontved *et al.*, 2012; Grontved and Hu, 2011; Tang-Peronard *et al.*, 2011). Recent research has shown that physical activity and high aerobic fitness (VO_{2peak}) level are associated not only with insulin sensitivity, obesity and other metabolic risk factors, but also with improved cognitive function in relation to biological markers (brain derived neurotrophic factor, BDNF), and cognitive tests (Aberg *et al.*, 2009). Furthermore, it has been found that BDNF is closely associated with the metabolic risk factors (Tyler *et al.*, 2002; Krabbe *et al.*, 2007). These apparently very different parameters, obesity, physical activity, fitness and cognitive function, seem to be interlinked. Associations between physical activity, fitness, obesity and CVD risk factors such as insulin resistance are well known, while knowledge of the association between the physical activity and cognitive function and biological mechanisms behind this association is increasing fast.

School-based interventions have shown that it is possible to improve CVD risk factor profile in children with an adverse risk factor profile (Kriemler *et al.*, 2010; Heath *et al.*, 2012). Despite that, the number of physical education (PE) lessons has decreased in Denmark since the 1960s from four lessons a week to only two lessons. The national guideline for physical activity for children is 60 min per day of moderate intensity PA (Pedersen and Andersen, 2011), but still the political will to increase PA in school has been limited. The main reason is probably that the purpose of the school system is primarily to teach children academic skills. The reluctance from teachers teaching other subjects and politicians to increase PE might be based on the concerns that taking time from theoretical subjects will decrease the abilities in these subjects.

The scientific knowledge about the association between PA or physical performance and cognitive function in children is still deficient and inconclusive (Chaddock *et al.*, 2011; Biddle and Asare, 2011). It is therefore of utmost importance to obtain more knowledge both about implementation of PA and benefits of PA on cognitive function in different age groups in order to implement preventive strategies in the school system. In order to do so knowledge about biological mechanisms of how PA exerts the effects on cognitive function and how this can be measured is needed.

4.2 INCREASING PA, DECREASING SEDENTARY BEHAVIOUR AND COGNITIVE FUNCTION

Besides metabolic benefits, regular physical activity may also improve cognitive function and prevent cognitive impairment (Aberg *et al.*, 2009). A convincing study including >1.2 million Swedish men has shown that more fit young men performed better in intelligence tests conducted before entry into military service, and they also got better jobs later and higher salaries than their less fit peers (Aberg *et al.*, 2009). This was even true in monozygotic twins (Figure 4.1). Although physical activity has relatively broad effects across a variety of cognitive functions, the benefits of physical exercise in older adults seem to be larger for executive functions (EF) (e.g. inhibitory control, working memory, planning, scheduling) (Kramer and Erickson, 2007).

Recent research in youth also suggests the fitness-cognition association is larger for tasks or task components that require extensive amounts of cognitive control (Chaddock *et al.*, 2011). Executive functions are associated with scholastic achievement. EFs predict both math and reading ability throughout the school years (Diamond, 2013).

A.   Combined intelligence

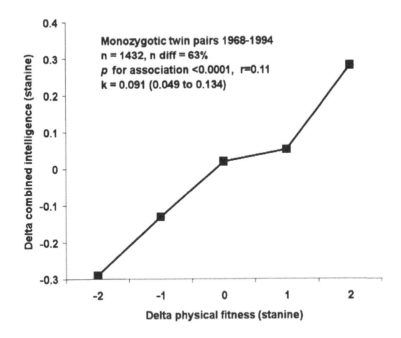

Figure 4.1 Dose-response relationship between aerobic fitness and cognitive function in monozygotic young adults / adults twins (Aberg *et al.*, 2009).

4.3 BIOLOGICAL PLAUSIBILITY

At the systems level, electrophysiological and neuroimaging studies have suggested that physical activity benefits cognitive performance by increasing neuroelectric activity, brain volume, and blood flow in the brain (Hillman *et al.*, 2008). At the molecular and cellular level, evidence from animal research has shown that exercise increases the availability of neural growth factors (e.g. BDNF, IGF-1) and supports synaptic plasticity, neurogenesis and angiogenesis in the brain (Cotman and Berchtold, 2002; Ratey and Loehr, 2011). Several human studies have shown that the synthesis of BDNF is increased during and following physical activity (Rasmussen *et al.*, 2009; Erickson *et al.*, 2011; Ferris *et al.*, 2007). Training induced increases in BDNF might explain some of the observed alterations in cognitive parameters since BDNF facilitates neuronal regenerative capacity and synaptic plasticity (Santos *et al.*, 2010). In support of this, Erickson *et al.* (2011) reported an increase in the volume of hippocampus following physical activity and this increase was associated with both increased serum BDNF as well as improved memory (Erickson *et al.*, 2011). The brain contributes to most of the plasma BDNF in healthy humans, which suggests that circulating levels of BDNF in plasma may reflect levels in the brain (Rasmussen *et al.*, 2009b).

Circulating levels of BDNF in plasma in humans reflects levels in hippocampus and BDNF is produced during an acute bout of exercise as well as the level being higher in fit subjects compared to unfit. Furthermore, levels of BDNF are closely related to insulin resistance (Krabbe *et al.*, 2007), which causes clustering of CVD risk factors and obesity. It is logic to extend our metabolic research in children with research in cognitive function and BDNF. A systematic review from our group focused on the effect of physical activity on BDNF and cognitive function is in press in the Scandinavian Journal of Medicine and Science in Sports (Huang *et al.*, 2013).

4.4 SCHOOL-BASED PHYSICAL ACTIVITY INTERVENTIONS

During the last decade our group has conducted three large school-based interventions with different amounts and intensities of increased physical activity with the aim of finding the balance between success of implementation and the effect on health. The political will to make the intervention compulsory is probably larger with smaller alterations to the existing curriculum, but the health effect is also smaller.

Our first intervention was the Copenhagen Schoolchild Intervention Study (CoSCIS) (Bugge *et al.*, 2012). In this study we increased physical education lessons from two to four, improved facilities and conducted a training programme for teachers. The study assessed short-term and long-term effects of a 3-yr controlled school-based physical activity (PA) intervention on fatness, cardiorespiratory fitness (VO_{2peak}) and CVD risk factors in children. The study involved 18 schools (10 intervention and 8 controls) and included a follow-up 4 yr after the end of intervention. The analyses included 696, 6- to 7-yr-old children at baseline, 612 after intervention (aged 9.5 yr) and 441 at follow-up (aged 13.4 yr). Anthropometrics and systolic blood pressure (SBP) were measured. VO_{2peak} was directly measured, and PA was assessed using accelerometry. Fasting blood samples were analyzed for CVD risk factors. A composite risk score was computed from z-scores of SBP, triglycerides, total cholesterol-to-HDL cholesterol ratio, homeostatic model assessment (HOMA score), skinfolds, and inverse VO_{2peak}. The HOMA score of the intervention group of boys had a smaller increase from baseline to after intervention compared with control boys ($P = 0.004$). From baseline to follow-up intervention group, boys had a smaller increase in SBP compared with control boys ($P = 0.010$). There were no other significant differences between groups. We did find positive changes in SBP and HOMA score in boys but not in PA, VO_{2peak}, fatness, and the other measured CVD risk factors. Our results indicated that a doubling of PE and providing training and equipment only revealed small improvements and may not be sufficient to induce major improvements in CVD risk factors in a normal population.

Based on our experience from CoSCIS we later performed an intervention where exposure was strengthened substantially. Physical activity was increased to 1 hour each school day over two consecutive schools-years, and emphasis was put on high intensity in part of the activities (Resaland *et al.*, 2011). The intervention was conducted at one school (I-school, n=125) and one control school (C-school, n=131). The PA lessons were planned, organized and led by expert PE teachers and they were not restricted to PE, but also included PA integrated in other lessons such as math and language lessons. In the C-school, children were offered the normal 45 min of PE twice weekly. The intervention resulted in a greater beneficial development in systolic (P=0.003) and diastolic (P=0.002) blood pressure, total cholesterol-to-high-density lipoprotein cholesterol ratio (P=0.011), triglyceride (P=0.030) and VO_{2peak} (P<0.001) in I-school children than in C-school children. No significant differences were observed in waist circumference, body mass index and the HOMA score between the two groups. Furthermore, the intervention, primarily carried out at moderate intensity, had the strongest impact in children with the least favourable starting point. In conclusion, the daily school-based PA intervention revealed substantial beneficial modifications in children's CVD risk profile and the higher effect may be related to longer duration of physical activities, a high intensity, and that PA was implemented by expert PE teachers.

Currently, we are testing an intervention with an exposure in between these two interventions, because it may be more plausible for politicians to change the school curriculum to three double PE lessons than a whole hour of physical activity every day. Preliminary results of health effect of the intervention look promising, and the political awareness of children's health has increased since we performed our first intervention in the school. It is therefore likely such change in school curriculum may occur. Further, the evidence that physical activity affects neural growth and cognitive skills is growing, and this may be a key argument in the discussion of future school curriculum. Future studies should aim at improving the understanding of the effects of different PA modes and intensities on cognitive function as well as metabolic CVD risk in children. This could help us design effective interventions to prevent adverse outcomes in the broader population and enable successful implementation.

4.5 REFERENCES

Aberg, M.A., Pedersen, N.L., Toren, K., Svartengren, M., Backstrand, B., Johnsson, T., Cooper-Kuhn, C.M., Aberg, N.D., Nilsson, M. and Kuhn, H.G., 2009, Cardiovascular fitness is associated with cognition in young adulthood. *Proceedings of the National Academy of Sciences*, **106**, pp 20906–20911.

Biddle, S.J. and Asare, M., 2011, Physical activity and mental health in children and adolescents: a review of reviews. *British Journal of Sports Medicine*, **45**, pp, 886–895.

Bugge, A., El-Naaman, B., Dencker, M., Froberg, K., Holme, I.M., McMurray, R.G. and Andersen L.B., 2012, Effects of a three-year intervention: the Copenhagen School Child Intervention Study. *Medicine and Science in Sports and Exercise*, **44**, pp, 1310–1317.

Chaddock, L., Pontifex, M.B., Hillman, C.H. and Kramer, A.F., 2011, A review of the relation of aerobic fitness and physical activity to brain structure and function in children. *Journal of International Neuropsychology and Sociology*, **17**, pp, 975–985.

Cotman, C.W. and Berchtold, N.C., 2002, Exercise: a behavioral intervention to enhance brain health and plasticity. *Trends in Neuroscience*, **25**, pp. 295–301.

Diamond, A. 2013, Executive function. *Annual Review of Psychology* **64**, pp. 135–168.

Erickson, K.I., Voss, M.W., Prakash, R.S., Basak, C., Szabo, A., Chaddock, L., Kim, J.S., Heo, S., Alves, H., White, S.M., Wojcicki, T.R., Mailey, E., Vieira, V.J., Martin, S.A., Pence, B.D., Woods, J.A., McAuley, E. and Krmer, A.F., 2011, Exercise training increases size of hippocampus and improves memory. *Proceedings of the National Academy of Sciences*, **108**, pp, 3017–3022.

Ferris, L.T., Williams, J.S. and Shen, C.L., 2007, The effect of acute exercise on serum brain-derived neurotrophic factor levels and cognitive function. *Medicine and Science in Sports and Exercise*, **39**, pp, 728–734.

Grontved, A. and Hu, F.B., 2011, Television viewing and risk of type 2 diabetes, cardiovascular disease, and all-cause mortality: a meta-analysis. *The Journal of American Medical Association*, **305**, pp, 2448–2455.

Grontved, A., Ried-Larsen, M., Moller, N. C., Kristensen, P. L., Wedderkopp, N., Froberg, K., Hu, F.B., Ekelund, U. and Andersen L.B., 2012, Youth screen-time behaviour is associated with cardiovascular risk in young adulthood: the European Youth Heart Study. *European Journal of Preventive Cardiology*, doi: 2047487312454760.

Heath, G. W., Parra, D. C., Sarmiento, O. L., Andersen, L. B., Owen, N., Goenka, S., Montes, F. and Brownson, R.C. 2012, Evidence-based intervention in physical activity: lessons from around the world. *Lancet*, **380**, pp, 272–281.

Hillman, C.H., Erickson, K.I. and Kramer, A.F., 2008, Be smart, exercise your heart: exercise effects on brain and cognition. *Nature Review of Neuroscience*, **9**, pp, 58–65.

Huang, T., Larsen, K.T., Ried-Larsen, M., Møller, N.C. and Andersen, L.B., 2013, The effects of physical activity and exercise on brain-derived neurotrophic factor in healthy humans: A review. *Scandinavian Journal of Medicine and Science in Sports*, doi: 10.1111/sms.12069.

Krabbe, K. S., Nielsen, A. R., Krogh-Madsen, R., Plomgaard, P., Rasmussen, P., Erikstrup, C., Fisher, C.P., Lindegaard, B., Petersen, A.M., Taudorf, S., Secher, N.H., Pilegaard, H., Bruunsgaard, H. and Pedersen, B.K., 2007, Brain-derived neurotrophic factor (BDNF) and type 2 diabetes. *Diabetologia,* **50**, pp, 431–438.

Kramer, A.F. and Erickson, K.I., 2007, Capitalizing on cortical plasticity: influence of physical activity on cognition and brain function. *Trends in Cognitive Science*, **11**, pp, 342–348.

Kriemler, S., Zahner, L., Schindler, C., Meyer, U., Hartmann, T., Hebestreit, H., Brunner-La Rocca, H.P., van Mechelen, W. and Puder J.J., 2010, Effect of school based physical activity programme (KISS) on fitness and adiposity in primary schoolchildren: cluster randomised controlled trial. *British Medical Journal*, **340**, pp, c785.

Lee, I. M., Shiroma, E.J., Lobelo, F., Puska, P., Blair, S.N. and Katzmarzyk, P.T., 2012, Effect of physical inactivity on major non-communicable diseases worldwide: an analysis of burden of disease and life expectancy. *Lancet*, **380**, pp, 219–229.

Pedersen, B.K. and Andersen, L.B., 2011, *Fysisk aktivitet: håndbog om forebyggelse og behandling*, (København: Rosendahls-Schultz Grafisk A/S).

Rasmussen, P., Brassard, P., Adser, H., Pedersen, M. V., Leick, L., Hart, E., Secher, N.H., Pedersen, B.K. and Pilegaard, H., 2009, Evidence for a release of brain-derived neurotrophic factor from the brain during exercise. *Experimental Physiology*, **94**, pp, 1062–1069.

Ratey, J.J. and Loehr, J.E., 2011, The positive impact of physical activity on cognition during adulthood: a review of underlying mechanisms, evidence and recommendations. *Reviews of Neuroscience*, **22**, pp, 171–185.

Resaland, G.K., Anderssen, S.A., Holme, I.M., Mamen, A. and Andersen, L.B., 2011, Effects of a 2-year school-based daily physical activity intervention on cardiovascular disease risk factors: the Sogndal school-intervention study. *Scandinavian Journal of Medicine in Science and Sports*, **21**, pp, 122–131.

Santos, A.R., Comprido, D. and Duarte, C.B., 2010, Regulation of local translation at the synapse by BDNF. *Progress in Neurobiology*, **92**, pp, 505–516.

Tang-Peronard, J.L., Andersen, H.R., Jensen, T.K. and Heitmann, B.L., 2011, Endocrine-disrupting chemicals and obesity development in humans: a review. *Obesity Reviews*, **12**, pp, 622-636.

Tyler, W.J., Alonso, M., Bramham, C.R., and Pozzo-Miller, L.D., 2002, From acquisition to consolidation: on the role of brain-derived neurotrophic factor signaling in hippocampal-dependent learning. *Learning and Memory*, **9**, pp, 224–237.

THE COMPANIONSHIP OF SEDENTARY BEHAVIOUR, PHYSICAL ACTIVITY, FITNESS, AND HEALTH- FINDINGS FROM THE EYHS (EUROPEAN YOUTH HEART STUDY)

L.B. Sardinha

Faculty of Human Kinetics – Technical University of Lisbon, Portugal

The European Youth Heart Study (EYHS) is a multi-centre, international study, addressing the prevalence and aetiology of cardiovascular disease (CVD) risk factors in children aged 9 and 15 years with a mixed cross-sectional and longitudinal design with data collection every 6 years including new young cohorts and retest of previous cohorts in Denmark, Portugal, Norway and Estonia. Later Iceland and Spain joined the study. The first assessments started in 1997 and a 6- and 12-year follow-up have been finished in Denmark, 6-year follow-up in Norway, Portugal and Iceland, and Portugal is currently collecting 12-year follow-up. Sedentary and physical activity behaviours were objectively assessed with accelerometers. Blood samples were drawn for analysis of traditional CVD risk factors, genetic mapping and a possibility to analyze new biomarkers. Assessments included also measurements of dietary intake, physical fitness including cardiorespiratory fitness (CRF), muscular strength, skinfold measurements and a comprehensive questionnaire for both children and parents. This short book chapter summarizes the major findings related to sedentary behavior, physical activity and physical fitness. The findings of the EYHS include cross-sectional and prospective observational data.

5.1 SEDENTARY BEHAVIOUR

During the past decades the increasing of sedentary behaviours, such as television watching and playing electronic games, may have contributed to increase the incidence of metabolic and CVD risk factors in children, including disturbed insulin and glucose metabolism, hypertension, general and abdominal obesity, and dyslipidaemia.

A cross-sectional analysis of data from the EYHS, revealed that, on average, European children spent 262 min/day in sedentary activity (van Sluijs *et al.*, 2010). Additionally, sedentary time increased substantially with increasing age, indicating that early intervention is needed to prevent this increase and the development of health problems associated with sedentary behaviour. Since sedentary activity is associated with a variety of behavioural and social factors, and associations are different for different countries, a single strategy aimed at reducing time spent in sedentary activity in youth is therefore unlikely to be effective across Europe as the target populations and behaviours of focus differ between countries (van Sluijs *et al.*, 2010). No associations between mode of transportation to school, outdoor play after school, participation in sport and exercise in clubs, and TV viewing with percent time sedentary were observed, suggesting that correlates associated with sedentary behaviour are likely to differ from those associated with physical activity (Nilsson *et al.*, 2009). Besides environment factors, it has been hypothesized that sedentary behaviour may be related to lower birth weight. Data from the different centers of the EYHS showed that birth weight did not affect sedentary behaviour (Ridgway *et al.*, 2011c).

Major dimensions of sedentary behaviour are TV viewing and computer games. Children and adolescents that have more autonomy over their own behaviour are more likely to watch more than 2 h of TV after school and spend more than an hour per day playing computer games (Jago *et al.*, 2008a). This TV viewing behaviour was associated with adiposity (Ekelund *et al.*, 2006). However, after adjustment for physical activity and other covariates, the association of TV viewing with clustered metabolic risk [the sum of four skin folds, hypertension (average of systolic blood pressure and diastolic blood pressure), hyperglycaemia (fasting plasma glucose), insulin resistance (fasting insulin), inverted fasting HDL cholesterol, and hypertriglyceridaemia] was no longer significant. These results suggest that TV viewing and physical activity may be separate entities and differently associated with adiposity and metabolic risk. The association between TV viewing and clustered metabolic risk was mediated by adiposity, whereas physical activity was associated with individual and clustered metabolic-risk indicators independently of obesity. As illustrated in figure 5.1, time spent sedentary was significantly and positively associated with fasting insulin and HOMA-IR in healthy Portuguese children after adjusting for total or central fat mass as measured with DXA, and time spent in moderate-and vigorous intensity physical activity (MVPA) and overall physical activity (Sardinha *et al.*, 2008a).

A prospective cohort study among Danish men and women, followed for up to 12 years, revealed that TV viewing and total screen time in adolescence were positively associated with adiposity, triglycerides, and metabolic syndrome z-score in young adulthood. Individuals who increased their TV viewing, computer use, or total screen time with more than 2 hours/day from adolescence to young adulthood had 0.90, 0.95, and 1.40 kg/m^2 higher body mass index, respectively, in young adulthood compared with individuals who remained stable or decreased their viewing time. Insulin and metabolic syndrome z-scores were also higher among individuals who increased their TV viewing, computer use, or total screen time more than 2 hours/day compared with individuals who remained stable or decreased their viewing time (Grontved *et al.*, 2012).

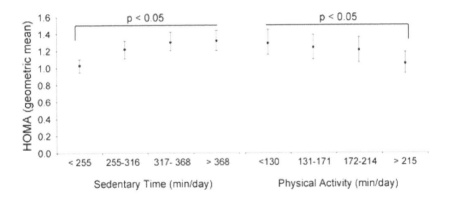

Figure 5.1 Adjusted geometric means of HOMA-IR stratified by quartiles of time spent sedentary (p for trend = 0.043) and time spent at MVPA (p for trend = 0.11) in 9- to 10-year-old Portuguese children (n= 308). Post hoc analyses revealed significant differences ($p < 0.05$) between the first and fourth quartile for time spent sedentary and at moderate and vigorous intensity. Data are adjusted for sex, sexual maturity, birth weight, and fat mass (Adapted from Sardinha *et al.*, 2008a).

Taken together, the cross-sectional and longitudinal findings suggest that screen-viewing behaviours of the entire family are likely to be important for changing youth screen-viewing. Preventive action against obesity and metabolic risk in children may need to target TV viewing and physical activity separately. Therefore, reducing sedentary behaviour and increasing the amount of time spent in MVPA may have beneficial effects on insulin resistance in healthy children. The development and implementation of multidimensional strategies focused on reducing sedentary behaviours and increasing overall involvement in different types of moderate-intensity activity are critically important in the primary prevention of metabolic disorders in children in order to improve young adulthood health.

5.2 PHYSICAL ACTIVITY

Lower birth weight has been associated with reduced physical performance, including muscle strength, muscle endurance and aerobic fitness in both childhood and adulthood and it has been suggested that this lower physical capacity may lead to reduced levels of physical activity. A survey using combined analysis of three European cohorts, indicated that there was no evidence for an association between birth weight and total physical activity or time spent in MVPA (Ridgway *et al.*, 2011c). Overall there was no evidence for an association between birth weight and sedentary time. Further, higher birth weight was found to be associated with higher fat mass index and greater waist circumference, adjusted for sex, age-group, sexual maturity, height, and socioeconomic status. Lower birth weight was associated with higher fasting insulin only after further adjustment for adolescent waist circumference and height (Ridgway *et al.*, 2011b). However, there was no evidence that physical activity or aerobic fitness can moderate the associations among higher birth weight and increased fat mass and metabolic risk in youth.

Influences on young peoples' physical activity are multi-factorial. A variety of psychological, social and physical environmental correlates of physical activity for young people have been identified. Data from a cross-sectional study among Norwegian boys and girls shows that there are psycho-social and environmental correlates of location-specific physical activity. Dependent of location (a) school commuting, b) informal games play at school and c) organized sport, structured exercise and games play in leisure time), psycho-social and environmental correlates explained between 15 and 55 percent of the variance in physical activity. The impact of peer support, enjoyment and perceived competence in physical activity generalized across the three locations. Enjoyment of physical education classes, parental support and teacher support, in contrast, confined to particular location-specific forms of physical activity. Generally, behavioural beliefs and environmental factors represented marginal correlates of all location-specific forms of activity (Ommundsen *et al.*, 2006). Frequency of outdoor play after school was found as a significant correlate for daily time in MVPA in 9-year-olds, while this correlate is attenuated in favour of participation in sport and exercise in clubs in 15-year-olds (Nilsson *et al.*, 2009).

After adjustment for sex, study location, sexual maturity, birth weight, and parental BMI, time spent at MVPA and time (min/d) spent at vigorous physical activity were independently associated with body fatness. Sex, study location, sexual maturity, birth weight, and parental BMI explained 29% of the variation in body fatness. Children who accumulated less than 1 h of moderate physical activity/d were significantly fatter than were those who accumulated more than 2 h/d. (Ekelund *et al.*, 2004).

Clustering of CVD risk factors has recently proved a better measure of cardiovascular health in children than single risk factors. A cross-sectional study of children from Denmark, Estonia, and Portugal reported that odds ratios for having clustered risk for ascending quintiles of physical activity were 3.29 (95% CI 1.96–5.52), 3.13 (1.87–5.25), 2.51 (1.47–4.26), and 2.03 (1.18–3.50), respectively, compared with the most active quintile. Risk factors included in the composite risk factor score (mean of Z scores) were systolic blood pressure, triglyceride, total cholesterol/HDL ratio, insulin resistance, sum of four skinfolds, and aerobic fitness. The first to the third quintile of physical activity had a raised risk in all analyses. The mean time spent above 2000 counts per minute (cpm) in the fourth quintile was 116 min per day in 9-year-olds and 88 min per day in 15-year-old children. It was found that, achieving 90 min of daily activity might be necessary for children to prevent insulin resistance, which seems to be the central feature for clustering of CVD risk factors (Andersen *et al.*, 2006). Figure 5.2 depicts the graded relationship between physical activity intensity quintiles and CVD Z-score.

Further cross-sectional analysis showed that physical activity and CRF were separately and independently associated with individual and clustered metabolic risk factors in children (Ekelund *et al.*, 2007). Total physical activity and all other subcomponents of physical activity were significantly associated with clustered metabolic risk. After excluding waist circumference from the summary score and further adjustment for waist circumference as a confounding factor, the magnitude of the association between CRF and clustered metabolic risk was attenuated, whereas the association with total physical activity was unchanged. Increased MVPA in adolescent boys was also found to be associated with better vascular health as assessed by improved arterial stiffness (Ried-Larsen *et al.*, 2013). Recently it was observed that maintaining the adolescent MVPA level or increases therein was associated with lower arterial stiffness compared to those that decline in MVPA level. This association was independent of a range of confounders, such as TV viewing, parental education, family history of CVD, soft drink and vegetable consumption (Grontved *et al.*, in press b). Furthermore, adiposity did not mediate this association, suggesting that MVPA could have a preventive effect on the general population, not only the overweight.

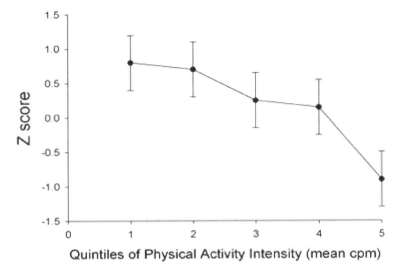

Figure 5.2 Mean *Z* score in every quintile of average physical activity intensity. Vertical bars=95% CI. (Andersen *et al.*, 2006: License permission 3153560906548; Content publisher: Elsevier; Content publication: *The Lancet*).

Besides being associated with the prevention of clustering of CVD risk factors, physical activity is an important predictor of bone health. Several previous studies in children and adolescents have reported positive associations between physical activity and bone density and architecture in boys and in girls. A cross-sectional study including Portuguese children demonstrated that vigorous intensity emerged as the main physical activity predictor of femoral neck strength but did not explain gender differences. Recommending daily vigorous physical activity for at least ~25 minutes seems to improve (10%–14%) femoral neck bone health in children (Sardinha *et al.*, 2008b).

Prospective observational analysis including 15-year old students from the Danish arm of the EYHS reported a physical activity declining from 45 minutes >3000 counts per minute in 1997 to 35 minutes >3000 cpm in 2003 (Jago et al., 2008b). Longitudinal regression analyses showed that a change in minutes >3000 cpm was negatively associated with fasting insulin levels and HOMA-IR in 2003. Results demonstrated that a 6-year decline in physical activity was associated with higher insulin and HOMA-IR levels, suggesting that preventing an age-related decline in physical activity may be an effective means of preventing youth insulin resistance.

In conclusion, birth weight may not be an important biological determinant of habitual physical activity in children and adolescents. The accumulated amount of time spent at MVPA is related to body fatness in children; however, this relation is weak, the explained variance was less than 1%. These data suggests that physical activity levels should be higher than the current international guidelines of at least 1 hour per day of physical activity of at least moderate intensity to prevent clustering of CVD risk factors. Vascular and bone health are improved by MVPA and more intense physical activity levels, respectively. Decrease in MVPA tends to have deleterious effects on biomarkers that are related to cardiovascular health and diabetes. These results suggest that fitness and activity affect metabolic risk through different pathways

5.3. PHYSICAL FITNESS

Health-related fitness cut-offs for children and adolescents allow the identification of target populations for health promotion policies and disease prevention at early ages. CRF is easy and relatively cheap to measure, and yet it is an accurate tool for screening children with clustering of CVD risk factors. Lower birth weight was associated with lower CRF, after adjusting for sex, age group, country, sexual maturity and socio-economic status, but introduction of fat free mass as a covariate in the model reduced the association between birth weight and CRF (Ridgway et al., 2011a). Adegboye et al. (2011) defined optimal cut-points for low CRF and evaluated its accuracy to predict clustering of risk factors for CVD in children and adolescents from EYHS. In girls, the optimal cut-offs for identifying individuals at risk were: 37.4 $mlO_2/min/kg$ (9-year-old) and 33.0 $mlO_2/min/kg$ (15-year-old). In boys, the optimal cut-offs were 43.6 $mlO_2/min/kg$ (9-year-old) and 46.0 $mlO_2/min/kg$ (15-year-old). Specificity (range 79.3–86.4%) was markedly higher than sensitivity (range 29.7–55.6%) for all cut-offs. Positive predictive values ranged from 19% to 41% and negative predictive values ranged from 88% to 90%. The diagnostic accuracy for identifying children at risk, measured by the area under the curve, was significantly higher than what would be expected by chance for all cut-offs. Recently it was observed that in 15-year-old adolescent boys with a higher CRF (just above this cut-off point of 46.0 $mlO_2/min/kg$) had lower arterial stiffness compared to the least fit boys, which further supports that this seems to be an adequate cut-off for an healthy CRF for adolescent boys (Ried-Larsen et al., 2013).

Results from 9- and 15-yr-olds from Denmark reported that physical fitness was weakly related to single CVD risk factors except sum of skinfolds where the relationship was strong (Wedderkopp *et al.*, 2003). Low fitness increased the risk of having three or more CVD risk factors. An odds ratio (OR) of 24.1 was found in the low fit group. Children and adolescents from Denmark, Portugal, Estonia, and Norway demonstrate a curvilinear relation between CRF and health parameters, including waist circumference, skinfolds, and blood pressure (Klasson-Heggebo *et al.*, 2006). Additionally, Anderssen *et al.* (2007) revealed a strong association between CRF and the clustering of CVD risk factors, as described earlier by Wedderkopp *et al.* (2003). The OR for clustering in each quartile of fitness, using the quartile with the highest fitness as reference, were 13.0, 4.8, and 2.5, respectively, after adjusting for country, age, sex, socio-economic status, pubertal stage, family history of CVD and diabetes. In stratified analyses by age group, sex and country, similar strong patterns were observed. Later, it was reported that physical activity, CRF and fatness (skinfold and waist circumference) were all independently associated with clustered CVD risk (summed z-score of the CVD risk factors systolic blood pressure, triglyceride, total cholesterol: HDL ratio, HOMA score and aerobic fitness) in these children (Andersen *et al.*, 2008). Results from a cohort study including 9- and 15-yr-olds from all regions of Norway found that low muscle fitness is associated with clustered metabolic risk, independent of CRF, and after adjustment for age, sex, and pubertal stage. Independent of muscle fitness, an inverse association was found between CRF and clustered metabolic risk. Moreover, the OR for having clustered risk in the least fit quartile compared with the most fit quartile were 7.2 and 17.3 for muscle fitness and CRF, respectively. This study found that muscle strength and CRF were independently associated with metabolic risk in youth (Steene-Johannessen *et al.*, 2009).

Changes in CRF are a significant predictor of changes in body fat percentage from childhood to adolescence, even after controlling for confounding factors such as physical activity, sex, and maturity (Ornelas *et al.*, 2011). A cohort study of Portuguese children show that while CRF significantly increased among boys and decreased in girls, the percentage of body fat decreased over time in boys and increased among girls. Alone, CRF explained 39%, 26%, and 25% of the total variance in waist circumference, fat mass, and trunk skinfold, respectively. Adjusting for physical activity, sex, and maturation changes, CRF remained a significant predictor of these body composition variables. Prospective observational analysis on the Danish cohorts showed that greater isometric strength of abdomen and back in youth was associated with lower levels of CVD risk factors in young adulthood independent of CRF, adiposity, socio-demographic and lifestyle factors (Figure 5.3). Each 1 SD difference in isometric muscle strength in youth was inversely associated with BMI, triglyceride, diastolic blood pressure, and a composite CVD risk factor score in young adulthood in multivariable adjusted analyses including CRF. Each 1 SD difference in isometric muscle strength in youth was significantly associated with 0.59 lower odds of general overweight/obesity in young adulthood and was marginally associated with incident raised of blood pressure, raised triglyceride and low HDL-C (Grontved *et al.*, in press b). Lower isometric muscle strength and CRF in youth were also independently associated with adverse levels of fasting insulin, insulin sensitivity, and beta-cell function in young adulthood (Grontved *et al.*, in press a).

In summary, low CRF is strongly associated with the clustering of CVD risk factors in children independent of country, age and sex. High levels of CRF are recognized to have wide ranging health benefits not only in terms of direct benefits observed in childhood, such as lower obesity risk and improved metabolic and vascular function, but also in terms of reduced disease risk in later life. The greatest benefit may be achieved when increasing CRF from low to moderate, mainly in those children and adolescents who are the least physically fit. Increasing CRF and muscle strength should both be targets in youth prevention strategies to prevent insulin resistance and beta-cell dysfunction and improve CVD risk factors and body composition phenotypes in young adults.

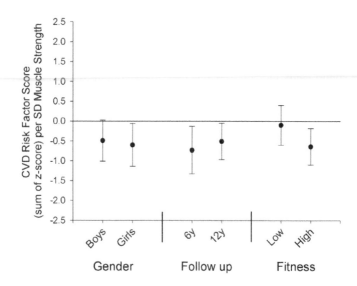

Figure 5.3 Isometric muscle strength in youth and composite cardiovascular risk factor score in young adulthood stratified by cardiorespiratory fitness (below and above the median, sex specific), follow-up time (6- or 12 years), and sex. (Adapted from Grontved *et al.*, in press b).

5.4 CONCLUSIONS

Key findings from both the cross-sectional and prospective observational data strongly suggest that sedentary behaviour, physical activity, CRF, and muscle strength are relevant behaviours and attributes that influence several dimensions of health in children and adolescents, with latter influence on young adulthood. Figure 5.4 depicts the key findings so far from the EYHS, including the potential independent effect of sedentary behaviour and physical activity on physical fitness.

Each of the exposures has some independent effects on different outcomes, and also combined effects that tend to have an increased magnitude, with a major contribution for the challenge that our society is currently facing, the battle against the ominous enemy of chronic disease. Reduced sedentary behaviour, and increased physical activity, CRF, and muscle strength may represent the common soil for a lifelong healthy life starting as early as in childhood.

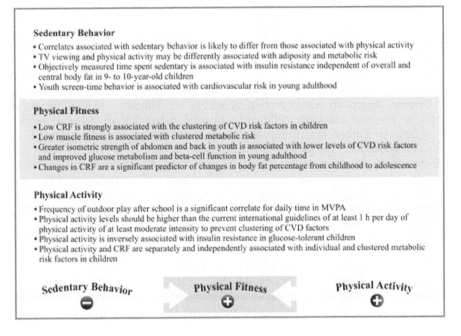

Sedentary Behavior
- Correlates associated with sedentary behavior is likely to differ from those associated with physical activity
- TV viewing and physical activity may be differently associated with adiposity and metabolic risk
- Objectively measured time spent sedentary is associated with insulin resistance independent of overall and central body fat in 9- to 10-year-old children
- Youth screen-time behavior is associated with cardiovascular risk in young adulthood

Physical Fitness
- Low CRF is strongly associated with the clustering of CVD risk factors in children
- Low muscle fitness is associated with clustered metabolic risk
- Greater isometric strength of abdomen and back in youth is associated with lower levels of CVD risk factors and improved glucose metabolism and beta-cell function in young adulthood
- Changes in CRF are a significant predictor of changes in body fat percentage from childhood to adolescence

Physical Activity
- Frequency of outdoor play after school is a significant correlate for daily time in MVPA
- Physical activity levels should be higher than the current international guidelines of at least 1 h per day of physical activity of at least moderate intensity to prevent clustering of CVD factors
- Physical activity is inversely associated with insulin resistance in glucose-tolerant children
- Physical activity and CRF are separately and independently associated with individual and clustered metabolic risk factors in children

Sedentary Behavior ⊖   Physical Fitness ⊕   Physical Activity ⊕

Figure 5.4 Summary of key findings from the EYHS.

5.5 REFERENCES

Adegboye, A.R., Anderssen, S.A., Froberg, K., Sardinha, L.B., Heitmann, B.L., Steene-Johannessen, J., Kolle, E. and Andersen, L.B., 2011, Recommended aerobic fitness level for metabolic health in children and adolescents: a study of diagnostic accuracy. *British Journal of Sports Medicine,* **45**, pp. 722–728.

Andersen, L.B., Harro, M., Sardinha, L.B., Froberg, K., Ekelund, U., Brage, S. and Anderssen, S.A., 2006, Physical activity and clustered cardiovascular risk in children: a cross-sectional study (The European Youth Heart Study). *Lancet,* **368**, pp. 299–304.

Andersen, L.B., Sardinha, L.B., Froberg, K., Riddoch, C.J., Page, A.S. and Anderssen, S.A., 2008, Fitness, fatness and clustering of cardiovascular risk factors in children from Denmark, Estonia and Portugal: the European Youth Heart Study. *International Journal of Pediatric Obesity,* **3**, pp. S58–66.

Anderssen, S.A., Cooper, A.R., Riddoch, C., Sardinha, L.B., Harro, M., Brage, S. and Andersen, L.B., 2007, Low cardiorespiratory fitness is a strong predictor for clustering of cardiovascular disease risk factors in children independent of country, age and sex. *European Journal of Preventive Cardiology,* **14**, pp. 526–531.

Ekelund, U., Anderssen, S.A., Froberg, K., Sardinha, L.B., Andersen, L.B. and Brage, S., 2007, Independent associations of physical activity and cardiorespiratory fitness with metabolic risk factors in children: the European youth heart study. *Diabetologia,* **50**, pp. 1832–1840.

Ekelund, U., Brage, S., Froberg, K., Harro, M., Anderssen, S.A., Sardinha, L.B., Riddoch, C. and Andersen, L.B., 2006, TV viewing and physical activity are independently associated with metabolic risk in children: the European Youth Heart Study. *PLOS Medicine,* **3**, doi: 10.1371/journal.pmed.0030488.

Ekelund, U., Sardinha, L.B., Anderssen, S.A., Harro, M., Franks, P.W., Brage, S., Cooper, A.R., Andersen, L.B., Riddoch, C. and Froberg, K., 2004, Associations between objectively assessed physical activity and indicators of body fatness in 9- to 10-y-old European children: a population-based study from 4 distinct regions in Europe (the European Youth Heart Study). *American Journal of Clinical Nutrition,* **80**, pp. 584–590.

Grontved, A., Ried-Larsen, M., Ekelund, U., Froberg, K., Brage, S. and Andersen, L.B., Independent and combined association of muscle strength and cardiorespiratory fitness in youth with insulin resistance and beta-cell function in young adulthood (EYHS) *Diabetes Care,* doi: 10.2337/dc12-2252

Grontved, A., Ried-Larsen, M., Moller, A., Kristensen, P.L., Froberg, K., Brage, S. and Andersen, L.B., Muscle strength in youth and cardiovascular risk in young adulthood (The European Youth Heart Study). *British Journal of Sports Medicine,* doi: 10.1136/bjsports-2012-091907.

Grontved, A., Ried-Larsen, M., Moller, N.C., Kristensen, P.L., Wedderkopp, N., Froberg, K., Hu, F.B., Ekelund, U. and Andersen, L.B., 2012, Youth screen-time behaviour is associated with cardiovascular risk in young adulthood: the European Youth Heart Study. *European Journal of Preventive Cardiology,* doi: 10.1177/2047487312454760.

Jago, R., Page, A., Froberg, K., Sardinha, L.B., Klasson-Heggebo, L. and Andersen, L.B., 2008a, Screen-viewing and the home TV environment: the European Youth Heart Study. *Preventive Medicine,* **47**, pp. 525–529.

Jago, R., Wedderkopp, N., Kristensen, P.L., Moller, N.C., Andersen, L.B., Cooper, A.R. and Froberg, K., 2008b, Six-year change in youth physical activity and effect on fasting insulin and HOMA-IR. *American Journal of Preventive Medicine,* **35**, pp. 554–560.

Klasson-Heggebo, L., Andersen, L.B., Wennlof, A.H., Sardinha, L.B., Harro, M., Froberg, K. and Anderssen, S.A., 2006, Graded associations between cardiorespiratory fitness, fatness, and blood pressure in children and adolescents. *British Journal of Sports Medicine,* **40**, pp. 25-29.

Nilsson, A., Andersen, L.B., Ommundsen, Y., Froberg, K., Sardinha, L.B., Piehl-Aulin, K. and Ekelund, U., 2009, Correlates of objectively assessed physical activity and sedentary time in children: a cross-sectional study (The European Youth Heart Study). *BMC Public Health,* **9**, pp. 322.

Ommundsen, Y., Klasson-Heggebo, L. and Anderssen, S.A., 2006, Psycho-social and environmental correlates of location-specific physical activity among 9- and 15- year-old Norwegian boys and girls: the European Youth Heart Study. *International Journal of Behavioral Nutrition and Physical Activity,* **3**, pp. 32.

Ornelas, R.T., Silva, A.M., Minderico, C.S. and Sardinha, L.B., 2011, Changes in cardiorespiratory fitness predict changes in body composition from childhood to adolescence: findings from the European Youth Heart Study. *Physician and Sportsmedicine,* **39**, pp. 78–86.

Ridgway, C.L., Brage, S., Anderssen, S., Sardinha, L.B., Andersen, L.B. and Ekelund, U., 2011a, Fat-free mass mediates the association between birth weight and aerobic fitness in youth. *International Journal of Pediatric Obesity,* **6**, doi: 10.3109/17477166.2010.526225

Ridgway, C.L., Brage, S., Anderssen, S.A., Sardinha, L.B., Andersen, L.B. and Ekelund, U., 2011b, Do physical activity and aerobic fitness moderate the association between birth weight and metabolic risk in youth?: the European Youth Heart Study. *Diabetes Care,* **34**, pp. 187–192.

Ridgway, C.L., Brage, S., Sharp, S.J., Corder, K., Westgate, K.L., van Sluijs, E.M., Goodyer, I.M., Hallal, P.C., Anderssen, S.A., Sardinha, L.B., Andersen, L.B. and Ekelund, U., 2011c, Does birth weight influence physical activity in youth? A combined analysis of four studies using objectively measured physical activity. *PLoS One,* **6**, 10.1371/journal.pone.0016125.

Ried-Larsen, M., Grontved, A., Froberg, K., Ekelund, U. and Andersen, L.B., 2013, Physical activity intensity and subclinical atherosclerosis in Danish adolescents: The European Youth Heart Study. *Scandinavian Journal of Medicine and Science in Sports.* Doi: 10.1111/sms.12046.

Sardinha, L.B., Andersen, L.B., Anderssen, S.A., Quiterio, A.L., Ornelas, R., Froberg, K., Riddoch, C.J. and Ekelund, U., 2008a, Objectively measured time spent sedentary is associated with insulin resistance independent of overall and central body fat in 9- to 10-year-old Portuguese children. *Diabetes Care,* **31**, pp. 569–575.

Sardinha, L.B., Baptista, F. and Ekelund, U., 2008b, Objectively measured physical activity and bone strength in 9-year-old boys and girls. *Pediatrics,* **122,** doi: 10.1542/peds.2007-2573.

Steene-Johannessen, J., Anderssen, S.A., Kolle, E. and Andersen, L.B., 2009, Low muscle fitness is associated with metabolic risk in youth. *Medicine and Science in Sports and Exercise,* **41**, pp. 1361–1367.

van Sluijs, E.M., Page, A., Ommundsen, Y. and Griffin, S.J., 2010, Behavioural and social correlates of sedentary time in young people. *British Journal of Sports Medicine,* **44**, pp. 747–755.

Wedderkopp, N., Froberg, K., Hansen, H.S., Riddoch, C. and Andersen, L., 2003, Cardiovascular risk factors cluster in children and adolescents with low physical fitness: The European Youth Heart Study (EYHS). *Pediatric Exercise Science,* **15**, pp. 419–427.

CHAPTER NUMBER 6

GENETICS OF PHYSICAL ACTIVITY: A BRIEF SUMMARY

J. Maia[1], D. Santos[1], R. Chaves[1], T. Gomes[1], F. Santos[1], M. Souza[1], A. Borges[1], S. Pereira[1], R. Garganta[1], D. Freitas[2], M. Thomis[3], and V. Diego[4]

[1]CIFID, Faculty of Sport, University of Porto, Portugal; [2]Department of Physical Education and Sport, University of Madeira, Portugal; [3]Department of Kinesiology, Faculty of Kinesiology and Rehabilitation Sciences, Katholieke Universiteit Leuven, Belgium; [4]Texas Biomedical Research Center, USA

6.1 INTRODUCTION

Moderate-to-high levels of physical activity (PA) are now established as conditional lifestyle factors to have a healthy, rewarding, and long life. It is also widely acknowledged that people vary, worldwide, in their PA habits and sports participation. This inter-individual heterogeneity is very well captured by a simple statistic – the variance. The answer to the question – why is there such a wealth of variation within and between populations in their PA levels and patterns? – is not as straightforward as it seems at first glance. Fortunately, the variance can be partitioned and its components "explained" by so-called determinants or correlates studied by Physical Activity Epidemiologists or, by contrast, the labours of Genetic Epidemiologists. The first camp mainly works with individual data where the assumption of independence of observations is mandatory; the second one samples twins and/or nuclear/extended families in which the non-independence due to familial relationships is modeled rather than assuming independence. Fortunately, recent reviews are available within each camp (de Vilhena e Santos *et al.*, 2012). In this brief summary, we will address the topic as follows: firstly, the stepwise approach offered by Genetic Epidemiology (GE) to study PA variation and covariation within and between family members will be presented; secondly, a brief summary about familial data will be done using what we might call a "psychology oriented agenda"; thirdly, GE data will be offered; finally, we will briefly address the Portuguese Healthy Families Study.

6.2 GENETIC EPIDEMIOLOGY FRAMEWORK

When answering the "simple" question – why do people vary in their PA levels and patterns? – Genetic epidemiologists usually sample families and/or twins, and use a series of steps with increasing complexity. Bouchard *et al.* (1997) (initially suggested a top-down and a bottom-up approach). Very briefly, five major steps are usually considered. In step one, some measure of familial aggregation is obtained – odds ratios or correlations – intraclass and interclass intra-trait or inter-traits among family members. In step two, the major question is – how much of the total variation is accounted for by genetic factors? A variance components summary measure is calculated, namely the heritability (h^2, which is defined as the ratio of the additive genetic variance to the total phenotypic variance). In step three, the question is – where in the genome are quantitative trait loci located responsible for the previously detected signal? The initial way was to conduct a genome-wide linkage study to identify chromosomal regions that may harbour the responsible genes. Once the zone has been fine mapped, so-called candidate genes are identified given their putative physiological mechanisms connected with PA, and a classical case-control association study (fourth step) is usually done. In the last decade, linkage analysis was superseded by a genome-wide association study (GWAS) approach in which thousands of unrelated subjects are genotyped for a few hundreds of thousands of genetic markers (usually SNPs) to discover new gene variants that are associated with any phenotypic expression of PA. However, the GWAS approach was generally plagued by the so-called "missing heritability" problem (Manolio *et al.*, 2009). The leading explanation for this missing heritability phenomenon is that the GWAS approach, because of its emphasis on large samples of unrelated subjects, was relatively incapable of detecting rare variation (Blangero, 2004; Blangero *et al.*, 2013; Blangero and Kent, 2011; Schork *et al.*, 2009). For this reason, there has been a call to return to GE studies employing families, and for the development of variance components methods for the efficient detection of rare variants (Blangero *et al.*, 2013).

6.3 AVAILABLE INFORMATION

6.3.1 Familial Aggregation

A consistent line of research uses what could be called a "psychology oriented agenda" where family studies are conducted without any consideration of genetic factors, mainly using social learning and practices, behaviours associated with PA, parental role modeling, support, ethnicity, encouragement, attitudes towards PA, and system of beliefs towards PA. In this type of research, parental roles in their children's physical activity (PA) has been consistently reported, although study design, sampling, data analysis and conclusions vary in many ways (Dregval and Petrauskiene, 2009; Gustafson and Rhodes, 2006). Parents have a significant influence in their children's PA levels and patterns, usually through a complex network of interrelationships where role modeling, support, encouragement, and attitudes/beliefs sharing are appropriate. However, the effect-size of these associations is not always consistent in magnitude and sign (de Vilhena e Santos *et al.*, 2012).

Table 6.1 A brief summary of familial aggregation results in PA levels

Author, Year, Country	Main Results
Adkins *et al.* (2004) USA	Parental PA (r=0.45) and support (r=0.26) associated with daughter's PA
Nichols-English *et al.* (2006) USA	Mother's PA was not associated with daughter's PA
Madsen *et al.* (2009) USA	Girls whose parents exercise more than 3 times/week were about 50% more active than girls with sedentary parents
Raudsepp and Viira (2000) Estonia	Correlation between parents and older sibling's PA with adolescents' moderate (sibs: r=0.285), vigorous (father-son: r=0.304; father-daughter: r=0.253; sibs: r=0.331), and very vigorous (father-son: r=0.377; father-daughter: r=0.302; mother-daughter: r=0.256; sibs: r=0.351) PA.
Vilhjalmsson and Kristjansdottir (2003) Iceland	Correlation between mothers' (r=0.104) and older daughters'(r=0.056) PA with girls' PA
Wagner *et al.* (2004) France	Association between parental engagement in sports and children's PA, with the following odds ratios: 1.48 (mother-son), 1.80 (mother-daughter), 1.36 (father-son), 1.41 (father-daughter), 1.97 (parents-offspring), and 1.56 (parents-offspring).
Teixeira e Seabra *et al.* (2004) Portugal	Association between parental and children sports participation, with the following odds ratios: 1.7-2.5 (father-son), 1.8-3.0 (father-daughter), 1.3-4.5 (mother-son), and 2.9-5.1 (mother-daughter)
Jacobi *et al.* (2011) France	Correlation between siblings' ($0.24 \leq r \leq 0.31$), parents' (mother-offspring: $0.15 \leq r \leq 0.25$; father-offspring: $0.00 \leq r \leq 0.05$), and children's PA
Wu and Pender (2002) Taiwan	Parental influence did not have direct effects on children's PA

Table 6.1 reports a small, but relevant, sample of studies conducted in last decade. In general, the studies reported a familial aggregation of PA, but with a high variance in its magnitude. For example, Adkins *et al.* (2004) reported a correlation between parental and siblings' PA of 0.45, whereas Jacobi *et al.* (2011) showed no correlation at all ($0.00 \leq r \leq 0.05$) for the dyad father-offspring. Furthermore, two studies reported a significant positive role of birth order, i.e., older siblings have important roles in their later born siblings' PA (Raudsepp and Viira, 2000; Vilhjalmsson and Kristjansdottir, 2003), with values varying from $0.06 \leq r \leq 0.35$. On the other hand, two other studies found no significant not only any significant role

for siblings' birth-order, nor any association among family member's PA (Nichols-English *et al.*, 2006; Wu and Pender, 2002). In summary, it is not possible yet to accurately determine which family member most influences siblings' PA levels, although we may say that there is a relevant familial aggregation of PA, where parents and older siblings play their roles. This reinforces the idea that the family is a very important social institution, highly relevant when considering the development of intervention strategies for PA promotion.

6.3.2 Genetic Epidemiology Information

There are not many studies using nuclear or extended families to identify the presence of genetic factors governing PA variation. Heritability estimates have generally been on the low end of the spectrum, with estimates at 0 (Perusse *et al.*, 1989), 9% (Mitchell *et al.*, 2003; Storti, 2007), and 19% (Blangero and Kent, 2011). One family study, however, reported a heritability of 60% (Butte *et al.*, 2006). It is probably that the higher genetic contribution in this latter study was found because PA was objectively assessed. On the opposite side, the use of questionnaires resulted in a maximum value of 29%. However, one must recognize that, so far, only two (Butte *et al.*, 2006; Cai *et al.*, 2006) studies monitored families' PA using accelerometry.

Twin studies are widely used to estimate the amount of genetic and environmental effects on PA. As is well known, monozygotic twins (MZ) share the same genes identical by descent and dizygotic twins (DZ) share, on average, 50% of their genes identical by descent; thus greater MZ resemblance is expected. Moreover, in contrast with family designs (unless objective measures of families' environments are available; e.g. as was implemented in Mitchell *et al.*, 2003), twin designs fraction the total variance in three basic components: shared environmental (c^2), unique environmental (e^2) and additive genetic factors (a^2). Available information suggests that MZ PA correlations [0.39 (Franks *et al.*, 2005) to 0.98 (Beunen and Thomis, 1999)] are greater than DZ correlations [-0.02 to 0.72 (Boomsma *et al.*, 1989)]. Additive genetic effects and c^2 present a similar pattern with a wide range of results for different PA phenotypes ranging from 0.00 (Joosen *et al.*, 2005; Stubbe *et al.*, 2005) to 0.85 (Stubbe *et al.*, 2005), and 0.00 (De Moor *et al.*, 2007b; De Moor *et al.*, 2007c; Duncan *et al.*, 2008; Eriksson *et al.*, 2006; Joosen *et al.*, 2005; Spinath *et al.*, 2002) to 0.84 (Stubbe *et al.*, 2005), respectively. Unique environmental (e^2) results are also well dispersed: 0.12 (Koopmans *et al.*, 1994) to 0.72 (McCaffery *et al.*, 2009). Table 6.2 presents a sample of recent data.

Table 6.2 A brief summary of twin results in PA levels

Author, Year, Country	Main results
Duncan *et al.* (2008) USA	PA 60 min cut-point: rMZ= 0.43, rDZ= 0.30, a^2= 0.45; e^2= 0.55 PA 150 min cut-point: rMZ= 0.30, rDZ= 0.25, c^2= 0.28; e^2= 0.72
Wood *et al.* (2008) United Kingdom	rMZ= 0.72, rDZ= 0.58, a^2= 0.92; c^2=0.00; e^2 = 0.08
McCaffery *et al.* (2009) USA	a^2= 0.10; c^2= 0.18; e^2= 0.72
Aaltonen *et al.* (2010) Finland	Baseline: rMZ=0.54, rDZ=0.24, a^2=0.44; e^2=0.56, $a^2_\male$=0.47; $e^2_\male$=0.54, $a^2_\female$=0.42; $e^2_\female$=0.56 Follow-up: rMZ=0.43, rDZ=0.15, h^2= 0.34; e^2=0.66, $h^2_\male$=0.38; $e^2_\male$=0.63 $h^2_\female$= 0.31; $e^2_\female$=0.67
Fisher *et al.* (2010) England	Total PA: rMZ= 0.76, rDZ= 0.71, c^2= 0.73; e^2= 0.27 Moderate-to-Vigorous PA: rMZ= 0.69, rDZ= 0.52, c^2= 0.61; e^2= 0.39

Only a very small amount of studies used the genome-wide linkage approach to identify chromosomal regions harboring candidate genes responsible for the familial clustering in PA levels; furthermore, their sample sizes varied from 767 (Simonen *et al.*, 2003a) to 4488 subjects (De Moor *et al.*, 2007b), using distinct genetic markers spacing and density. In summary, no common markers were discovered across studies. Suggestive linkages were found with markers nearby different candidate activity-related genes: gene encoding *ETBR* gene, *MC4R*, *UCP1*, *FABP2*, *CASR*, *SLC9A9* (but see Table 6.3).

As previously presented, association studies usually follow a case-control design and report on a candidate gene associated with a particular PA phenotype. In summary, different genes have been associated with PA traits, although results are quite dispersed. *FTO rs9939609* gene polymorphism is known for its impact on fat mass regulation (Scuteri *et al.*, 2007), but the two studies (Berentzen *et al.*, 2008; Liu *et al.*, 2010) investigating its influence on PA failed to demonstrate a significant and positive effect. *ACE* gene (I/D polymorphism) is linked to cardiovascular homeostasis through angiotensin II formation and bradykinin inactivation Wang and Staessen (2000). Fuentes *et al.* (2002) hypothesized that it could exert some influence on PA but found no association. This was in opposition to Winnicki *et al.* (2004) results that found a strong relationship with PA. *LEPR* gene regulates adipose-tissue mass through hypothalamus effects on fullness and energy use. The administration of leptin in animals produces the activation of the sympathetic nervous system (SNS) (Tang-Christensen *et al.*, 1999) that has been associated with measurements of spontaneous PA (Christin *et al.*, 1993). Stefan *et al.* (2002) and Richert *et al.* (2007) results may reflect this evidence with a significant influence of *Gln223Arg* polymorphism on PA levels. The remaining studies focused their attention in different genes leading to less clear results in terms of their influence on PA. The *MC4R* gene plays an important role in the physiology of obesity (Larsen *et al.*, 2005) and has been linked to energy expenditure (Cole *et al.*, 2010). A significant association with higher levels of PA was demonstrated by Loos *et al.* (2005). The *DRD2* gene is involved in the amount of movement (in mice) and the rewarding system, as well as in motor control (Gingrich and Caron, 1993), making it an obvious candidate gene for PA. However, Simonen *et al.* (2003a) only found an association between *DRD2* and PA as assessed by recall questionnaire. Table 6.4 presents recent data.

Table 6.3 A brief summary of linkage results in PA levels

Author, Year, Country	Main results
Simonen *et al.* (2003b) U.S.A.	Locus: *13q22-q3; Phenotype – Total PA; Genetic Marker – D13S317* Locus: *4q28.2; Phenotype* – MVPA; *Genetic Marker – UCP1* Locus: *7p11.2; Phenotype – MVPA; Genetic Marker – IGFBP1* Locus: *9q31.1; Phenotype – MVPA ; Genetic Marker – D9S938* Locus: *13q22-q31; Phenotype – MVPA; Genetic Marker – D13S317* Locus: *11p15; Phenotype – Time spent in PA; Genetic Marker – C11P15_3* Locus: *15q13.3; Phenotype – Time spent in PA; Genetic Marker – D15S165*
Cai *et al.* (2006) U.S.A.	Locus: TPA; *Phenotype – 18q; Genetic Marker – D18S64* Locus: *18q; Phenotype – LPA; Genetic Marker – D18S1102-D18S474* Locus: *18q; Phenotype* – MPA; *Genetic Marker – D18S64* Locus: *18q; Phenotype* – VPA; *Genetic Marker – D18S64*
De Moor *et al.* (2007a) Netherlands	Locus: *19p13.3; Phenotype* – Exercise Participation; *Genetic Marker – D19S247*
De Moor *et al.* (2007b) Great Britain	Locus: *3q24; Phenotype* – Athlete Status; *Genetic Marker – D3S1569* Locus: *4q32.3; Phenotype* – Athlete Status; *Genetic Marker – D4S1597*

In 2009, De Moor *et al.* (2009) performed the only GWAS available, so far, in the literature. The goal was to identify genetic variants associated with adult leisure-time exercise behaviour in 1644 unrelated Dutch and 978 American adults of European ancestry. The analysis uncovered 37 novel SNPs for exercise participation that gather in three different genomic regions, leading the authors to suggest that PA is under the influence of many genetic variants with small effect sizes.

Table 6.4 A brief summary of Association studies in PA levels

Author, Year, Country	Main results
Berentzen *et al.* (2008) Norway	Phenotype: Leisure-time PA; Sample: Obese; Locus – *16q12.2*; Gene – *FTO*; Polymorphism – *rs9939609*; D/D – 26.4% TT; D/R – 45% TA; R/R – 28.6% AA;
	Phenotype: Leisure-time PA; Sample: Controls; Locus – *16q12.2*; Gene – *FTO*; Polymorphism – *rs9939609*; D/D – 35.6% TT; D/R – 47.2% TA; R/R – 17.2% AA;
Hakanen *et al.* (2009) Finland	Phenotype: PA; Locus – *16q12.2*; Gene – *FTO*; Polymorphism – *rs9939609*; D/D – 31.9% TT; D/R – 26.4% TA; R/R – 28.5% AA;
Cole *et al.* (2010) USA	Phenotype: PA; Locus – *1704*; Gene – *MC4R*; Polymorphism – *MC4R*;
	Phenotype: Awake time in vigorous activity; Locus – 602; Gene – *MC4R*; Polymorphism – *MC4R*;
Liu *et al.* (2010) Europe and USA	Phenotype: Vigorous PA; Locus – *16q12.2*; Gene – *FTO*; Polymorphism – *rs9939609*; D/D – 181 TT; D/R – 359 AT; R/R – 204 AA;

6.4 PORTUGUESE HEALTHY FAMILY STUDY

In 2005, the Portuguese Healthy Family Study (*Estudo de Famílias Saudáveis Portuguesas*) was launched, aiming at describing and exploring the complex relationships of their physical activity habits, body composition, physical fitness, nutritional behaviours, metabolic syndrome, and bone health. Nuclear families from mainland, Azores and Madeira islands were sampled. In phase 1, only physical activity was assessed in about 12.385 subjects (3.378 families). In 2009 phase 2 started in a smaller sample of about 1.363 subjects (515 families), all of them were assessed in all domains previously mentioned. In 2009–2010 phase 3 started with a mixed-longitudinal study with 12 to 16 year old students and their families during a three-year period. In 2010 phase 4 was conducted in a specific locality, Vouzela region (Active Vouzela study), where primary and secondary school children and adolescents and their families were enrolled, and measured in all variables. A co-partner of this project is the GEAFAS study which was launched in Madeira, sampling three generation families whose siblings had to be twins covering the same range of variables, in addition to DNA collection from all subjects. In the next two sections, a very brief summary of some results will be presented.

6.4.1 Familial Clustering in Physical Activity Levels

A number of studies are being written and submitted within the GE framework, using Generalised Estimating Equations (GEE) and Maximum Likelihood (ML) techniques to uncover correlation patterns within families, to estimate heritability and its stability over different classes of siblings' ages, to verify the presence of sex-specific genetic factors in diverse PA expressions, to test genotype-by-environment interactions in PA and their distinct effects in metabolic syndrome (MS) indicators, to test pleiotropic effects in PA, body composition and MS, and much more. Furthermore, sibling analysis study using objective PA measures and a wealth of covariates including nutritional behaviours, MS indicators, body composition, physical fitness, birth weight, and other important psychological variables is being written using variance components as the analytical technique. Another research avenue deals with multilevel modeling to disclose complex network of relationships within and between families using individuals, dyads and family levels. Finally, a very brief use of geographic information systems (GIS) linking sports facilities, potential uses to promote PA, and families at risk are presented.

6.4.2 GIS, Sports Facilities and Families at Risk (Active Vouzela Study)

The MS is a recognizable cluster of risk factors associated with cardiovascular diseases (ATP III, 2001). Epidemiology and public health researchers have documented the association between built environment, MS, obesity, physical inactivity, and healthy lifestyle (Dengel *et al.*, 2009; Thornton *et al.*, 2011), suggesting that reduced opportunities for PA in the neighbourhood may impact on population health. Although it is difficult to clearly assess the built environment and its association to health aspects, GIS are proposed as a modern tool to manipulate, analyse, and present health information linked to a geographic location, as well as to integrate spatial information and thus develop precise measures of the built environment.

We hypothesize that proximity to PA/sports facilities resources may have a protective effect to MS risk within families. The study sample comprised 220 families from the central region of Portugal (Vouzela). MS indicators included serum glucose, total cholesterol, triglycerides, systolic blood pressure and waist circumference. Firstly, all 71 sports facilities were georeferenced by geographic coordinates, using Google Earth and zip code/address information. Buffer distances of sports facilities ranged 500 meters. Secondly, MS risk within families was defined according to two criteria: (i) families with two or more members having (ii) 2 or more risk factors. Prevalence of families with MS risk was 26.4% ($n_f=58$), from which 51.7% live outside sport facilities' proximities, while 54.3% of families without cardiometabolic risk live near sport facilities' proximities, i.e., inside a 500 meters' buffer. We plan to employ a recently developed variance components approach (Williams-Blangero *et al.*, 2012) that explicitly models the GIS data as a spatial environmental variance component. This may help to clarify the relative importance of genetic and environmental effects on PA traits in relation to MS risk.

6.5 ACKNOWLEDGEMENTS

Fundação para a Ciência e Tecnologia (PTDC/DES/67569/2006 FCOMP-01-0124-FEDEB-09608).

6.6 REFERENCES

Adkins, S., Sherwood, N.E., Story, M. and Davis, M., 2004, Physical activity among African-American girls: The role of parents and the home environment. *Obesity Research,* **12**, pp, S38–45.

Berentzen, T., Kring, S.I., Holst, C., Zimmermann, E., Jess, T., Hansen, T. and Sorensen, T.I., 2008, Lack of association of fatness-related FTO gene variants with energy expenditure or physical activity. *Journal of Clinical Endocrinology and Metabolism, 93*, pp, 2904–2908.

Beunen, G. and Thomis, M., 1999, Genetic determinants of sports participation and daily physical activity. *International Journal of Obesity and Related Metabolic Disorders, 23*, pp, S55–63.

Blangero, J. and Kent, J.W.Jr., 2011, Characterizing the Extent of Human Genetic Variation for Performance-Related Traits. In *Genetic and Molecular Aspects of Sport Performance*, Vol. 18, edited by Bouchard C. and Hoffman E.P. (Oxford: Wiley-Blackwell), pp. 33–45.

Blangero, J., 2004, Localization and identification of human quantitative trait loci: king harvest has surely come. *Current Opinion in Genetics and Development, 14*, pp, 233–240.

Blangero, J., Diego, V.P., Dyer, T.D., Almeida, M., Peralta, J., Kent, J.W., Jr. and Goring, H.H., 2013, A kernel of truth: statistical advances in polygenic variance component models for complex human pedigrees. *Advances in Genetics,* **81**, pp, 1–31.

Boomsma, D.I., van den Bree, M.B., Orlebeke, J.F. and Molenaar, P.C., 1989, Resemblances of parents and twins in sports participation and heart rate. *Behavior Genetics,* **19**, pp, 123–141.

Bouchard, C., Malina, R. and Pérusse, L., 1997, *Genetics of Fitness and Physical Performance.* (Champaign: Human Kinetics).

Butte, N.F., Cai, G., Cole, S.A. and Comuzzie, A.G., 2006, Viva la Familia Study: genetic and environmental contributions to childhood obesity and its comorbidities in the Hispanic population. *American Journal of Clinical Nutrition,* **84**, pp, 646–654.

Cai, G., Cole, S.A., Butte, N., Bacino, C., Diego, V., Tan, K. and Comuzzie, A.G., 2006, A quantitative trait locus on chromosome 18q for physical activity and dietary intake in Hispanic children. *Obesity (Silver Spring),* **14**, pp, 1596 1–1604.

Christin, L., O'Connell, M., Bogardus, C., Danforth, E.Jr. and Ravussin, E., 1993, Norepinephrine turnover and energy expenditure in Pima Indian and white men. *Metabolism,* **42**, pp, 723–729.

Cole, S.A., Butte, N.F., Voruganti, V.S., Cai, G., Haack, K., Kent, J.W.Jr. and Gibbs, R.A., 2010, Evidence that multiple genetic variants of MC4R play a functional role in the regulation of energy expenditure and appetite in Hispanic children. *American Journal of Clinical Nutrition,* **91**, pp, 191–199.

De Moor, M.H., Liu, Y.J., Boomsma, D.I., Li, J., Hamilton, J.J., Hottenga, J.J. and Deng, H.W., 2009, Genome-wide association study of exercise behavior in Dutch and American adults. *Medicine and Science in Sports and Exercise,* **41**, pp, 1887–1895.

De Moor, M.H., Posthuma, D., Hottenga, J.J., Willemsen, G., Boomsma, D.I. and De Geus, E.J., 2007, Genome-wide linkage scan for exercise participation in Dutch sibling pairs. *European Journal of Human Genetics,* **15**, pp, 1252–1259.

De Moor, M.H., Spector, T.D., Cherkas, L.F., Falchi, M., Hottenga, J.J., Boomsma, D.I. and De Geus, E.J., 2007b, Genome-wide linkage scan for athlete status in 700 British female DZ twin pairs. *Twin Research Human Genetics,* **10**, pp, 812–820.

De Moor, M.H., Stubbe, J.H., Boomsma, D.I. and De Geus, E.J., 2007c, Exercise participation and self-rated health: do common genes explain the association? *European Journal of Epidemiology,* **22**, pp, 27–32.

de Vilhena e Santos, D.M., Katzmarzyk, P.T., Seabra, A.F. and Maia, J.A., 2012, Genetics of physical activity and physical inactivity in humans. *Behavior Genetics,* **42**, pp, 559–578.

Dengel, D.R., Hearst, M.O., Harmon, J.H., Forsyth, A. and Lytle, L.A., 2009, Does the built environment relate to the metabolic syndrome in adolescents? *Health Place,* **15**, pp, 946–951.

Dregval, L. and Petrauskiene, A., 2009, Associations between physical activity of primary school first-graders during leisure time and family socioeconomic status. *Medicina (Kaunas),* **45**, pp, 549–556.

Duncan, G.E., Goldberg, J., Noonan, C., Moudon, A.V., Hurvitz, P. and Buchwald, D. (2008). Unique environmental effects on physical activity participation: A twin study. *PLoS One,* **3**, doi: 10.1371/journal.pone.0002019.

Eriksson, M., Rasmussen, F., and Tynelius, P., 2006, Genetic factors in physical activity and the equal environment assumption-- the Swedish young male twins study. *Behavior Genetics,* **36**, pp 238–247.

Expert Panel on Detection, E. and Treatment of High Blood Cholesterol, A., 2001, Executive Summary of The Third Report of The National Cholesterol Education Program (NCEP) Expert Panel on Detection, Evaluation, And Treatment of High Blood Cholesterol In Adults (Adult Treatment Panel III). *Journal of the American Medical Associantion,* **285**, pp, 2486–2497.

Fisher, A., van Jaarsveld, C.H., Llewellyn, C.H. and Wardle, J., 2010, Environmental influences on children's physical activity: quantitative estimates using a twin design. *PLoS One,* **5**, doi: 10.1371/journal.pone.0010110.

Franks, P.W., Ravussin, E., Hanson, R.L., Harper, I.T., Allison, D.B., Knowler, W.C. and Salbe, A.D., 2005, Habitual physical activity in children: the role of genes and the environment. *American Journal of Clinical Nutrition,* **82**, pp, 901–908.

Fuentes, R.M., Perola, M., Nissinen, A. and Tuomilehto, J., 2002, ACE gene and physical activity, blood pressure, and hypertension: a population study in Finland. *Journal of Applied Physiology,* **92**, pp, 2508–2512.

Gingrich, J.A. and Caron, M.G., 1993, Recent advances in the molecular biology of dopamine receptors. *Annual Review of Neuroscience,* **16**, pp, 299–321.

Gustafson, S.L. and Rhodes, R.E., 2006, Parental correlates of physical activity in children and early adolescents. *Sports Medicine,* **36**, pp, 79–97.

Hakanen, M., Raitakari, O.T., Lehtimaki, T., Peltonen, N., Pahkala, K., Sillanmaki, L., and Ronnemaa, T., 2009, FTO genotype is associated with body mass index after the age of seven years but not with energy intake or leisure-time physical activity. *Journal of Clinical Endocrinology and Metabolism,* **94**, pp, 1281–1287.

Jacobi, D., Caille, A., Borys, J.M., Lommez, A., Couet, C., Charles, M. A. and Oppert, J.M., 2011, Parent-offspring correlations in pedometer-assessed physical activity. *PLoS One,* **6**, doi: 10.1371/journal.pone.0029195PONE-D-11-19286 [pii].

Joosen, A.M., Gielen, M., Vlietinck, R. and Westerterp, K.R., 2005, Genetic analysis of physical activity in twins. *American Journal of Clinical Nutrition,* **82**, pp, 1253–1259.

Koopmans, J.R., Lorenz, J.P.V.D. and Boomsma, D.I., 1994, Smoking and sports participation. In *Factors in Coronary Heart Disease.* edited by Faire U. and Berg K. (Dordrecht: Kluwer Academic), pp. 217–235.

Larsen, L.H., Echwald, S.M., Sorensen, T.I., Andersen, T., Wulff, B.S. and Pedersen, O., 2005, Prevalence of mutations and functional analyses of melanocortin 4 receptor variants identified among 750 men with juvenile-onset obesity. *Journal of Clinical Endocrinology Metabolism,* **90**, pp, 219–224.

Liu, G.F., Zhu, H.D., Lagou, V., Gutin, B., Stallmann-Jorgensen, I.S., Treiber, F.A. and Snieder, H., 2010, FTO variant rs9939609 is associated with body mass index and waist circumference, but not with energy intake or physical activity in European- and African-American youth. *BMC Medical Genetics,* doi: 10.1186/1471-2350-11-57.

Loos, R.J., Rankinen, T., Tremblay, A., Perusse, L., Chagnon, Y. and Bouchard, C., 2005, Melanocortin-4 receptor gene and physical activity in the Quebec Family Study. *International Journal of Obesity,* **29**, pp, 420–428.

Madsen, K.A., McCulloch, C.E. and Crawford, P.B., 2009, Parent modelling: perceptions of parents' physical activity predict girls' activity throughout adolescence. *Journal of Pediatrics,* **154**, pp, 278–283.

Manolio, T.A., Collins, F.S., Cox, N.J., Goldstein, D.B., Hindorff, L.A., Hunter, D.J. and Visscher, P.M., 2009, Finding the missing heritability of complex diseases. *Nature,* **461**, pp, 747–753.

McCaffery, J.M., Papandonatos, G.D., Bond, D.S., Lyons, M.J. and Wing, R.R., 2009, Gene X environment interaction of vigorous exercise and body mass index among male Vietnam-era twins. *American Journal of Clinical Nutrition,* **89**, pp, 1011–1018.

Mitchell, B.D., Rainwater, D.L., Hsueh, W.C., Kennedy, A.J., Stern, M.P. and Maccluer, J.W., 2003, Familial aggregation of nutrient intake and physical activity: results from the San Antonio Family Heart Study. *Annals of Epidemiology,* **13**, pp, 128–135.

Nichols-English, G.J., Lemmon, C.R., Litaker, M.S., Cartee, S.G., Yin, Z., Gutin, B., and Barbeau, P., 2006, Relations of black mothers' and daughters' body fatness, physical activity beliefs and behavior. *Ethnicity and Disease,* **16**, pp, 172–179.

Perusse, L., Tremblay, A., Leblanc, C. and Bouchard, C., 1989, Genetic and environmental influences on level of habitual physical activity and exercise participation. *American Journal of Epidemiology,* **129**, pp, 1012–1022.

Raudsepp, L. and Viira, R., 2000, Sociocultural correlates of physical activity in adolescents. *Pediatric Exercise Science,* **12**, pp, 51–60.

Richert, L., Chevalley, T., Manen, D., Bonjour, J.P., Rizzoli, R. and Ferrari, S., 2007, Bone mass in prepubertal boys is associated with a Gln223Arg amino acid substitution in the leptin receptor. *Journal of Clinical and Endocrinol Metabolism,* **92**, pp, 4380–4386.

Schork, N.J., Murray, S.S., Frazer, K.A. and Topol, E.J., 2009, Common vs. rare allele hypotheses for complex diseases. *Current Opinion in Genetic and Development,* **19**, pp, 212–219.

Scuteri, A., Sanna, S., Chen, W.M., Uda, M., Albai, G., Strait, J. and Abecasis, G.R., 2007, Genome-wide association scan shows genetic variants in the FTO gene are associated with obesity-related traits. *PLoS Genetic,* **3**, doi: 10.1371/journal.pgen.0030115.

Simonen, R.L., Rankinen, T., Perusse, L., Leon, A.S., Skinner, J.S., Wilmore, J.H. and Bouchard, C., 2003a, A dopamine D2 receptor gene polymorphism and physical activity in two family studies. *Physiology and Behavior,* **78**, pp, 751–757.

Simonen, R.L., Rankinen, T., Perusse, L., Rice, T., Rao, D.C., Chagnon, Y. and Quebec Family, S., 2003b, Genome-wide linkage scan for physical activity levels in the Quebec Family study. *Medicine and Science in Sports and Exercise,* **35**, pp, 1355–1359.

Spinath, F.M., Wolf, H., Angleitner, A., Borkenau, P. and Riemann, R., 2002, Genetic and environmental influences on objectively assessed activity in adults. *Personality and Individual Differences,* **33**, pp, 633–645.

Stefan, N., Vozarova, B., Del Parigi, A., Ossowski, V., Thompson, D.B., Hanson, R.L. and Tataranni, P.A., 2002, The Gln223Arg polymorphism of the leptin receptor in Pima Indians: influence on energy expenditure, physical activity and lipid metabolism. *International Journal of Obesity and Related Metabolic Disorders,* **26**, pp, 1629–1632.

Storti, K.L., 2007, *Familial Aggregation of Physical Activity,* Doctor of Philosophy, (Pittsburgh: University of Pittsburgh).

Stubbe, J.H., Boomsma, D.I. and De Geus, E.J., 2005, Sports participation during adolescence: a shift from environmental to genetic factors. *Medicine and Science in Sports and Exercise,* **37**, pp, 563–570.

Tang-Christensen, M., Havel, P.J., Jacobs, R.R., Larsen, P.J. and Cameron, J.L., 1999, Central administration of leptin inhibits food intake and activates the sympathetic nervous system in rhesus macaques. *Journal of Clinical Endocrinology and Metabolism,* **84**, pp, 711–717.

Teixeira e Seabra, A.F., Mendonça, D.M.d.M.V.d. and Maia, J.A.R., 2004, Agregação familiar nos hábitos de prática desportiva: um estudo em crianças e jovens dos 10 aos 19 anos de idade. *Revista Brasileira de Ciência e Movimento,* **12**, pp, 7–14.

Thornton, L.E., Pearce, J.R. and Kavanagh, A.M., 2011, Using Geographic Information Systems (GIS) to assess the role of the built environment in influencing obesity: a glossary. *International Journal of Behavioral Nutrion and Physical Activity,* **8**, pp, 71.

Vilhjalmsson, R. and Kristjansdottir, G., 2003, Gender differences in physical activity in older children and adolescents: the central role of organized sport. *Social Science and Medicine,* **56**, pp, 363–374.

Wagner, A., Klein-Platat, C., Arveiler, D., Haan, M.C., Schlienger, J.L. and Simon, C., 2004, Parent-child physical activity relationships in 12-year old

French students do not depend on family socioeconomic status. *Diabetes and Metabolism,* **30**, pp, 359–366.

Wang, J. G. and Staessen, J.A., 2000, Genetic polymorphisms in the renin-angiotensin system: relevance for susceptibility to cardiovascular disease. *European Journal of Pharmacology,* **410**, pp, 289–302.

Williams-Blangero, S., Criscione, C.D., VandeBerg, J.L., Correa-Oliveira, R., Williams, K.D., Subedi, J. and Blangero, J., 2012, Host genetics and population structure effects on parasitic disease. *Philosophical Transactions of the Royal Society: Biological Sciences,* **367**, pp, 887–894.

Winnicki, M., Accurso, V., Hoffmann, M., Pawlowski, R., Dorigatti, F., Santonastaso, M. and Group, H.S., 2004, Physical activity and angiotensin-converting enzyme gene polymorphism in mild hypertensives. *American Journal of Medical Genetics,* **125**, pp, 38–44.

Wood, A.C., Rijsdijk, F., Saudino, K.J., Asherson, P. and Kuntsi, J., 2008, High heritability for a composite index of children's activity level measures. *Behavior Genetics,* **38**, pp, 266–276.

Wu, T.Y. and Pender, N., 2002, Determinants of physical activity among Taiwanese adolescents: an application of the health promotion model. *Research in Nursing and Health,* **25**, pp, 25–36.

TRAINING AND TESTING ELITE YOUNG ATHLETES

N. Armstrong

Children's Health and Exercise Research Centre, University of Exeter, UK

7.1 INTRODUCTION

The elite young athlete is one who has superior athletic talent, undergoes specialized training, receives expert coaching and is exposed to early competition (Mountjoy *et al.,* 2008). It is not unusual to see 2 year-old children in gymnasium initiation programmes and training time increases with age with, for example, elite young gymnasts training for 30 hours or more each week. Participation in organized competitive sport often begins as early as 6–7 years of age and by their teens some young athletes have experienced several years of intensive training and high-level competition.

Participation in most sports requires a foundation of aerobic fitness and in several sports aerobic fitness is the most important physiological component of performance. During childhood and adolescence aerobic fitness increases with age, growth and maturation but can be further enhanced through endurance training. Endurance training consists of a structured exercise programme that is sustained for a sufficient length of time and at sufficient intensity and frequency to induce an improvement in aerobic fitness. Well-structured endurance training programmes with elite young athletes include regular testing to monitor performance.

This chapter will outline the development of aerobic fitness during childhood and adolescence and examine what we know of endurance training and aerobic fitness testing in youth, with particular reference to elite young athletes.

7.2 AEROBIC FITNESS

Aerobic fitness can be defined as the ability to deliver oxygen to the muscles and to utilize it to generate energy to support muscle activity during exercise. Peak oxygen uptake (peak VO_2), the highest rate at which oxygen can be consumed during exercise, is widely recognized as the best single measure of young people's aerobic fitness (Armstrong *et al.,* 2008). A high peak VO_2 is a pre-requisite of elite performance in many sports but in some sports the ability to sustain submaximal exercise is paramount and blood lactate (BLa) accumulation during exercise provides a useful indicator of aerobic fitness (Armstrong and Welsman, 2008). In other sports the ability to engage in rapid changes of pace is as important as achieving maximal aerobic power or sustaining submaximal performance. In this case it is the transient kinetics of VO_2 which best describe the relevant component of aerobic fitness (Armstrong and Barker, 2009).

7.2.1 Peak Oxygen Uptake

In boys, peak VO_2 (l/min) increases with age in an almost linear manner with a ~150% increase over the age range 8–16 years. Girls' data show a similar but less consistent trend with a tendency to level-off at ~14 years and an increase in peak VO_2 of ~80% from 8–16 years. Boys' values are ~10% higher than those of girls during childhood, probably due to the boys' greater maximal stroke volumes (SVs). During adolescence greater increases in boys' muscle mass and haemoglobin concentration drive the gender difference in peak VO_2 to ~35–40%. When peak VO_2 is expressed in ratio with body mass (ml/kg/min) a different picture emerges with boys' values remaining essentially unchanged with age at ~48–50 ml/kg/min and girls' values declining from ~45–35 ml/kg/min during adolescence. The reporting of peak VO_2 in ratio with body mass is relevant in the context of sports in which body mass is supported and moved but it has clouded the physiological understanding of peak VO_2 during growth and maturation. With body mass appropriately controlled for using allometry or multi-level modelling, boys' peak VO_2 is shown to increase through childhood and adolescence into young adulthood and girls' values to increase at least until puberty and possibly into young adulthood. This analysis is in conflict with expressing peak VO_2 in ratio with body mass but clearly demonstrates that maturation is independently associated with increases in peak VO_2 above those explained by age and body size (Armstrong *et al.*, 2008).

7.2.2 Blood Lactate Accumulation

BLa accumulation during exercise must be interpreted with caution and should not be assumed to reflect a direct relationship with muscle lactate production. Gender differences and maturation effects independent of age remain to be substantiated but children have consistently been shown to accumulate less BLa than adults at the same relative exercise intensity or relative VO_2. However, the lower exercise-induced BLa accumulation in children than in adults may reflect faster removal from the blood, and/or a smaller muscle mass with a higher percentage of type I muscle fibres rather than lower muscle lactate production (Armstrong and Welsman, 2008).

7.2.3 Oxygen Uptake Kinetics

During childhood and adolescence the time constant (τ) of the exponential increase in VO_2 at the onset of both moderate and heavy intensity exercise slows with age. There are no gender differences in the τ during the transition from rest to moderate intensity exercise but boys have a faster τ than girls at the onset of heavy intensity exercise. During youth peak VO_2 is not related to the VO_2 τ during the transition to either moderate or heavy intensity exercise probably because peak VO_2 is largely dependent on oxygen delivery to the muscles whereas VO_2 kinetics appear to be more reliant on oxygen utilization by the muscles (Armstrong and Barker, 2009).

7.3 ENDURANCE TRAINING

7.3.1 Peak Oxygen Uptake and Training

Elite young athletes normally have higher peak VO_2 values than their non-sporting peers but as almost all studies report cross-sectional comparisons the extent to which this difference is due to initial selection for sport, subsequent training or both is unknown. In addition, most studies report peak VO_2 using the ratio standard (ml/kg/min) which favours small people so direct comparisons of the aerobic fitness of, say, gymnasts and hockey players using this methodology are fundamentally flawed. Nevertheless, mean peak VO_2 values of >60 ml/kg/min and >50 ml/kg/min for trained boys and girls respectively are regularly reported and individual values >75 ml/kg/min for trained boys are not unknown (Armstrong and Barker, 2011).

There is no compelling evidence to suggest that maximal arterial-venous oxygen difference or maximal heart rate (HR) is enhanced with training during youth. However, the literature is consistent in reporting trained young athletes to have higher maximal SVs than their untrained peers (Rowland *et al.*, 2002). These findings are supported by a prospective study of 10–11-year-olds in which a 13 week endurance training programme resulted in a rise in peak VO_2 brought about solely by an increase in maximal SV in both boys and girls. The boys increased their peak VO_2 to a greater extent than the girls (15% versus 8%) only because of a higher maximal SV improvement (15% versus 11%) (Obert *et al.*, 2003).

The mechanisms underlying a training-induced increase in maximal SV are unclear. Data on young people are sparse and inconsistent with some studies reporting significant increases in cardiac dimensions with training (Obert *et al.*, 1998, 2003) and others observing no changes (George *et al.*, 2005). Estimates of shortening fraction and ejection fraction at rest appear to be similar in both trained and untrained children (Obert *et al.*, 1998) but trained children have been reported to increase their shortening fraction more during maximal exercise than untrained children (Oyen *et al.*, 1990). It also seems reasonable to suggest that SV might be enhanced through a more effective peripheral muscle pump and/or plasma volume expansion increasing venous return but empirical support of this hypothesis is not currently available (Armstrong and Barker, 2011).

7.3.2 Blood Lactate Accumulation and Training

BLa accumulation during exercise has been reported to be lower in trained young runners than in similarly aged untrained children (van Huss *et al.*, 1988). The primary mechanism in adults appears to be an increase in oxidative capacity but the mechanisms underpinning training-induced changes in BLa accumulation during youth remain to be proven. High intensity endurance training has been demonstrated to result in lower BLa accumulation post-training than at the same pre-training exercise intensity or VO_2 (Massicote and MacNab, 1974) whereas no changes in BLa accumulation have been observed following low intensity endurance training (Ekblom, 1969). The lactate threshold (TLAC), the point at which BLa increases non-linearly during incremental exercise, is a useful indicator of aerobic fitness and in trained young athletes it occurs at a higher percentage of peakVO_2 than in their untrained peers (Fernhall et al., 1996). The assessment and interpretation of BLa accumulation during childhood and adolescence is challenging and non-invasive equivalents of the TLAC, such as the ventilation threshold (TVENT), are commonly used to avoid taking blood (Fawkner et al, 2002). The TVENT expressed either as a percentage of peak VO_2 or as a running velocity has been demonstrated to correlate well with middle distance running performance in prepubertal athletes although the correlation might be slightly weaker than that with peak VO_2 (Fernhall et al., 1996).

Changes in the maximal lactate steady state (MLSS), the highest exercise intensity that can be sustained without a progressive accumulation of BLa, have been used to monitor adult athletes' training and performance. No well-controlled study appears to have directly measured MLSS in elite young athletes and examined its relationship with performance although fixed BLa reference values, such as 2.5 or 4mM, have been used as surrogates of the MLSS to monitor both training and performance. The running speed corresponding to a BLa accumulation of 4mM has been reported to increase following a training programme (Rotstein et al., 1986) and to be correlated with 2 and 3 mile run performance in adolescent runners (Fernhall et al., 1996). Similarly, a BLa accumulation of 2.5mM has been shown to be correlated with 1500m run performance in adolescent runners (Almarwaey et al., 2003). However, the interpretation of data on young people's lactate reference values is confounded by differences in methodology (Armstrong and Welsman, 2008).

7.3.3 Oxygen Uptake Kinetics and Training

A training-induced speeding of the VO_2 τ could enhance sports performance by resisting fatigue through a reduced depletion of intra-muscular high-energy phosphates and a lower accumulation of hydrogen ions and inorganic phosphate in the muscle. However, knowledge of training effects on VO_2 kinetics during youth is restricted to a limited number of cross-sectional studies. Comparisons of prepubertal swimmers with their untrained peers have reported no significant differences in the VO_2 τ during the transition from rest to either moderate or heavy intensity leg exercise (Cleuziou et al., 2002) but trained prepubertal swimmers have been observed to demonstrate faster VO_2 kinetics at the onset of heavy intensity arm exercise (Winlove et al., 2010). In contrast, a study of 14-year-old pubertal girls reported a significantly faster VO_2 kinetic response to the onset of heavy exercise in trained swimmers than in an untrained group during both leg and arm exercise (McNarry et al., 2011). The authors attributed the conflicting results in prepubertal and pubertal girls to both a greater stage of maturation and a longer history of training in the pubertal girls. In the only other published study to date, 15 year-old boys from a Premier League football academy were observed to demonstrate a faster VO_2 kinetic response to the onset of moderate intensity exercise than age-matched controls (Marwood et al., 2010). More research using new technologies, such as magnetic resonance spectroscopy (MRS) and near infrared spectroscopy (**NIRS**), is needed to establish the mechanisms underlying speeded VO_2 kinetic responses following training. Both oxygen delivery and oxygen utilization are likely to be enhanced by training but as the VO_2 kinetic response is independent of increases in peak VO_2 during youth enhanced oxygen utilization by the muscles might be the primary mechanism (Armstrong and Barker, 2009).

7.3.4 Exercise Prescription

Peak VO_2 is the only component of young people's aerobic fitness on which there are sufficient data to estimate a dose-response relationship with endurance training. Genetic influences on the responsiveness of peak VO_2 to endurance training are not well-understood but it appears that, as with adults, there is a continuum from high responders to non-responders. It has been estimated that ~45% of the training-induced change in peak VO_2 is due to heritability (Danis *et al.*, 2003). It has been hypothesized that there is a maturational threshold below which the effects of training will be minimal (Gilliam and Freedson, 1968) but more recent research has demonstrated that this is clearly not the case. Early studies suggesting that prepubertal children do not respond to training or girls are less receptive to training than boys are confounded by training programmes using less than optimum intensity exercise. To induce significant changes in peak VO_2 the relative intensity of the exercise needs to be within the HR range 85–90% of maximum (i.e. ~170–180 beats/min) which is higher than that which has been shown to be effective with adults. There appear to be no age, maturation or gender effects on the magnitude of peak VO_2 responses to training during youth although changes tend to be smaller than those observed with adults. Following a 12 week training programme consisting of 3–4 sessions per week, for 40 minutes per session, an increase in peak VO_2 of ~8–9% would be expected in healthy children and adolescents (Armstrong and Barker, 2011).

There are too few rigorously determined data to specifically analyze the dose-response effects of endurance training on elite young athletes but there is no evidence to suggest that they would respond in a significantly different manner to other healthy young people. Two similar studies of 14- and 16-year-old elite soccer players employed interval training programmes of 2 sessions per week, for 8 weeks and 10 weeks respectively. The exercise sessions were soccer-specific with HR maintained in the range 90–95% of maximum in both studies and significant increases in peak VO_2 of 12% and 9% respectively were reported. Unfortunately, neither study included a control group for comparison (Chamari *et al.*, 2005; McMillan *et al.*, 2005).

Assuming that they are not non-responders to training, greater increases in peak VO_2 are likely following the long-term, specific training programmes experienced by elite young athletes. For example, Obert *et al.* (1996) determined the peak VO_2 of five 9-year-old girl swimmers on a swim bench before and after a 52 week training programme which consisted of 10, 60–90 minute sessions per week with HR in the range 85–90% of maximum. They reported a significant 29% increase in the peak VO_2 (ml/kg/min) of the trained girls and no change in the peak VO_2 of an untrained control group over the same time period.

7.3.5 The Unexplained Underperformance Syndrome

The positive effects of training are well-documented but elite young athletes training for 20–30 hours per week over several years might find themselves victims of a syndrome often termed overtraining but perhaps more accurately viewed as the unexplained underperformance syndrome (UPS). UPS occurs where frequent competition, high intensity training and non-sport specific stressors, perhaps associated with growth and development, combine to negatively affect the performance of the elite young athlete. During episodes of UPS the young athlete might experience decreased interest in training and competition, frustration with lack of improvement, inability to concentrate, depression, short temper, decreased self-confidence, increased conflicts with coach and/or parents, and high levels of stress. There are few data on the prevalence of UPS during youth but recent surveys indicate ~30% of elite young athletes have experienced the UPS with a higher prevalence in individual sports than in team sports and in girls than in boys. The sensitive management of the UPS involves moderate levels of aerobic exercise, possibly cross-training, together with an emphasis on skill-based work. Full training and competition should be re-introduced progressively with attention being paid to rest periods and incremental increases in levels of competition (Winsley and Matos, 2011).

7.4 EXERCISE TESTING

Winter *et al.* (2007) provide a compelling case that regular assessments should be an integral part of an athlete's training and scientific support programme. Assessments should evaluate strengths and weaknesses, inform and evaluate the effectiveness of training programmes, provide motivation and measurable goals, assist in talent identification and the prediction of future performance, and enhance knowledge and understanding of sport and exercise. It has been recommended that physiological assessment and support should be provided every 3 months, thus allowing sufficient time for the adaptations from training to manifest themselves (Davison *et al.,* 2009). The testing frequency should, however, be discussed and agreed with the coach and focus around key periods in the athlete's training cycle and competition schedule. Performance tests involving elite young athletes must also take into account the influence of growth and maturation and the different rates of individual biological clocks. Unfortunately, most methods of estimating maturation are intrusive, invasive or ethically questionable although Mirwald *et al.* (2002) have developed a useful means of estimating maturity from anthropometric measures. An understanding and appropriate quantification of measurement error is essential to monitor young people's fitness and performance on a longitudinal basis (Atkinson and Nevill, 2007).

Laboratory determinations of physiological variables during youth are well-documented and reliable but the interpretation of performance data in relation to body size remains shrouded with controversy and in a sporting context it is prudent to analyse, interpret and monitor data using both the ratio and allometric methods

(Welsman and Armstrong, 2008). Ideally laboratory exercise tests should be sport-specific and simulate the type of exercise used in competition. Most laboratory tests of peak VO_2 are performed on treadmills or cycle ergometers but more specialised machines such as rowing and kayaking ergometers, swim benches and swimming flumes are also available. Peak VO_2 determined during treadmill running has been shown to be a stable measure of aerobic fitness which is generally protocol independent although wide differences have been observed across different ergometers. For example, treadmill running determinations of peak VO_2 produce values ~8–10, ~15 and ~33% higher than those determined on cycle, rowing and swim bench ergometers respectively (Armstrong and Welsman, 2008; Barker and Armstrong, 2011).

Laboratory measurement of peak VO_2 is impractical for use with large groups and a plethora of field tests to estimate peak VO_2 have emerged but these tests generally have limited application to elite young athletes. Innovative sports–specific field tests to estimate peak VO_2 have been developed (e.g. Chamari et al., 2005) but despite their attractiveness their power to predict peak VO_2 is low to moderate and not an adequate replacement for a laboratory assessment of peak VO_2 (Armstrong and Welsman, 2008; Barker and Armstrong, 2011).

BLa monitoring is not limited to laboratory use and BLa profiles are regularly used to monitor fitness and inform training intensities in athletics, cycling and swimming. Training zones (or intensity domains) using TLAC to discriminate between moderate and heavy exercise, MLSS as the physiological marker of the beginning of very heavy exercise and peak VO_2 as the lower threshold of severe exercise are commonly used and have been shown to be reliable with young athletes in sports such as cycling (Monfort-Steiger et al., 2005).

VO_2 kinetics during youth has been determined in the laboratory during running on a treadmill, upright cycling and arm ergometry. Although the overall shape of the VO_2 response is independent of the type of ergometry the τ varies with the mode of exercise and it has been suggested that the more specific the exercise to the sport the more likely the detection of training-induced changes (Winlove et al., 2101). The regular monitoring of the VO_2 kinetics of elite young athletes in training has not been reported.

7.5 CONCLUSION

Elite young athletes undergoing intensive training and high frequency participation in sports competition from an early age are a special population worthy of study. However, data on training-induced changes in aerobic fitness, appropriate exercise prescriptions and the UPS are relatively sparse compared with data on adult athletes. Elite young athletes are not mini-adults and techniques used with adults for the assessment and interpretation of performance are often neither ethical nor appropriate for use with young people. Recent technological developments (e.g. MRS and NIRS) have opened up new avenues of research in paediatric exercise science and need to be applied to the study of elite young athletes.

Elite young athletes deserve to have the opportunity to fulfil their potential in accordance with their health and well-being. Paediatric exercise scientists and coaches therefore need to understand fully the impact of growth, age, maturation and training on performance and be able to incorporate this knowledge into the design, execution and monitoring of their training programmes.

7.6 REFERENCES

Almarwaey, O.A., Jones, A.M. and Tolfrey, K., 2003, Physiological correlates with endurance running performance in trained adolescents. *Medicine and Science in Sports and Exercise*, **35,** pp. 480–487.

Armstrong, N. and Barker, A.R., 2009, Oxygen uptake kinetics in children and adolescents: A review. *Pediatric Exercise Science,* **21**, pp. 130–147.

Armstrong, N. and Barker, A.R., 2011, Endurance training and elite young athletes. In *The Elite Young Athlete*, edited by Armstrong, N. and McManus, A.M. (Basel: Karger), pp. 59–83.

Armstrong, N., McManus, A.M. and Welsman, J.R., 2008, Aerobic fitness. In *Paediatric Exercise Science and Medicine,* edited by Armstrong, N. and van Mechelen, W. (Oxford: Oxford University Press), pp. 269–282.

Armstrong, N. and Welsman, J.R., 2008, Aerobic fitness. In *Paediatric Exercise Science and Medicine,* edited by Armstrong, N. and Van Mechelen, W. (Oxford: Oxford University Press), pp. 97–108.

Atkinson, G. and Nevill, A.M., 2007, Method agreement and measurement error in the physiology of exercise. In *Sport and Exercise Physiology Testing Guidelines*, edited by Winter, E.M., Bromley, P.D., Davison, R.C.R., Jones, A.M. and Mercer, T.H., (London: Routledge), pp. 41–48.

Barker, A.R. and Armstrong, N., 2011, Exercise testing elite young athletes. In *The Elite Young Athlete*, edited by Armstrong, N. and McManus, A.M. (Basel: Karger), pp.106–125.

Chamari, K., Hachana, Y., Kaouech, F., Jeddi, R., Moussa-Chamari, I. and Wisleff, U., 2005, Endurance training and testing with the ball in young elite soccer players. *British Journal of Sports Medicine*, **39,** pp. 24–25.

Cleuziou, C., Lecoq, A.M., Candau, R., Courteix, D., Guenon, P. and Obert, P., 2002, Kinetics of oxygen uptake at the onset of moderate and heavy exercise in trained and untrained pre-pubertal children. *Science and Sports,* **17**, pp. 291–296.

Danis, A., Kyriazis, Y. and Klissouras, V., 2003, The effect of training in male pre-pubertal and pubertal monozygotic twins. *European Journal of Applied Physiology*, **89**, pp. 309–318.

Davison, R.R., van Someron, K.A. and Jones, A.M., 2009, Physiological monitoring of the Olympic athlete. *Journal of Sport Sciences,* 27, pp. 1–10.

Ekblom, B., 1969, Effect of physical training in adolescent boys. *Journal of Applied Physiology*, **27,** pp. 350–355.

Fawkner, S.G., Armstrong, N., Childs, D.J. and Welsman, J.R., 2002, Reliability of the visually assessed ventilatory threshold and V-Slope in children. *Pediatric Exercise Science,* **14**, pp.181–193.

Fernhall, B., Korht, W., Burkett, L.N. and Walters, S., 1996, Relationship between the lactate threshold and cross-country run performance in high school male and female runners. *Pediatric Exercise Science*, **8**, pp. 37–47.

George, K.P., Gates, K.E. and Tolfrey, K., 2005, Impact of aerobic training on left ventricular morphology and function in pre-pubescent children. *Ergonomics,* **48,** pp. 1378–1379.

Gilliam, T.B. and Freedson, P., 1980, Effects of a 12 week physical fitness programme on peak VO_2, body composition and blood lipids in 7–9-year-old children. *International Journal of Sports Medicine,* **1,** pp. 73–78.

Marwood, S., Roche, D., Rowland, T., Garrard, M. and Unnithan, V., 2010, Faster pulmonary oxygen uptake kinetics in trained versus untrained male adolescents. *Medicine and Science in Sports and Exercise,* **42,** pp. 127–134.

Massicote, D.R. and MacNab, R.B.J., 1974, Cardiorespiratory adaptations to training at specific intensities in children. *Medicine and Science in Sports,* **6,** pp. 242–246.

McMillan, K., Helgerud, J., Macdonald, R. and Hoff, J., 2005, Physiological adaptations to soccer specific endurance training in professional youth soccer players. *British Journal of Sports Medicine,* **39,** pp. 273–277.

McNarry, M.A., Welsman, J.R. and Jones, A.M., 2011, Influence of training status and exercise modality on pulmonary oxygen uptake kinetics in pubertal girls. *European Journal of Applied Physiology,* **111,** pp. 621–631.

Mirwald, R.L., Baxter-Jones, A.D., Bailey, D.A. and Buenen, G. P., 2002, An assessment of maturity from anthropometric measurements. *Medicine and Science in Sports and Exercise,* **34,** pp. 689–694.

Montfort-Steiger, V., Williams, C.A. and Armstrong, N., 2005, The reproducibility of an endurance performance test in adolescent cyclists. *European Journal of Applied Physiology,* **94,** pp. 618–625.

Mountjoy, M., Armstrong, N., Bizzini, L., Blimkie, C., Evans, J., Gerrard, D., Hangen, J., Knoll, K., Micheli, L., Sangenis, P. and van Mechelen, W., 2008, IOC consensus statement: 'training the elite young athlete'. *British Journal of Sports Medicine,* **42,** pp.163–164.

Obert, P., Courteix, D., Lecoq, A-M. and Guenon, P., 1996, Effect of long-term intense swimming training on the upper body peak oxygen uptake of pre-pubertal girls. *European Journal of Applied Physiology,* **73,** pp. 136–143.

Obert, P., Mandigouts, S., Nottin, A., Vinet., N'Guyen, L.D. and Lecoq, A-M., 2003, Cardiovascular responses to endurance training in children: Effect of gender. *European Journal of Clinical Investigation,* **33,** pp. 199–208.

Obert, P., Stecken, F., Courteix, D., Lecoq, A.M. and Guenon, P., 1998, Effect of long term endurance training on left ventricular structure and diastolic function in pre-pubertal children. *International Journal of Sports Medicine,* **19,** pp 149–154.

Oyen, E-M., Scuster, S. and Brode, P.E., 1990, Dynamic exercise echocardiography of the left ventricle in physically trained children compared to untrained healthy children. *International Journal of Cardiology,* **29,** pp. 29–33.

Rotstein, A., Dotan, R., Bar-Or, O. and Tenebaum, G., 1986, Effect of training on anaerobic threshold, maximal aerobic power and anaerobic performance of preadolescent boys. *International Journal of Sports Medicine,* **7,** pp. 281–286.

Rowland, T.W., Unnithan V., Fernhall, B., Baynard, T. and Lange, C., 2002, Left ventricular responses to dynamic exercise in young cyclists. *Medicine and Science in Sports and Exercise,* **34,** pp. 637–642.

Van Huss, W.D., Evans, S.A., Kurowshki, T., Andersen, D.J. Allen, R. and Stephens, K., 1988, Physiological characteristics of male and female age-group runners. In *Competitive Sports for Children and Youth*, edited by Brown, E.W. and Branta, C.F. (Champaign, IL: Human Kinetics), pp. 143–158.

Welsman, J.R. and Armstrong, N., 2008, Interpreting exercise performance data in relation to body size. In *Paediatric Exercise Science and Medicine,* edited by Armstrong, N. and van Mechelen, W. (Oxford: Oxford University Press), pp. 13–21.

Winlove, M.A., Jones, A.M. and Welsman, J.R., 2010, Influence of training status and exercise modality on pulmonary oxygen uptake kinetics in pre-pubertal girls. *European Journal of Applied Physiology,* **108**, pp. 1169–1179.

Winsley, R.J. and Matos, N., 2011, Overtraining and elite young athletes. In *The Elite Young Athlete*, edited by Armstrong, N. and McManus, A.M. (Basel: Karger), pp. 106–125.

Winter, E.M., Bromley, P.D., Davison, R.C.R., Jones, A.M. and Mercer, T.H., 2007, Rationale. In *Sport and Exercise Physiology Testing Guidelines*, edited by Winter, E.M., Bromley, P.D., Davison, R.C.R., Jones, A.M. and Mercer, T.H., (London: Routledge), pp. 7–10.

Part III

Physiology

MODERATE EXERCISE, ENERGY INTAKE RESTRICTION AND POSTPRANDIAL TRIACYLGLYCEROL IN HEALTHY GIRLS

K. Tolfrey, A.E. Thackray, and L.A. Barrett
Loughborough University, UK

8.1 INTRODUCTION

Elevated postprandial triacylglycerol (TAG) concentrations have been implicated in the development of atherosclerosis (Zilversmit, 1979), and are established as an independent risk factor for future cardiovascular diseases in adults (Nordestgaard et al., 2007). The process of atherosclerosis is initiated during childhood and adolescence, prompting preventative interventions that may delay atherosclerotic progression early in life (McGill et al., 2000). Accumulating evidence in boys demonstrates the TAG lowering effect of moderate intensity exercise interventions (e.g., Tolfrey et al., 2012). It is possible that the energy deficit associated with a single session of exercise may be responsible for the attenuation in postprandial [TAG]. Replacing the exercise-induced energy deficit has been shown to diminish or even eliminate the reduction in postprandial [TAG] in men (Burton et al., 2008). Although an exercise-induced energy deficit appears to reduce postprandial [TAG] to a greater extent than a diet-induced deficit (Gill and Hardman, 2000; Maraki et al., 2010), attenuations in postprandial [TAG] have been reported following a single day of energy-intake restriction in young, healthy women (Maraki et al., 2010). However, we are not aware of studies that have examined the effect of energy-intake restriction on postprandial [TAG] in young people. Therefore, the aim of this study was to compare the effect of an isoenergetic mild energy deficit, induced by acute moderate intensity exercise or food energy-intake restriction on postprandial [TAG] in healthy, active girls.

8.2 METHODS

Complete data were available for 11 healthy, active girls (mean (SD) age 12.1(0.6) years; 42.1(5.8) kg; 47(6) mL.kg^{-1}.min^{-1}). Informed assent was provided by all participants and consent by parents. Following treadmill habituation, peak oxygen uptake (peak $\dot{V}O_2$) was determined using an incremental uphill treadmill protocol. Participants completed three, 2 day experimental conditions in a counterbalanced crossover design. On day one, participants either rested (CON), walked at 60% peak $\dot{V}O_2$ inducing a net energy expenditure of 1.46(0.01) MJ (EX) or restricted food energy-intake by 1.47(0.18) MJ (ER). On day two, capillary blood samples were taken in the fasted state and at pre-determined intervals throughout the 6.5 h postprandial period while participants rested. Participants consumed a standardised breakfast immediately after the fasting sample at 08:00 (1.5 g fat, 1.8 g carbohydrate, 0.4 g protein and 93 kJ energy per kg body mass). A standardised lunch was consumed at 12:00 (1.0 g fat, 1.9 g carbohydrate, 0.6 g protein and 79 kJ energy per kg body mass).

Data were analysed using the IBM SPSS statistics software for Windows version 19 (IBM Corporation, New York, USA). The trapezium rule was used to calculate the area under the plasma concentration versus time curve for TAG (TAUC-TAG), glucose (TAUC-glucose) and insulin (TAUC-insulin). Fasting and TAUC responses were compared using separate one-way within measures ANOVA. Differences in postprandial [TAG] were examined using separate 3 x 7 (condition by time) within-measures ANOVA. Interpretation of data was based on 95% confidence intervals (95% CI) and effect sizes (ES) for the absolute differences. In the absence of an empirical clinical anchor, an ES of 0.2 was considered the minimum important difference in all outcome measures, 0.5 moderate and 0.8 large (Cohen, 1988). Results are presented as mean (SD).

8.3 RESULTS

Energy intake on Day 1 of CON, ER and EX were 7.45(1.35), 5.94(1.30) and 7.37(1.28) MJ respectively, resulting in an energy deficit of 1.51(0.23) MJ in ER and 1.55(0.21) MJ in EX relative to CON. The diet- and exercise-induced energy deficits were not different from each other (95% CI -0.07 to 0.15, ES = 0.19). Compared with CON, fasting plasma [TAG] was lower after ER (95% CI   -0.22 to -0.01, ES = 0.42) and EX (95% CI -0.38 to -0.19, ES = 1.33); EX was also lower than ER (95% CI -0.30 to -0.03, ES = 0.66) (Table 8.1). The main effect for condition revealed differences in postprandial [TAG] over time (ES = 0.50) (Figure 8.1). The TAUC-TAG was considerably lower after EX than CON (95% CI -2.89 to -0.86, ES = 0.80), with small differences between ER and CON (95% CI -1.85 to 0.16, ES = 0.27) and EX and ER (95% CI -2.48 to 0.42, ES = 0.40) (Table 8.1).

Fasting plasma [glucose] was lower compared with CON after both ER (95% CI -0.29 to -0.02, ES = 0.59) and EX (95% CI -0.34 to -0.05, ES = 0.80); the difference between EX and ER was small (95% CI -0.17 to 0.09, ES = 0.20) (Table 8.1). Differences in postprandial plasma [glucose] across conditions over time were small (main effect condition ES = 0.39). The only meaningful difference in TAUC-glucose was seen between EX and ER (95% CI -0.12 to 2.88, ES = 0.48) (Table 8.1). Fasting plasma [insulin] was lower following ER than CON (95% CI -22.9 to 0.1, ES = 0.47) and EX than CON (95% CI -29.8 to -4.0, ES = 0.77); a small difference was seen between EX and ER (-18.3 to 7.3, ES = 0.30) (Table 8.1). Differences in postprandial plasma [insulin] across conditions were trivial (main effect condition ES = 0.09). No meaningful differences were evident in TAUC-insulin across the conditions (ES = 0.04 to 0.12) (Table 8.1).

Table 8.1 Fasting and total area under the concentration versus time curve (TAUC) for plasma [triacylglycerol], [glucose] and [insulin] in the control condition (CON), energy-intake restriction condition (ER) and exercise condition (EX).

	CON	ER	EX
Fasting triacylglycerol (mmol.L^{-1})	0.97 (0.24)	0.86 (0.31)	0.69 (0.17)
Fasting glucose (mmol.L^{-1})	5.55 (0.29)	5.40 (0.22)	5.36 (0.19)
Fasting insulin (pmol.L^{-1})	59.5 (27.2)	48.2 (21.0)	42.7 (14.9)
TAUC-TAG (mmol.L^{-1} 6.5 h)	8.55 (2.89)	7.70 (3.26)	6.67 (1.63)
TAUC-glucose (mmol.L^{-1} 6.5 h)	40.8 (3.1)	39.9 (3.1)	41.3 (2.7)
TAUC-insulin (pmol.L^{-1} 6.5 h)	1552 (448)	1488 (634)	1508 (412)

All values are mean (SD).

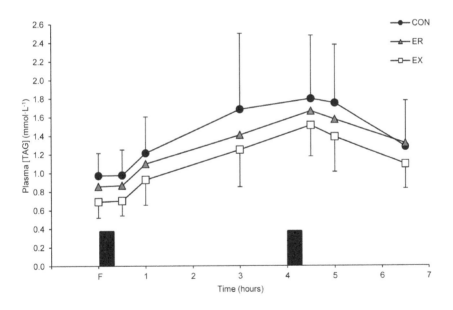

Figure 8.1 Fasting (F) and postprandial plasma triacylglycerol (TAG) concentration for the control condition (CON), energy-intake restriction condition (ER) and exercise condition (EX). Black rectangles indicate consumption of the breakfast (08:00) and lunch (12:00) meals.

8.4 CONCLUSION

The main finding from the present study was that an exercise-induced energy deficit elicits a greater reduction in fasting and postprandial [TAG] than an isoenergetic diet-induced deficit in healthy, active girls. This suggests that the origin of the acute energy deficit influences the magnitude of change in fasting and postprandial [TAG], consistent with previous studies in adults (Gill and Hardman, 2000; Maraki *et al.*, 2010). Although acute moderate intensity exercise has been shown to attenuate postprandial [TAG] in adolescent boys previously (e.g., Tolfrey *et al.*, 2012), the small attenuation seen due to acute energy-intake restriction is a novel finding in this population. Furthermore, we also reported that the fasting [glucose] and [insulin] were reduced to a greater extent following the exercise than the energy-intake restriction condition. Therefore, exercise prescription may promote greater acute benefits in lipid, glucose and insulin metabolism than dietary restriction in healthy, active girls.

8.5 REFERENCES

Burton, F.L., Malkova, D., Caslake, M.J. and Gill, J.M.R., 2008, Energy replacement attenuates the effects of prior moderate exercise on postprandial metabolism in overweight/obese men. *International Journal of Obesity*, **32**, pp. 481–489.

Cohen, J., 1988, *Statistical power analysis for behavioural sciences*, (Hillsdale (NJ): Lawrence Erlbaum Associates).

Gill, J.M.R. and Hardman, A.E., 2000, Postprandial lipemia: effects of exercise and restriction of energy intake compared. *The American Journal of Clinical Nutrition*, **71**, pp. 465–471.

Maraki, M., Magkos, F., Christodoulou, N., Aggelopoulou, N., Skenderi, K. P., Panagiotakos, D., Kavouras, S.A. and Sidossis, L.S., 2010, One day of moderate energy deficit reduces fasting and postprandial triacylglycerolemia in women: the role of calorie restriction and exercise. *Clinical Nutrition*, **29**, pp. 459–463.

McGill, H.C., McMahan, C.A., Herderick, E.E., Malcom, G.T., Tracy, R.E. and Strong, J.P., 2000, Origin of atherosclerosis in childhood and adolescence. *The American Journal of Clinical Nutrition*, **72**, pp. S1307–1315.

Nordestgaard, B.G., Benn, M., Schnohr, P. and Tybjærg-Hansen, A., 2007, Nonfasting triglycerides and risk of myocardial infarction, ischemic heart disease, and death in men and women. *Journal of the American Medical Association*, **298**, pp. 299–308.

Tolfrey, K., Bentley, C., Goad, M., Varley, J., Willis, S. and Barrett, L., 2012, Effect of energy expenditure on postprandial triacylglycerol in adolescent boys. *European Journal of Applied Physiology*, **112**, pp. 23–31.

Zilversmit, D.B., 1979, Atherogenesis: a postprandial phenomenon. *Circulation*, **60**, pp. 473–485.

TRAINING INCREASES ANABOLIC AND REDUCES INFLAMMATORY RESPONSE TO A SINGLE PRACTICE IN MALE VOLLEYBALL PLAYERS

A. Eliakim[1], S. Portal[2], Y. Meckel[3], and D. Nemet[1]

[1]Pediatric Department, Child Health and Sport Center, Meir Medical Center, Sackler School of Medicine, Tel-Aviv University, Israel; [2]School of Nutritional Sciences, Hebrew University of Jerusalem, Israel; [3]Zinman College of Physical Education and Sport Sciences, Wingate Institute, Israel

9.1 INTRODUCTION

Exercise-induced changes in anabolic-catabolic hormonal balance and circulating inflammatory cytokines are used frequently by adolescent athletes and coaches to optimize training (Eliakim and Nemet, 2010). A unique feature of exercise is that it leads often to simultaneous increase of antagonistic mediators. For example, exercise stimulates anabolic components of the growth hormone (GH) $\rightarrow$ IGF-I (insulin-like growth factor-I) axis, and in the same time, it may elevate catabolic pro-inflammatory cytokines such as Interlukin-6 (IL-6), IL-1 and TNF-α (Nemet and Eliakim, 2010). The balance between the anabolic and inflammatory/catabolic response to exercise will dictate training efficiency and the health implications of exercise. If the anabolic response dominates, exercise will probably lead to increased muscle mass and improved fitness. In contrast, a greater catabolic response, particularly if prolonged and/or combined with inadequate nutrition, may lead to overtraining. While hormonal response to a single exercise bout was determined previously, the effect of prolonged training on the response to a single exercise in adolescent athletes was less studied. This is important because studies on the effect of fitness on hormonal responses to exercise yielded conflicting results (Eliakim and Nemet, 2008). Moreover, it is particularly important in adolescent athletes since puberty is characterized by rapid linear and muscle mass growth, and by spontaneous spurt of anabolic hormones. We previously demonstrated that prolonged training was associated with reduced catabolic response to a single practice in elite adolescent female volleyball players (Eliakim *et al.*, 2013). The aim of the present study was to examine the effects of similar training on the hormonal and inflammatory response to a single volleyball practice in elite *male* adolescent players.

9.2 METHODS

Fourteen healthy, male, elite, national team level, Israeli junior volleyball players (age 16.3±1.1 years, Tanner stage for pubic hair 4–5) participated in the study. All participants were members of the Israeli national junior volleyball team. The study was performed during the first 7 weeks of the volleyball season. Participants trained 18–22 hours per week. Training involved tactic and technical drills emphasizing volleyball skills and team strategies (~ 20% of the time), power and speed drills with and without the ball (~25% of the time), and interval sessions (~25% of the time). About 15% of the time consisted of endurance-type training (i.e. long-distance running). The additional 15% of the time consisted of resistance training using mainly circuit training with free weights at 65–75% of 1RM.

Standard, calibrated scales and stadiometers were used to determine height, weight, and BMI. Fat percentage was calculated from skinfolds measurements. Fitness assessment, included anaerobic (vertical jump and the Wingate Anaerobic Test) and aerobic measures (VO_2 max predicted by the 20m shuttle-run). The practice consisted of 20 min dynamic warm-up which included jogging, stretching and running drills at sub-maximal speed (up to 80% of maximal speed), and additional 20 min of volleyball drills. The main part of the practice included seven repetitions of seven consecutive sprints from the back of the volleyball court to the net, maximal jump and a hit of the volleyball over the net in the end of each sprint. Each repetition lasted about 1.5 min with 1min rest to collect the balls between repetitions. Blood samples were collected before and immediately after the 60 min volleyball practice, before and after 7 weeks of training. Measurements included the anabolic hormones GH, IGF-I, IGF binding protein-3 and testosterone, the catabolic hormone cortisol, the pro-inflammatory marker IL-6, and the anti-inflammatory marker IL-1 receptor antagonist, using commercially available kits.

A two-way repeated measure ANOVA (with Bonferroni post hoc test) was used to compare the effect of training on exercise practice associated changes. Statistical significance was set at $p<0.05$. Data presented as mean ± standard deviation (SD).

9.3 RESULTS

Training led to significant improvement of anaerobic properties and predicted VO_2max (Table 9.1). Volleyball practice, both before and after the training intervention, was associated with a significant increase of serum lactate, GH, testosterone and IL-6 levels. GH response to the same relative intensity volleyball practice was significantly increased, and the IL-6 response was significantly reduced at the end compared to before the training intervention (Table 9.2, Figure 9.1).

Table 9.1 Anthropometric and fitness characteristics of the participants. (*p<0.05).

	Pre training	Post training
Height (cm)	190.9±4.1	191.1±4.4
Weight (kg)	77.4±9.7	78.9±9.7*
BMI (kg/m^2)	21.2±2.4	21.6±2.3*
Fat (%)	13.5±3.9	13.2±5.0
VO$_2$ max (ml/kg/min)	44.8±6.1	48.0±4.0*
Anaerobic peak power (Watt/kg)	13.7±0.9	14.8±1.1*
Anaerobic mean power (Watt/kg)	9.5±0.7	10.0±0.9*
Vertical Jump (m)	3.17±0.06	3.21±0.09

Table 9.2 Training effect on hormonal and inflammatory response to a single volleyball practice.* p<0.05 pre vs post practice; † p<0.05 pre vs post training.

	Pre Training		Post Training	
	Pre practice	Post practice	Pre practice	Post practice
GH (ng/ml)	0.2±0.2	2.7±2.4*	0.3±0.5	5.0±3.1*†
IGF-I (ng/ml)	506.7±125.7	522.3±96.6	498.7±114.5	503.9±129.7
IGFBP-3 (ng/ml)	6026±883	5987±1362	5169±1546	5850±976*
Testosterone (ng/ml)	6.2±3.5	7.3±3.6*	6.4±1.9	8.3±5.5*
Cortisol (mcg/L)	20.8±6.6	22.1±6.1	23.0±4.1	22.7±8.5
IL-6 (pg/ml)	1.2±0.6	3.1±1.7*	1.0±0.6	1.6±1.0*†
IL1ra (pg/ml)	296.4±85.8	319.8±83.7	344.1±136.2	366.6±212.7
Lactate (nmol/L)	3.1±0.7	5.7±1.3*	2.3±0.6	4.8±0.7*

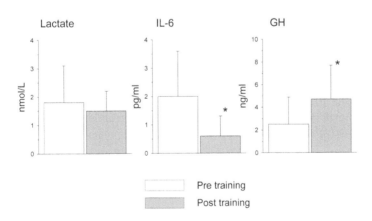

Figure 9.1 Effect of training on serum lactate, GH and IL-6 response to a single volleyball practice.

9.4 DISCUSSION

Training during the initial phases of the volleyball training season was associated with significant improvements in both anaerobic and aerobic properties. As previously described (Eliakim *et al.,* 2009), prior to the training intervention, a single, typical volleyball practice was associated with a significant increase of the anabolic hormones GH and testosterone, and the pro-inflammatory marker IL-6. Changes in GH and testosterone may indicate exercise-associated anabolic adaptations, and IL-6 increase may suggest its important role in micro-traumatic muscle damage repair following volleyball training. The main finding of the present study is that following 7 weeks of training during the early volleyball season, GH was significantly increased and IL-6 significantly reduced in response to the same relative intensity volleyball practice. The results are consistent with our previous findings that training was associated with reduced catabolic response to a single volleyball practice in elite adolescent female players (Eliakim *et al.,* 2013). Overall, this suggests that in addition to the training-related effect on improved anaerobic and aerobic properties, part of the training adaptation includes improved anabolic and reduced inflammatory response to exercise. Changes in anabolic-catabolic balance and inflammatory cytokines can be used by athletes and coaches to determine training intensity also in team sports like volleyball.

9.5 REFERENCES

Eliakim, A. and Nemet, D., 2008, Exercise provocation test for growth hormone secretion. *Pediatric Exercise Science*, **20**, pp. 370–378.

Eliakim, A. and Nemet, D., 2010, Exercise training, physical fitness and the growth hormone-insulin-like growth factor-I axis and cytokine balance. *Medicine and Sport Science*, **55**, pp. 128–140.

Eliakim, A., Portal, S., Zadik, Z., Meckel, Y. and Nemet, D., 2013, Training reduces catabolic and inflammatory response to a single practice in female volleyball players. *Journal of Strength Condition and Research*, In Press.

Eliakim, A., Portal, S., Zadik, Z., Rabinowitz, J., Adler-Portal, D., Cooper, D. M., Zaldivar, F. and Nemet, D., 2009, The effect of volleyball training on anabolic hormones and inflammatory markers in elite male and female adolescent players. *Journal of Strength and Conditioning Research*, **23**, pp. 1553–1559.

Nemet, D. and Eliakim, A., 2010, Growth hormone-insulin-like growth factor-I and inflammatory response to single exercise bout in children and adolescents. *Medicine and Sport Science*, **55**, pp. 141–155.

THERMOREGULATORY RESPONSES OF ARTISTIC GYMNAST YOUNG ATHLETES AND NON-ATHLETE GIRLS DURING EXERCISE IN HEAT

G.T. Leites[1,2], P.L. Sehl[1], G.S. Cunha[1,3], A. Detoni Filho[1], and F. Meyer [1]

[1]Federal University of Rio Grande do Sul, Brazil; [2]McMaster University, Canada; [3]Federal Institute of Education, Science and Technology Farroupilha, Brazil

10.1 INTRODUCTION

Artistic gymnast (AG) young athletes may restrict fluid intake during training and competitions as it is assumed that avoiding body mass increase helps performance. It is also unclear whether the intensive physical training of AG athletes since prepubescent years improves thermoregulatory responses to exercise. It is then possible that a persistent hypohydration state combined with physical adaptations make thermoregulatory responses of AG athletes different from those of non-athletic girls during a continuous exercise.   The purpose of this study was to compare rectal temperature (T_{re}), heart rate (HR) and sweating responses between AG young athletes and non-athlete girls during cycling at similar relative intensity both in a heat (HC) and in thermoneutral (TC) environment conditions.

10.2 METHODS

Fourteen prepubescent and heat-acclimatized girls participated in the study and they were either in the AG group (n=7) or in the non-athletic – but physically active – group (n=7). As inclusion criteria, the girls had not been diagnosed with any chronic disease. They were not using any medication that would affect their cardiovascular or thermoregulatory responses. This study was approved by the Research Ethics Committee of the Federal University of Rio Grande do Sul. The participants and their guardians were informed and freely signed consent forms.

10.2.1 Preliminary Session

Physical activity was assessed using the Physical Activity Questionnaire for Older Children (PAQ-C) (Crocker et al., 1997). Stage 1 of biological maturation was confirmed through observation of breast and pubic area (Tanner, 1962). Height and body mass were assessed and the body surface area (BSA) was determined using the Dubois and Dubois equation (Dubois and Dubois, 1916). To determine VO_2 peak, a gradual exercise test was conducted on a cycle ergometer (Ergo Fit 167, Toledo, Spain, 5–watt resolution) using the McMaster protocol and open circuit indirect calorimetry (O_2 and CO_2 analyzer Medgraphics CPX/D, breath by breath, Minnesota, USA). Body composition was obtained from Dual-energy X-ray absorptiometry (DXA).

10.2.2 Experimental Session

The experimental sessions occurred in the morning, and the girls ate a standardized breakfast. The experimental protocol was identical for the two sessions except for the environmental conditions (HC or TC) in which the order was randomized. Prior to exercise, body mass was measured, a HR monitor (Polar Electro Oy, S610, Finland) was put on and then a flexible rectal thermometer (Physitemp Instruments, Inc., Ret-1, Clifton, New Jersey, USA) was inserted 10–12 cm beyond the anal sphincter.

The girls cycled at a load (W) corresponding to ~55% of the VO_2 peak, at a cadence between 60 and 80 rpm, for 30 min in the heat (35oC and 40% RH) and in the thermoneutral (24°C and 50% RH) condition, inside an environmental chamber (Russells Technical Products, Holland). After 15 min of cycling, VO_2 was measured for 3 min to check exercise intensity. Tre and HR were measured every 5 min. Cycling was interrupted if two of the following events occurred simultaneously: Tre > 39°C, HR ≥ 200 bpm, symptoms of heat exhaustion (nausea, disorientation, headache, and dizziness), and inability to maintain a cycling frequency below 60 rpm.

During cycling, refrigerated water (~15°C) was available for consumption ad libitum. The bottle was weighed (Ohaus Compact Scale, CS2000, New Jersey, USA) before and after cycling to calculate volume intake. After the girls had urinated and dried out their bodies, body mass was measured to calculate sweat volume (Δ body mass before and after cycling corrected for water intake while exercising). The sweat volume was then divided by BSA.

10.2.3 Statistical Analysis

Data showed normal distribution and results were described as mean and SD. The ANOVA two-way test was used to compare the groups over time. For independent samples, Student's t-test was used for the intergroup comparisons; when interaction (group vs. time). The significance level adopted was 5%.

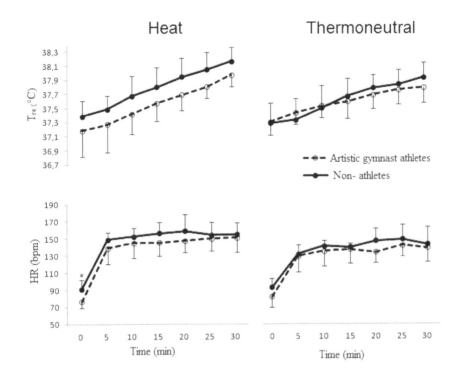

Figure 10.1 Rectal temperature (T_{re}) and heat rate (HR) during cycling in both environmental conditions (mean ± SD). $^*P<0.05$.

10.3 RESULTS

Artistic gymnast young athletes and non-athletic girls were similar in age (8.7±1.3 and 9.4±1.5 yrs-old, respectively), height (129.5±0.06 and 132.5±0.09 cm), body mass (24.5±4.3 and 26.5±5.1 kg), BSA (0.038±0.003 and 0.036±0.002 m2.kg-1) and free fat mass (20.2±3.0 and 20.1±3.1 kg). Body fat (%) was lower in AG athletes than non-athletic girls (13.3±4.3 and 20.3±3.7, P=0.01). According to PAC-C all girls are physically active (>3). Peak VO2 was similar between groups (47.5±7.5 and 46.8±10.1 mL.kg^{-1}.min^{-1}), as well HRmax (183±12 and 189±13 bpm) and maximal work rate (89.2±13.3 and 85.7±19.6 W). During cycling, VO2 as a % of their individual VO2 peak and the work load were similar between the athletes (546±2.1% and 35.0±3.5 W) and non-athletes (54.4±3.7% and 37.5±12.5 W) in the HC and in the TC (54.4±2.8% and 36.5±10.3 W for the athletes and 54.3±2.8% and 33.7±2.5 W and 54.9±3.5% and 36.6±10.0 W for the non-athletes girls), demonstrating that groups cycled at similar intensity relative to their VO2 peak.

Tre and HR responses by group and thermal environments are present in Figure 10.1. Tre was similar between athletes and non-athletes at each moment and the final Tre was 38.0°C±0.2 and 38.2±0.2°C in the heat, and 37.8±0.2°C and

37.9±0.2°C in thermoneutral environment. The magnitude of Tre increase was also similar between groups in both environmental conditions. Initial HR was lower in athletes (76±7 vs. 91±11 b, P=0.01), but, during cycling it became similar between groups in both environmental conditions.

Sweat volume (mL.m^{-2}) was similar between AG athletes and non-athletes (respectively, 144±107 and 190±134 in the HC and 234±210 and 166±182 in TC). Water intake was also similar between athletes and non-athletes (64±87 and 117±61 mL in HC, and 54±109 and 47±44 mL in TC), resulting therefore in similar body water balance (-81±71 and 77±107 mL in HC, and -161±219 and -130±228 mL). Dehydration was lower than 1% in both groups and conditions.

10.4 CONCLUSION

In the present study, prepubescent AG athletes showed similar T_{re} and sweating responses compared to physically active girls during continuous cycling at similar intensity either in the heat and thermoneutral conditions.

10.5 REFERENCES

Crocker, P.R., Bailey, D.A., Faulkner, R.A., Kowalski, K.C. and McGrath, R., 1997, Measuring general levels of physical activity: Preliminary evidence for the Physical Activity Questionnaire for Older Children. *Medicine and Science in Sports and Exercise*, **29**, pp. 1344–1349.

Dubois, D. and Dubois, E.F., 1916, Clinical calorimetry: a formula to estimate the approximate surface area if height and weight be known. *Archives of Internal Medicine*, **17**, pp. 863–871.

Tanner, J.M., 1962, *Growth at Adolescence*, 2nd ed., (Oxford: Blackwell Scientific Publication), pp.19–25.

CHAPTER NUMBER 11

LIPID PROFILE AND PRESENCE OF DYSLIPIDAEMIA IN PHYSICALLY ACTIVE AND INSUFFICIENTLY ACTIVE BRAZILIAN ADOLESCENTS

C.M. Tomeleri[1], D.P. Silva[1], M.S. Carnelossi[1], D. Venturini[1], A.M. Okino[1], D. S. Barbosa[1], J.A. Oliveira[1], E.R.V. Ronque[1], and E.S. Cyrino[1]

[1]Londrina State University, Brazil; Support: CNPq and CAPES.

11.1 INTRODUCTION

In recent decades, atherosclerotic disease (AD) has been among the leading causes of morbidity and mortality worldwide, and given its multifactorial trait, both its progression and severity is closely related to the presence and duration of a series of attributes called risk factors (Berenson *et al.*, 1998; Gerber and Zielinsky, 1997). With the exception of age, the dyslipidaemia characterized by a condition in which there is an abnormal lipid or lipoprotein concentration in the blood, is the most important risk factor for the development of atherosclerosis (Rabelo, 2001). It should be noted, however, that similar to other risk factors, the dyslipidaemia is often behavioural and therefore may be influenced the lifestyle adopted. Accordingly, the presence or absence of dyslipidaemia may be related to levels of physical activity (Kones, 2011). From this perspective, the objective of this study was to evaluate whether changes in lipid profiles differ between adolescents classified as physically active or insufficiently active.

11.2 METHOD

This study was approved by the local ethical committees and was a school based study, in which the sample was composed of adolescents (11–17 years-old) of both genders from Londrina, Brazil. Initially, 1,396 adolescents of both genders agreed to participate and returned the completed, signed consent form. However, 382 boys and girls were later excluded (e.g. absence from the fasting blood sample measurement; lack of 10–12 hours of fasting; absence on the day of the questionnaire). Therefore, after the field work, 1,014 adolescents (Boys: 42.2% and girls: 57.8%) composed the sample.

Physical activity (PA) was measured using the Baecke questionnaire (Baecke *et al.*, 1982), which has been validated for use with Brazilian adolescents (Guedes *et al.*, 2006). The questionnaire is related to sports activity during leisure time and considers physically active, young people to be those who reported more than 240 min / week (> 4 h / wk) of moderate or vigorous-intensity physical activity during the last 4 months. Biochemical parameters, including serum triglycerides (TG), total cholesterol (TC), high-density lipoprotein cholesterol (HDL-C), low-density lipoprotein cholesterol (LDL-C) were obtained after fasting for 10–12 hours, by a specialized laboratory at the University site following standard procedures. Lipid profile was examined using the cutoffs specific for adolescents identified by de Back *et al.* (2005) (i.e. TC ≥170 mg/dL, LDL ≥130 mg/dL, HDL<45 mg/dL and triglycerides ≥130 mg/dL).

For the general characteristics of the sample, descriptive statistics were used and data presented as means and standard deviations. Categorical data were presented as percentages and the Chi-square test was used to compare active and insufficiently active groups. In all analyses, SPSS version 17.0 was used with a significance level of 5%.

11.3 RESULTS

The general characteristics of the adolescents are presented in Table 11.1. There were differences between the sexes for the variables of height and age, with higher values for boys compared with girls (P <0.05). The only difference in mean lipid levels was in TG concentrations between the sexes, where values were approximately 13% higher for girls compared with boys (P <0.05). Between the active and insufficiently active groups, there was only a difference in mean HDL-C in boys. As for lipid abnormalities, as presented in Figure 11.1, the dyslipidaemia characterized by low HDL-C was different in the male active and insufficiently active groups. However, for girls differences were not observed for any of the lipid changes.

11.4 CONCLUSION

The results of this study suggest that lipid abnormalities do not differ between active and insufficiently active girls. However, differences in mean HDL cholesterol and the prevalence of this dyslipidaemia were observed between active and insufficiently active boys.

Table 11.1 General characteristics of the Brazilian adolescents, according to sex and physical activity.

	Boys			Girls		
	Active (*n*= 114)	Ins. Active (*n*= 314)	Total (*n*= 428)	Active (*n*= 71)	Ins. Active (*n*= 515)	Total (*n*= 586)
Age, y	13.1 ± 1.6	13.1 ± 1.4	13.1 ± 1.4	13.1 ± 1.6	12.8 ± 1.4	12.8 ±1.4 [a]
Weight, kg	48.7 ± 12.0	49.1 ± 14.5	48.7± 1.4	48.7 ±12.8	47.3 ±11.7	47.5 ±11.8
Height (m)	1.5 ± 0.1	1.5 ± 0.1	1.5 ± 0.1	1.5 ± 0.1	1.53 ± 0.1	1.5 ± 0.1 [a]
BMI, kg/m^2	19.8 ± 3.8	19.8 ± 4.0	19.8 ± 3.9	20.2 ± 4.5	19.8 ± 4.0	19.9 ± 4.1
TC, mg/dL	163.6±28.3	162.7±27.5	163.0 ±27.7	165.1±26.4	164.5±27.9	164.6±27.7
LDL, mg/dL	97.8±24.9	99.4±24.2	99.0±24.4	99.3±22.3	99.0±25.4	99.0±25.0
HDL, mg/dL	53.7 ± 13.2	50.8 ±14.3 [b]	51.6 ± 14.0	52.4± 10.8	52.2±12.7	52.2±12.5
TG, mg/dL	60.3±34.4	61.8±33.2	61.4±33.5	67.2±31.4	66.0±34.9	66.1±34.5 [a]

Note: mean ± standard deviation; [a] significance differences between sexes; [b] significance differences between groups active and insufficiently active (Ins. Active); BMI= body mass index; TC=total cholesterol; LDL=low density lipoprotein; HDL=high density lipoprotein; TG = triglycerides.

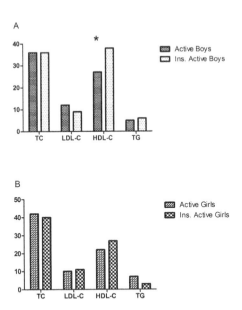

Figure 11.1 A = boys; B = Girls. Presence of dyslipidaemia between groups active and insufficiently active (Ins. Active). * Significance differences between groups active and ins. active.

11.5 REFERENCES

Baecke J.A.A., Burema J. and Frijters J.E.R., 1982, A short questionnaire for the measurement of habitual physical activity in epidemiological studies. *The American Journal of Clinical Nutrition*, **36**, pp. 936–942.

Berenson G.S., Srinivasan S.R., Bao W., Newman W.P., Tracy R.E. and Wattigney W.A., 1998, Association between multiple cardiovascular risk factors and atherosclerosis in children and young adults. The Bogalusa Heart Study. *The New England Journal of Medicine*, **338,** pp. 1650–1656.

de Back Giuliano I.C., Caramelli B., Pellanda L., Duncan L., Mattos S. and Fonseca F.H., 2005, Brazilian Society of Cardiology., I GUIDELINE OF PREVENTION OF ATHEROSCLEROSIS IN CHILDHOOD AND ADOLESCENCE. *Arquivos Brasileiros de Cardiologia,* **85.** PP. S4–36.

Gerber Z.R.S. and Zielinsky P., 1997, Risk factors of atherosclerosis in children. An epidemiologic study. *Arquivos Brasileiros de Cardiologia*, **69**, pp. 231–236.

Guedes D., Lopes C., Guedes J. and Stanganelli L., 2006, Reproducibility and validity of the Baecke questionnaire for assessing of the habitual physical activity in adolescents. *Revista Portuguesa de Ciências do Desporto,* **6**, pp. 265–274.

Kones R., 2011, Primary prevention of coronary heart disease: integration of new data, evolving views, revised goals, and role of rosuvastatin in management. A comprehensive survey. *Drug Design, Development and Therapy*, **5**, pp. 325–380.

Rabelo L.M., 2001, Atherosclerotic risk factors in adolescence. *Jornal de Pediatria,* **77**, pp.153–164.

BONE ULTRASOUND ATTENUATION OF CHILDREN WITH DOWN SYNDROME: RELATIONS WITH STATIC STABILOMETRIC CHARACTERISTICS

B. Ferry[1,4], M. Gavris[1,3], S. Serbanoiu[2], I. Hantiu[3], C. Tifrea[2] and D. Courteix[1]

[1]Clermont Université, Université Blaise Pascal, EA 3533, Laboratoire des Adaptations Métaboliques à l'Exercice en Conditions Physiologiques et Pathologiques, Clermont-Ferrand, France ; [2]Centre de Recherche Interdisciplinaire "Dr. Alexandru Partheniu", UNEFS Bucarest, Romania ; [3]Research Center on Human Performance, Oradea University, Romania; [4]Université Limoges, Faculté des Sciences et Techniques, STAPS, Limoges, France

12.1 INTRODUCTION

Down syndrome (DS), the most common genetic cause of developmental disability, is characterized by intellectual disability and musculoskeletal disorders (Sago *et al.*, 2000). Clinically, children with DS are described as having low tone which may affect muscle strength and motor skills. Many studies show that individuals with DS, particularly the males, have lower than normal bone mineral density (Angelopoulou *et al.*, 1999; Sepulveda *et al.*, 1995). It may be a cause of early onset osteoporosis. The significant increase in the life expectancy of individuals with Down syndrome (Englund *et al.*, 2013) could increase the prevalence of this disease. The amount of bone mass in adolescence is a key determinant of the amount of bone mass in adulthood. The ultimate target population for osteoporosis prophylaxis may indeed be the young, rather than the elderly. The clinical assessment of osteoporosis relies mainly on bone mineral density (BMD) measurements using dual-energy X-ray absorptiometry (DXA). DXA does not provide any information on bone structure and matrix factors. QUS variables, in addition to bone density (Brunader and Shelton, 2002), measure some characteristics of bone quality such as micro architecture, elasticity and density (Njeh *et al.*, 1997). The link existing between muscle and bone ("functional muscle-bone unit") is well described today (Schoenau and Fricke, 2006). The key idea is the analysis of bone parameters under consideration of muscle function. The muscle contraction places the greatest physiological load on bone, and so the strength of bone must adapt to muscle strength (Schoenau, 2006). It can be argued that a deficit of muscle contraction represents the major cause of bone weakness (secondary bone disease). Therefore, if muscle hypotonia is reported in subjects with Down syndrome, a resulting osteopenia would be observed. The purpose of this study was to assess the bone status of children with DS as well as their body stability as surrogate of muscle tonicity.

12.2 METHOD

A group of 89 children with Down syndrome (DS: 47 males, 42 females) aged between 7 and 19 years participated in this study. A sample of 97 healthy subjects (CTL: 46 males, 51 females) aged between 10 and 19 years, served as controls. Measurements were performed with support of the Special Olympics organization and the French Federation of Adapted Sport; they were conducted with the same ambulatory devices in France and Romania. The study was approved by Bucharest University (UNEFS) ethical committee and the medical department of Adapted Sport Federation in France. Parents and children were informed about the objectives and procedures. Written informed consent was obtained from all parents or subjects.

12.2.1 Bone Measurements

Ultrasound bone attenuation (BUA, dB/MHz) and speed of sound (SOS, m/s) were measured using an Achilles Insight device. The intra-operator coefficient of variation (CV) for BUA and SOS were 1.6% and 0.4% respectively. To verify the meaning of QUS data obtained at the calcaneus, we measured lumbar spine and hip bone mineral densities by DXA and bone QUS data in a sample of 70 healthy and osteoporotic subjects.

12.2.2 Stabilometric Measures

The measures were obtained by means of a 3-strain gauge platform with automatic weight correction (Stabilotest, PostureWin-Platform V328). The following parameters were used to assess the balance: the postural sway area (*Area*, mm^2), the Centre of Pressure's (CoP) total path length over the time (*Length*, mm), the variance of velocity (*VFY*), the average sway velocity (*aV*) and the CoP's total path length per unit surface (*LFS*). The measures were established at 51.2 s in standard conditions (eyes open only).

12.2.3 Statistical Analyses

Because all data did not respect the Gaussian distribution, non parametric tests were used and for a complex statistical analysis, the data were log-transformed. Pearson two-tailed correlations were performed to test the relationships between BMDs values and QUS data. Intra group differences were tested between the age groups using a non parametric Mann-Whitney *U* test. In order to assess the potential relationships between ultrasound measures, age and stabilometric performances, either Pearson or Spearman two-tailed correlations were calculated. Regressions were made between age and QUS or stabilometric data.

12.3 RESULTS

CTL total group and DS total group were similar in age and weight. Subjects with DS were smaller and had higher BMI than CTL group ($p<0.001$). When compared to CTL, subjects with DS had lower BUA (-4%) but similar SOS values. There was a positive correlation between age and BUA for the two groups, the regression slope of DS being significantly lower than that of CTL ($p<.001$). Whatever the over parameters (SOS and stabilometric values), there was no evolution with age in DS whereas there was a positive correlation between age and SOS, a negative one between age and all stabilometric parameters. The stabilometric parameters (Area, Length and LFS) were higher for DS than for CTL.

12.4 DISCUSSION AND CONCLUSION

The present results point out the significantly lower BUA values observed in children with Down syndrome. These values are associated to significant poorer stabilometric values. The fact that the speed of sound failed to differ between groups may be due to the age range of this population. The literature (Alwis *et al.*, 2010) suggested that the precision of QUS measurements is a function of age, especially in younger children (6 to 12 years in their study). Considering the link between BUA and BMD (Cortet *et al.*, 2004) and in accordance with previous studies (Sepulveda *et al.*, 1995), it can be suggested that individuals with Down syndrome had lower BMD than the controls. The less marked increase with age in BUA for the DS group reflects a disorder of bone maturation in this group.

According to the concept of "functional muscle-bone unit"(Frost and Schonau, 2000), bone mass and bone geometry are influenced by growth and muscle development in children and adolescents. Hypotonia reported in these subjects can result in reduced bone mass and alteration of bone matrix. The techniques commonly used to assess the muscle tone are highly subjective and give limited information about the state of the neuromuscular system. We chose to use stabilometric parameters as indexes of muscular tonicity because this device provides objective measures of body stability and tonicity. What is remarkable is that for all parameters the values expressed by the children with Down syndrome were unaffected by age. Stabilometric performances displayed by the controls were higher and showed an improvement of stability and tonicity with age. These improvements correlated negatively with age, suggesting that the lower the values, the higher the performances.

VFY, a parameter usually associated with a hyper- or hypo- muscle tone of the posterior chain (Vallier, 1985) was not correlated with BUA. If stabilometry is a method widely used by clinicians for measuring the balance and postural tonicity, it remains debatable as regards its relevance for measuring muscle tone.

In conclusion, the present results point out the bone parameter degradation observed in individuals with Down syndrome suggesting the need of a precocious monitoring of their bone status. Stabilometric performance does not appear to change with age for DS when they are improving for CTL. Such results support the fact that a postural practice could be proposed at the earliest age in DS population.

12.5 REFERENCES

Alwis, G., Rosengren, B., Nilsson, J.A., Stenevi-Lundgren, S., Sundberg, M., Sernbo, I., and Karlsson, M.K. 2010. Normative calcaneal quantitative ultrasound data as an estimation of skeletal development in Swedish children and adolescents. *Calcified Tissue International*, **87**, pp. 493–506.

Angelopoulou, N., Souftas, V., Sakadamis, A., and Mandroukas, K. 1999. Bone mineral density in adults with Down's syndrome. *European Radiology*, **9**, pp. 648–651.

Brunader, R., and Shelton, D.K. 2002. Radiologic bone assessment in the evaluation of osteoporosis. *American Family Physician*, **65**, pp.1357-1364.

Cortet, B., Boutry, N., Dubois, P., Legroux-Gerot, I., Cotten, A., and Marchandise, X. 2004. Does quantitative ultrasound of bone reflect more bone mineral density than bone microarchitecture? *Calcified Tissue International*, **74**, pp. 60–67.

Englund, A., Jonsson, B., Zander, C. S., Gustafsson, J., and Anneren, G. 2013. Changes in mortality and causes of death in the Swedish Down syndrome population. *American Journal of Medical Genetics* A, **161**, pp. 642–649.

Frost, H. M., and Schonau, E. 2000. The "muscle-bone unit" in children and adolescents: a 2000 overview. *Journal of Pediatric Endocrinology and Metabolism*, **13**, pp. 571–590.

Njeh, C. F., Boivin, C. M., and Langton, C. M. 1997. The role of ultrasound in the assessment of osteoporosis: a review. *Osteoporosis International*, **7**, pp. 7-22.

Sago, H., Carlson, E.J., Smith, D.J., Rubin, E.M., Crnic, L.S., Huang, T.T., and Epstein, C.J. 2000. Genetic dissection of region associated with behavioral abnormalities in mouse models for Down syndrome. *Pediatric Research*, **48**, pp. 606–613.

Schoenau, E. 2006. Bone mass increase in puberty: what makes it happen? *Hormone Research*, **65**, pp. 2–10.

Schoenau, E., and Fricke, O. 2006. Interaction between muscle and bone. *Hormone Research*, **66**, pp. 73–78.

Sepulveda, D., Allison, D.B., Gomez, J.E., Kreibich, K., Brown, R.A., Pierson, R.N., Jr., and Heymsfield, S.B. 1995. Low spinal and pelvic bone mineral density among individuals with Down syndrome. *American Journal Mental Retardation*, **100**, pp. 109–114.

Vallier, G. 1985. Corrélations stabilométriques et cliniques chez 60 adultes présentant un syndrome de déficience posturale. In Masson (Ed.), *Entrées du système postural fin*. Premières journée de posturologie clinique, directed by Gagey P.M. and Weber B. pp. 123–130.

Part IV

Neuromuscular Issues

ISOKINETIC STRENGTH OF LOWER LIMBS AND ITS DIFFERENCES DEPENDING ON GENDER, MUSCLE GROUP AND ANGULAR VELOCITY IN CHILDREN

M. Tomáš, Z. František, M. Lucia, and T. Jaroslav
Charles University, FPES, Czech Republic
[Project was supported by GACR P407/11/P784 and MSM 0021620864.]

13.1 INTRODUCTION

Strength is an important component of fitness in health and disease, because weak muscles may markedly limit a person's physical fitness and daily physical abilities. To assess muscle strength in youths, tests such as sit ups, number of push ups, curls, standing long jump, etc., are often used in practice. These tests require multijoint movements and therefore they do not evaluate strength of the isolated muscle group. Testing of isokinetic strength provides an objective approach in diagnostics and simpler quantification of muscular strength in children. Nevertheless, in this field there are many gaps dealing with its manifestation among youths (Degache *et al.*, 2010, Jones and Stratton, 2000). The goal of this study was to identify muscle strength of knee extensors (KE) and flexors (KF) in non-sporting primary school population and compare results in terms of intersexual differences, muscle group and speed of muscle contraction.

13.2 METHODS

The monitoring was carried out with 57 13 years old children not participating in regular sport activity (Boys: n = 31, height = 158.5±8.0 cm, weight = 53.0±12.6 kg, Girls: n=26, height = 158.6±6.3 cm, weight = 50.7±11.5 kg.

Maximum peak muscle torque (PT) of KE and KF with preferred leg during concentric contraction in angular velocities (60, 120, 180, 240 and $300° \cdot s^{-1}$) were assessed by Cybex dynamometer (Cybex NORM ®, Humac, CA, USA). All tested subjects completed a short warm-up (4 min of jogging and dynamic half squats (2 sets@15 repetitions). The testing protocol consisted of 3 maximum attempts.

Three way ANOVA (2x2x5) was used for assessment of the effect of independent variables [Gender (Boys, Girls), Muscle group (knee extensors, flexors), Angular velocity $(60–300°·s^{-1})$] and their interaction. Effect size coefficient was assessed using partial coefficient "Eta square" – η_p^2). Multiple comparisons of means were carried out using Bonferroni's *post-hoc* test.

13.3 RESULTS

Gender did not influence the PT of thigh muscles (p>0.05, $\eta_p^2 = 0.002$). At the lowest velocity boys achieved 1.56 ± 0.71 N·m·kg^{-1} and girls 1.70 ± 0.70 N·m·kg^{-1}. This difference of 8.2% was not significant ($t_{112} = 1.04$, p>0.05). On the contrary, at the highest velocity boys achieved 0.86 ± 0.41 N·m·kg^{-1} in comparison to girls 0.80 ± 0.40 N·m·kg^{-1}. This difference was not significant ($t_{112} = 0.79$, p>0.05). KE produced significantly higher PT in comparison to KF (p<0.01, $\eta_p^2 = 0.644$). At the lowest velocity, boys produced lower PT than girls (B: 2.13 ± 0.48 N·m·kg^{-1}; G: 2.31 ± 0.42 N·m·kg^{-1}). On the other hand, at the highest velocity, boys achieved better performance than girls by 5.1% (B: 1.17 ± 0.29 N·m·kg^{-1}; G: 1.11 ± 0.26 N·m·kg^{-1}) (Figure 13.1). At the lowest velocity boys produced lower strength of KF (0.99 ± 0.36 N·m·kg^{-1}) in comparison to girls (1.09 ± 0.24 N·m·kg^{-1}). At the velocity of $120°·s^{-1}$, both groups achieved the same performance (0.89 N·m·kg^{-1}) and from $180°.s^{-1}$ boys produced higher PT. At the velocity of $300°·s^{-1}$, boys achieved better performance than girls by 12.5%. Angular velocity significantly affected PT (p<0.01, $\eta_p^2 = 0.452$). *Post-hoc* tests revealed that after each increase of angular velocity significant decrease PT (p<0.01). Interactions of the monitored variables are presented in Table 13.1.

Table 13.1 Effect of independent variables on the examined dependent variable.

Independent variable	Type III Sum of Squares	df	Mean Square	F	Sig.	Partial Eta Squared
G	0.09	1	0.09	0.86	0.353	0.002
MG	99.06	1	99.06	993.79	0.000	0.644
AV	45.15	4	11.29	113.23	0.000	0.452
G * MG	0.11	1	0.11	1.09	0.296	0.002
G * AV	0.61	4	0.15	1.53	0.191	0.011
MG * AV	5.88	4	1.47	14.75	0.000	0.097
G * MG *A V	0,02	4	0.00	0.05	0.995	0.000
Error	54.83	550	0.10			
Total	1005.84	570				

Legend: G – Gender, MG – Muscle Group, AV – Angular Velocity.

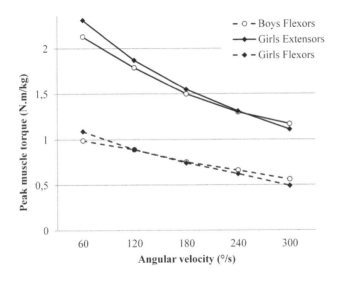

Figure 13.1 Comparison of peak torque of knee extensors and flexors in observed children.

13.4 DISCUSSION

Gender had no effect on the strength of KE and KF at any of velocity. The results are in line with results of study by De Ste Croix et al. (2002) who tested 10–14 year old children and present insignificant differences of PT in terms of gender. Lungren et al. (2011) reported insignificant differences of PT in a 12 year old population. These results can be caused by the fact that peak strength velocity occurs about a year after peak height velocity (11.4–12.2 years in girls and 13.4–14.4 years in boys). Therefore, 13–14 year old girls are more likely to be in phase of peak strength gains while the boys are likely to be still in peak height velocity phase (De Ste Croix et al., 1999). Muscle strength of KE and KF increases between 11th and 15th year in boys up to 50%. The most progressive increase occurs between 12th and 14th year (Degache et al., 2010). Development of muscle strength in youths depends on factors such as age, anthropometric parameters (body height, body weight) and sexual maturation (Beunen and Malina, 1988). Our results are inconsistent with the study by Deighan et al. (2009), who observed significant differences of PT from the perspective of gender in a 13 year old Chinese population. Degache et al., (2010) published with 13 year old sporting children the PT of KE 156.9 ± 31.6 N·m at $60°·s^{-1}$ and 110.59 ± 23.8 N·m at $180°·s^{-1}$. Concerning KF, they presented PT at the lowest velocity 97.5 ± 21.5 N.m and 87.9 ± 22.2 N·m in higher velocity. When compared to our study, non-sporting subjects produced lower PT at the lowest velocity by 27.8 % (113.3 ± 28.8 N·m) and at the higher velocity by 27.9 % (79.7 ± 19.6 N·m). Even greater differences were found in comparison of PT in KF when at lower velocity the sporting participants achieved higher PT by 46.0 % (52.6 ± 20.1 N·m) and at higher velocity by 55.6 % (39 ± 17.5 N·m). The above results show a positive effect of sport activity on the level of PT. We confirmed a significant decrease of PT for KE and KF occurred with increasing velocity (Maly et al., 2011).

13.5 CONCLUSION

The study did not show significant differences in the level of PT in KE and KF between boys and girls in a 13 year old non-sporting population normalized to participant's body weight. Girls achieved higher values of PT at lower velocities while boys at higher velocities. Speed of muscle contraction had a significant effect on the level of strength. Based on comparison of the results with available literature, a significant difference appears to be in the level of PT between physically active and inactive population. The definition of standards for assessment of strength of specific muscle groups for physically active and inactive population appears to be necessary.

13.6 REFERENCES

Beunen, G. and Malina, R.M., 1988, Growth and physical performance relative to timing of the adolescent spurt. *Exercise and Sports Sciences Reviews,* **16**, pp. 503–540.

Degache, F., Richard, R., Edouard, P., Oullion, R. and Calmels, P., 2010, The relationship between muscle strength and physiological age: A cross-sectional study in boys aged from 11 to 15. *Annals of Physical and Rehabilitation Medicine*, **53**, pp. 180–188.

Deighan, M.A., Nevill, A.M., Mafulli, N., Cheng, J.C. and Gleeson, N., 2009, Evaluation of knee peak torque in athletic and sedentary children. *Acta Orthopaedica et Traumatologica Turcica*, **43**, pp.484–490.

De Ste Croix, M.B.A., Armstrong, N. and Welsman, J.R., 1999, Concentric isokinetic leg strength in pre-teen, teenage and adult males and females. *Biology of Sport*, **16**, pp. 75–86.

De Ste Croix, M.B.A., Armstrong, N., Welsman, J.R. and Sharpe, P., 2002, Longitudinal changes in isokinetic leg strength in 10–14 year olds. *Annals of Human Biology*, **29**, pp. 50–62.

Jones, M.A. and Stratton, G., 2000, Muscle function assessment in children. *Acta Paediatrica*, 2000, **89**, pp. 753–761.

Lundgren, S., Nilsson, J.A., Ringsberg, K.A.M. and Karlsson, M.K., 2011, Normative data for test of neuromuscular performance and DXA-derived lean body mass and fat mass in pre-pubertal children. *Acta Paediatrica*, **100**, pp. 1359–1367.

Maly, T., Zahalka, F. and Mala, L., 2011, Differences between isokinetic strength characteristics of more and less successful professional soccer teams. *Journal of Physical Education and Sport,* **11**, pp. 306–312.

VOLUNTARY ACTIVATION OF THE ADDUCTOR POLLICIS IN CHILDREN: A PERIPHERAL MAGNETIC STIMULATION STUDY

V. Martin[1], V. Kluka[1], S. Garcia Vicencio[1], F. Maso[2], and S. Ratel[1]

[1]Université Blaise Pascal, France; [2] Centre de formation, ASM Rugby, France

14.1 INTRODUCTION

Although it is self-evident that young children produce less strength than adults during maximal voluntary contractions (MVC), it still remains unclear whether or not these differences persist when strength is normalized to dimensional changes throughout growth, *i.e.* whether there are significant differences in strength relative to muscle size between children and adults. More specifically, it remains to be elucidated whether age-related changes in absolute strength are simply due to the increase in muscle size or whether they can also be ascribed to differential qualitative factors (Bouchant *et al.,* 2011).

Among these qualitative factors, nervous factors have been frequently put forward. For instance, some studies suggest that children are not able to fully activate their motor units during MVC. However, few authors have conducted direct measurements of motor unit activation and consequently, no consensus has been reached regarding the voluntary activation (VA) capacities of children. Whilst Belanger and McComas (1989) found no difference in VA levels of the triceps surae between pre- and post-pubertal children, as estimated using the twitch interpolation technique, others reported lower activation scores on the triceps surae and knee extensors in pre-pubertal children when compared to their post-pubertal counterparts (Blimkie, 1989) and adults (Grosset *et al.,* 2008; O'Brien *et al.,* 2010). Such discrepancy may be partly ascribed to the confounding influence of the level of physical activity on VA levels, as this variable is highly sensitive to physical training.

Therefore, the purpose of this study was to compare, between children and adults, the VA of a hand muscle, the adductor pollicis, that is not influenced by the level of physical activity.

14.2 METHODS

Thirteen boys (age: 11.1 ± 0.3 yr) and eight adult men (age: 22.5 ± 2.2 yr) were involved in this study. None of the volunteers had any orthopaedic condition, or metallic prostheses that precluded involvement in the study. Written informed consent was obtained from the participants and/or their guardians. The local ethics committee approved the protocol.

After a 10-min passive warming-up under a heating lamp, the adductor pollicis muscle function was measured using single peripheral magnetic stimulations and isometric MVCs.

To isolate the contribution of the adductor pollicis, the hand and the wrist were placed in a supinated position and restrained with a plastic cast and Velcro straps. The force produced by the adductor pollicis muscle was measured with a strain gauge, connected to a metal ring, placed at the level of the interphalangeal joint of the thumb. The thumb was abducted and its metacarpophalangeal and interphalangeal joints fully extended.

Three to five MVC trials were performed until reproducible results were obtained. During MVCs, subjects were requested to produce a maximal effort, maintained for 3 seconds. Single stimulations were delivered through a 43-mm figure-of-height coil (1.6 T), connected to a magnetic stimulator (Magstim 200^2, UK), and positioned over the ulnar nerve, close to the ulnar styloid. These stimulations were delivered during (superimposed twitch) and 3s after the MVC (potentiated twitch, Pt), according to the twitch interpolation technique, to calculate VA. The best trial was retained for further analysis. Data were compared between children and adults with the student t-test for independent samples. The significance level was set at $P<0.05$.

14.3 RESULTS

As expected, the maximal voluntary isometric force of the adductor pollicis muscle was significantly lower in children as compared to their adult counterparts (66.8 ± 22.3 vs. 103.2 ± 15.9 N respectively; $P < 0.001$; Figure 14.1). Pt was also significantly lower in children (6.0 ± 3.1 vs. 10.4 ± 3.1 N; $P < 0.01$). Finally, the twitch interpolation technique revealed that the VA of the adductor pollicis was significantly lower in children than in adults (85.0 ± 9.9 vs. 94.8 ± 3.8 % respectively; $P < 0.05$; Figure 14.2).

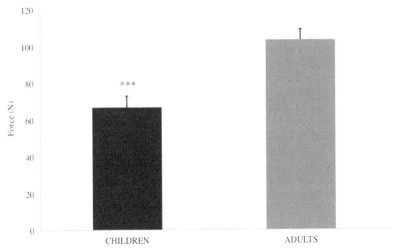

Figure 14.1 MVC force of the adductor pollicis in children and adults. Data are mean ± SE. Significantly different from adults: ***: P < 0.001.

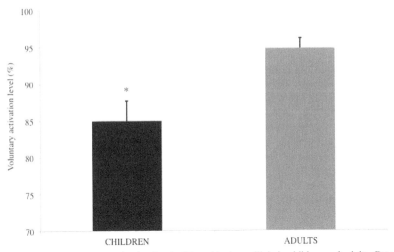

Figure 14.2 Voluntary activation level of the adductor pollicis in children and adults. Data are mean ± SE. Significantly different from adults: *: P < 0.05.

14.4 DISCUSSION

The results show that boys have a reduced ability to activate their adductor pollicis, as compared to adult men. This may partly explain the difference of MVC observed between children and adults, the other part being attributable to differences in muscle size and contractile properties, as suggested by the lower twitch amplitude in children.

Our voluntary activation results are consistent with other studies conducted on the triceps surae (Grosset *et al.*, 2008) and the knee extensor muscles (O'Brien *et al.*, 2010), showing a reduced VA in children as compared to adults. Interestingly, there was a 10% difference in VA values between children and adults, as previously reported by O'Brien *et al.* (2010).

The underlying factors of this reduced voluntary activation in children remain to be identified. O'Brien *et al.* (2012) suggested that children may have a reduced ability to fully recruit their motor units spatially and/or temporally due to the particular excitability of motoneurons. Grosset *et al.* (2007) did observe reduced stretch and T-reflexes in children but these results were mainly attributable to the reduced muscle-tendon stiffness in children. Accordingly, the H-reflex was not different from adults in this study. Alternatively, O'Brien *et al.* (2012) suggested that children may not have established the full motor pathways required to drive motor neurons to their maximal capacity. However, studies are lacking to support this hypothesis.

To conclude, this study has demonstrated a reduced ability of children to voluntarily activate their muscles. The application of magnetic stimulation over the peripheral nerves was well tolerated by the children. Indeed, this technique is not painful, contrary to electrical stimulation. The validity of this technique being established, this opens new perspectives for the evaluation of the development of neuromuscular function during growth.

14.5 REFERENCES

Belanger A.Y. and McComas A.J., 1989, Contractile properties of human skeletal muscle in childhood and adolescence. *European Journal of Applied Physiology and Occupational Physiology*, **58**, pp. 563–567.

Blimkie C.J., 1989, Age- and sex-associated variations in strength duing childhood: anthopometric, morphologic, neurologic, biomechanic, endocrinologic, genetic and physcial activity correlates. In *Perspectives In Exercise Science And Sport Medicine: Youth, Exercise And Sport*, edited by Gisolfi C.V. and Lamb D.R. (Indianapolis: Benchmark Press), pp. 99–163.

Bouchant A., Martin V., Maffiuletti N.A. and Ratel S., 2011, Can muscle size fully account for strength differences between children and adults? *Journal of Applied Physiology*, **110**, pp. 1748–1749.

Grosset J.F., Mora I., Lambertz D. and Perot C., 2008, Voluntary activation of the triceps surae in prepubertal children. *Journal of Electromyography and Kinesiology*, **18**, pp. 455–465.

Grosset J.F., Mora I., Lambertz D. and Perot C., 2007, Changes in stretch reflexes and muscle stiffness with age in prepubescent children. *Journal of Applied Physiology*, **102**, pp. 2352–2260.

O'Brien T.D., Reeves N.D,. Baltzopoulos V., Jones D.A. and Maganaris C.N., 2010, In vivo measurements of muscle specific tension in adults and children. *Exprimental Physiology*, **95**, pp. 202–210.

O'Brien T.D., Reeves N.D,. Baltzopoulos V., Jones D.A. and Maganaris C.N., 2012, Commentary on child-adult differences in muscle activation—a review. *Pediatric Exercise Science*, **24**, pp. 22–25.

CHANGES OF POSTURAL STABILITY WITH REGARD TO GENDER, AGE AND VISUAL CONTROL OF CHILDREN

Z. František, M. Tomáš, M. Lucia, and G. Tomáš
Charles University, FPES, Czech Republic
MSM 0021620864 and GACR P407/11/P784

15.1 INTRODUCTION

The aim of this study is to describe postural parameters and their changes with regard to age in the standing position with open and closed eyes and to describe differences between boys and girls of young school age. This study is focused on a group of children aged 7 – 11 years who are expected to manifest major changes in the parameters of postural stability. School age is a very important period for postural stability changes (Westcott *et al.*, 1997) and significant changes of postural stability parameters in this period have been described (Nolan *et al.* 2005). Orientation in space and a sense of balance are provided by interaction between the vestibular and sensory systems, vision and proprioception, especially (Shumway-Cook and Woollacott, 2001). Between the seventh and tenth year, postural control and balance are becoming similar to that in adults and children in this period are gradually shifting to a more accurate balance control strategy (Westcott *et al.*, 1997).There are several methods to evaluate postural stability by means of movement analysis of the centre of pressure (COP) by a foot in a standing position (Doyle *et al.*, 2007). Commonly used COP parameters in postural control studies are deviations in left right directions, Total Travelled Way (TTW) and standard deviation (SD) of velocity (Hadian *et al.*, 2008).

15.2 METHODS

The group of participants consisted of 210 children aged 7–11 years (age=9.4 ± 1.6 year, height= 139.1 ± 15.2 cm, weight=36.3 ± 9.2 kg). There were 105 girls and 105 boys (40 7-year-olds, 44 8-year-olds, 42 9-year-olds, 42 10-year-olds, 42 11-year-olds). There were the same number of boys and girls in every age group. All children in this study were healthy and had written parental consent. For measurement of postural stability we used FootScan device (RScan, Belguim). For measurements, we used standard tests (Kapteyn *et al.*, 1983) with time length of 30 s with sampling frequency 33 Hz. Evaluated parameters of COP included values of right left and front back displacements, velocity calculated as the change in position of COP with regard to scanning frequency and total trajectory of COP during the measurement (Total Traveled Way – TTW) (Palmier *et al.*, 2001). Monitored parameters of postural stability as a dependent variable were calculated using one way variance (Univariate ANOVA). Independent variables effect (age, gender, visual control) and interaction effect were evaluated by statistical significance (F-test) and by Effect size coefficient (partial coefficient "Eta square" - η_p^2). Multiple Comparison Procedure of monitored groups was realized by Bonferroni *post-hoc* test. Non-parametric *t*-test was used for inter-sexual postural stability comparison.

15.3 RESULTS

We confirmed a significant effect of children's age on postural stability parameters ($p<0.01$, $\eta_p^2 = 0.202$). Post-hoc tests did not approve significant differences between nearby age groups ($p>0.05$), (7 years vs. 8 years; 9 years vs. 10 years; 9 years vs. 11 years; 10 years vs. 11 years). The group of girls had significantly lower and better values of postural stability parameters against the group of boys ($p<0.01$, $\eta_p^2 = 0.031$).

Table 15.1 Statistical analysis of the observed variables and their interaction effect.

Source	Mean Square	F	Sig.	η_p^2
Age	219584.705	25.137	.000	.202
Gender	110150.612	12.609	.000	.031
Visual control	574251.225	65.737	.000	.142
Age*Gender	8236.194	.943	.439	.009
Age*Visual control	8349.221	.956	.432	.010
Gender*Visual control	212.236	.024	.876	.000
Age*Gender*Visual control	7121.865	.815	.516	.008
Error	8735.550			

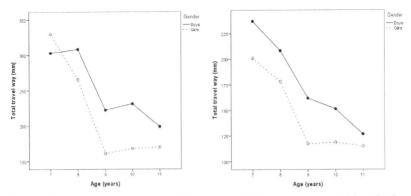

Figure 15.1 Comparison of postural stability parameter TTW between boys and girls – visual (left) and non visual control (right) according to the age.

Post-hoc tests confirmed significant differences of postural parameters between groups of girls and boys (p<0.05) in tests with visual control (8 years, 9 years, 10 years) and (p<0.05) and without visual control (9 years and 10 years). Visual control had a significant effect on children's postural stability (p<0.01, $\eta_p^2 = 0.142$). Interactive effect of independent variables had no significant effect on the selected postural stability parameters.

15.4 DISCUSSION

Postural parameters changes which are based on COP movement have been confirmed by other studies (Kirschenbaum *et al.*, 2001). Inter age differences were presented by Figura *et al.* (1991), who monitored a faster decrease of COP velocity in children between the sixth and eighth year of age than between the eighth and tenth year of age. Our TTW parameter while standing with eyes closed decreases throughout the whole monitored time period. Based on the developmental curve of TTW we may observe a decreasing value of the selected parameter and increasing quality of postural stability (Doyle *et al.*, 2007). Other authors found out a steeper decrease in mean velocity of fluctuations between the seventh and eighth year of age; after the eighth year of age, the decrease was, according to their results, slight and in older age, mean velocity of COP fluctuations even temporarily increased (Riach and Starkes, 1994). The decrease of COP movement in standing with eyes closed is shifted to a later age period. Explanation can be found in the fact that standing without visual control is more difficult. Stability in the standing position with eyes closed reaches the level similar to that of adults' probably later than in the standing position with eyes open. This may confirm the results of studies published previously. Figura *et al.* (1991) did not find any significant differences in bipedal standing with eyes open between ten-year-old children and adults. While standing with eyes closed, significant differences between 10 year-old children and adults have been found (Rival *et al.*, 2005). Movements of COP were lower in girls than in boys in our study. Significant differences between the samples of girls and boys have been demonstrated. This may indicate a better ability to maintain stability in girls. Another possible explanation may be girls' better ability to concentrate at the comparable age.

15.5 CONCLUSIONS

This study confirmed a decreasing level of monitored COP parameters while standing with open and closed eyes among children aged 7–11 years. The decrease is more pronounced in the first half of the monitored period. Postural stability of children while standing with eyes open is improving with age. This study confirmed the fact that visual control has a significant effect on children's postural stability. Postural stability of children while standing with eyes closed is improving with age. This study confirmed significant differences of postural parameters between groups of girls and boys in both tests with and without visual control. Generally, COP parameters are higher in a standing position with eyes closed. With the loss of visual information, postural stability of children aged 7–11 years is getting worse. Results cannot be generalized to the whole child population but an interesting trend appeared. Selection of children for this study was based on availability and it cannot be regarded as random.

15.6 REFERENCES

Doyle, R.J., Hsiao-Weckler, E.T., Ragan, B.G. and Rosengren, K.S., 2007, Generalizability of center of pressure measures of quiet standing. *Gait and Posture*, **25**, pp. 166–171.

Figura, F., Cama, G., Capranica, L., Guidetti, L. and Puejo, C. 1991, Assessment of static balance in children. *Journal of Sports Medicine and Physical Fitness*, **31**, pp. 235–242.

Hadian, M., Negahban, H., Talebian, S., Jafar, A.H., Sangari, M.A. and Hytonen, M., 1993, Postural Control and age. *Acta Otolaryngol (Stockh)*, **113**, 119–122.

Kapteyn, T.S., Bles, W., Njiokiktjien, C.J., Koddle, L., Massen, C.H. and Mol, J.M., 1983, Standardization in platform stabilometry being a part of posturography. *Agressologie*, **24**, pp. 321–326.

Kirschenbaum, N., Riach, C., L. and Starkes, J.L., 2001, Non-linear development of postural control and strategy use in young children: a longitudinal study. *Experimental Brain Research*, **140**, pp. 420–431.

Nolan, L., Grigorenko, A. and Thortensson, A., 2005, Balance control: sex and age differences in 9- to 16-year-olds. *Developmental Medicine and Child Neurology*, **47**, pp. 449–454.

Palmieri, R.M., Ingelsoll, C.D., Stone, M.B. and Krause, B.A., 2002, Center-of-presure used in the assessment of postural control. *Journal of Sport Rehabilitation*, **11**, pp. 51–66.

Riach, C.L. and Starkes, J.L., 1994, Velocity of centre of pressure excursions as an indicator of postural control systems in children. *Gait and Posture*, **2**, pp. 167–172.

Rival, C., Ceyte, H. and Olivier, I., 2005, Developmental changes of static standing balance in children. *Neuroscience Letters*, **376**, pp. 133–136.

Shumway-Cook, M. and Woollacott, M.H., 2001, *Normal postural control: Theory and practical applications*. Philadelphia: Lippincott Williams & Wilkins.

Westcott, S.L., Richardson, P.K. and Lowes, L.P., 1997, Evaluation of postural stability in children: current theories an assessment tools. *Physical Therapy*, **77**, pp. 629–645.

ADVANCEMENT IN THE INTERPRETATION OF ISOKINETIC RATIOS DERIVED FROM THE HAMSTRING AND QUADRICEPS

J.R. Pereira[1], V. Vaz[1], J. Valente-dos-Santos[1], M.J. Coelho-e Silva[1], R. Soles-Gonçalves[2], J. Páscoa-Pinheiro[1], A. Areces[3], and G. Atkinson[4]

[1]University of Coimbra, Portugal; [2]Polytechnic Institute of Coimbra, Portugal; [3]University of Corunna, Spain; [4]Teesside University, UK

16.1 INTRODUCTION

The most reported strength index of the muscles of the knee has been the concentric (CC) hamstring-quadriceps ratio. It has been reported that the ratio of absolute knee extension (KE) and flexion (KE) muscle force should exceed 0.66 (Aagaard *et al.*, 1998). Another popular ratio is derived from the eccentric (ECC) mode (i.e., KE_{ECC}/KF_{ECC}). During knee extension, the quadriceps contract concentrically (KE_{CC}) and the hamstrings contract eccentrically (KF_{ECC}). Conversely, the hamstrings contract concentrically (KF_{CC}) and the quadriceps eccentrically (KE_{ECC}) during the knee flexion. To accurately detect muscle imbalance about the knee joint, the hamstrings-quadriceps ratio can also be described as a KE_{ECC}/KE_{CC} ratio representing knee extension, or KF_{CC}/KF_{ECC} representing knee flexion. The simplicity of ratios makes them popular amongst researchers for 'normalizing' measurements of one variable with respect to another variable. Nevertheless, ratios are reliant on the assumption that the scaling exponent is a value of one in all datasets. One approach to deriving this exponent is to quantify the slope of the regression between logarithmically-transformed numerator and denominator in the ratio (Atkinson and Batterham, 2012). Differences between local and international adolescent roller hockey players in terms of the above mentioned ratios were noted in a previous report (Coelho-e-Silva *et al.*, 2012) and this study was designed to examine the application of more accurate allometric based indices of KE and KF muscle actions as alternatives to traditional ratios in adolescent hockey players.

16.2 METHODS

The sample comprised 73 competitive roller hockey players aged 14.5–16.5 years, who were classified as competing at local (n=41) and international (n=32) levels. Chronological age (CA) was calculated to the nearest 0.1 year and a radiograph of the left hand-wrist was taken to determine skeletal age (SA) using the Fels method (Roche et al., 1988). Fat-free mass was derived from fat mass obtained by the equation of Slaughter et al. (1988). Isokinetic knee extension and flexion were measured using a calibrated dynamometer (Biodex System 3, Shirley, NY, USA) at angular velocities of $60^\circ.s^{-1}$. Details regarding warm-up, positioning, encouragement, familiarisation, number of trials, and data quality were reported (Coelho-e-Silva et al., 2012). For each action, concentric and eccentric modes of knee flection and knee extension were considered and the best respective peak torques were retained. The following ratios were determined: KF_{CC}/KE_{CC}, KE_{ECC}/KF_{ECC}, KE_{ECC}/KE_{CC}, KF_{CC}/KF_{ECC} (Aagaard et al., 1998). Coefficients of correlation were calculated between peak torques, biological determinants (CA, SA, stature, body mass and fat-free mass), and the four ratios. Simple allometric models ($Y=a \cdot X^b \cdot \varepsilon$) were obtained from linear regressions of the logarithmic transformations, in the form of $\log (Y) = \log (a) + b \cdot \log (x) + \log (\varepsilon)$. Regression diagnostics were checked for each model (Nevill et al., 1992). Peak torques, traditional ratios and adjusted-indices were subsequently considered in comparisons of players by competitive levels. Significance level was set at 5%. Analyses were performed using SPSS version 17.0 software (SPSS,Chicago, IL).

16.3 RESULTS

Table 16.1 Coefficients of correlation between peak torques from concentric and eccentric modes of the knee flexion and knee extension (right portion) in the total sample of adolescent hockey players (n=73).

Variable	Correlation			
	KF_{ECC}	KE_{ECC}	KF_{CC}	KE_{CC}
CA (y)	+0.285*	+0.228	+0.375**	+0.320**
SA (y)	+0.493**	+0.443**	+0.492**	+0.541**
Stature (cm)	+0.313**	+0.342**	+0.459**	+0.465**
Body mass (kg)	+0.400**	+0.374**	+0.436**	+0.523**
FFM (kg)	+0.369	+0.250*	+0.406**	+0.492
$KF_{CC} \cdot KE_{CC}^{-1}$	-	-	+0.331**	+0.316**
$KE_{ECC} \cdot KF_{ECC}^{-1}$	-0.574**	+0.162		-
$KE_{ECC} \cdot KE_{CC}^{-1}$	-	+0.462	-	-0.365**
$KF_{CC} \cdot KF_{ECC}^{-1}$	-0.611	-		+0.076

Table 16.1 summarizes the correlation between peak torques, CA, SA, stature, body mass, fat-free mass and traditional ratios obtained from peak torques. Data suggests an interrelationship between traditional ratios and the magnitude of particular strength parameters. It was possible to obtain four allometric models, which are presented in Table 16.2 ($KF_{CC}/KE_{CC}^{0.777}$, $KE_{ECC}/KF_{ECC}^{0.517}$,

$KE_{ECC}/KE_{CC}^{0.650}$, $KF_{CC}/KF_{ECC}^{0.493}$). Comparisons between roller hockey players by competitive levels (Table 16.3) evidence a significant difference between groups for the peak torque of knee extension (concentric mode). International participants attained better performances on strength protocol and a significant difference between groups was noted for KE_{ECC}/KF_{CC}. International players presented a lower ratio. The effect of competitive level was also significant for two power functions: $KE_{ECC}.KE_{CC}^{-0.650}$ and $KF_{CC}.KF_{ECC}^{-0.493}$. International players attained lower values in the first of the two mentioned functions and higher values in the last function.

Table 16.2 Modelling the relationship between peak torques to obtain a parameter independent of strength magnitude (middle portion of the table) and correlation between peak torque (X) and scaled relationship between peak torques (right portion of the table).

Ratio (Y/X)	Model $Log(Y) = Log(a) + b \cdot Log(x)$		Correlation $(X, Y \cdot X^{-b})$
	b-exponent	95%CI	r
$KF_{CC} \cdot KE_{CC}^{-1}$	0.777	0.623 to 0.931	+0.002
$KE_{ECC} \cdot KF_{ECC}^{-1}$	0.517	0.374 to 0.661	+0.011
$KE_{ECC} \cdot KE_{CC}^{-1}$	0.650	0.444 to 0.856	+0.034
$KF_{CC} \cdot KF_{ECC}^{-1}$	0.493	0.361 to 0.625	+0.015

Table 16.3 Mean (± standard deviation) by stage competitive level (local x international) and results of analyses of variance to test the effect of competitive level on strength).

Variable	Competitive level		Student´s Test		
	Local (n=41)	International (n=32)	t	P	ES-r
PT KF_{ECC}	240.4 ± 62.0	251.8 ± 78.6	-0.694	0.490	0.082
PT KE_{ECC}	155.6 ± 35.8	148.7 ± 32.9	0.850	0.398	0.100
PT KF_{CC}	98.4 ± 23.2	108.0 ± 17.7	-1.951	0.055	0.226
PT KE_{CC}	168.1 ± 40.7	188.1± 25.5	-2.568	0.012	0.277
$KF_{CC} \cdot KE_{CC}^{-1}$	0.59 ± 0.10	0.58 ± 0.67	0.833	0.408	0.098
$KE_{ECC} \cdot KF_{ECC}^{-1}$	0.66 ± 0.10	0.63 ± 0.20	0.681	0.499	0.087
$KE_{ECC} \cdot KE_{CC}^{-1}$	0.94 ± 0.15	0.79 ± 0.15	4.059	0.000	0.434
$KF_{CC} \cdot KF_{ECC}^{-1}$	0.42 ± 0.06	0.46 ± 0.13	-1.813	0.077	0.226
$KF_{CC} \cdot KE_{CC}^{-0.777}$	1.85 ± 0.29	1.85 ± 0.21	-0.044	0.965	0.005
$KE_{ECC} \cdot KF_{ECC}^{-0.517}$	9.15 ± 1.38	8.70 ± 1.70	1.245	0.217	0.146
$KE_{ECC} \cdot KE_{CC}^{-0.650}$	5.58 ± 0.80	4.95 ± 0.94	3.092	0.003	0.344
$KF_{CC} \cdot KF_{ECC}^{-0.493}$	6.56 ± 1.03	7.19 ± 1.03	-2.603	0.011	0.295

16.4 DISCUSSION

A ratio is based on the assumption that the slope of the relationship between logarithmically-transformed numerator and denominator is a value of one (Atkinson and Batterham, 2012). If this is not so, then the ratio will scale inaccurately at the lower and higher ends of the range of measured values, leading to errors in interpreting measurements. There are other problems. When one normally distributed variable is divided by another normally distributed variable, it is unlikely that the resulting ratio is not normally distributed itself (Atkinson and Batterham, 2012). The cause of hamstring injuries is still unclear, although it has been suggested that muscle imbalance between the hamstring and quadriceps may predispose towards injury. A 'normal' KF_{CC}/KE_{CC} of >0.6 is frequently used as an injury prevention and rehabilitation tool (Baltzopoulos and Brodie, 1989) but the reasoning behind its use does not relate to functional movements seen during both daily living and sporting activities. This study added a new focus of discussion regarding the interpretation of ratios. It is suggested that allometrically-derived exponents provide more accurate information on potential muscle imbalance, because they are not dependent on the general magnitude of strength. Specifically, a simple ratio could underestimate muscle imbalance when general quadriceps strength is low and *vice versa*. Assessing muscle balance is considered important, but independently, the peak moment ratios and angle specific moment curves provide only a limited amount of information. A more functional approach to assess muscle balance is required and the best technique to examine the interrelationship between extensors and flexors should also be re-examined.

16.5 ACKNOWLEDGMENTS AND CONTRIBUTIONS

JRP was supervised by MJCS, VV and JVS. This output was prepared by MJCS and GA. Data collected by VV, JVS, RSG, MJCS. AA, JPP substantially contributed in the interpretation of data. GA critically reviewed the chapter. All authors approved the final version.

16.6 REFERENCES

Aagaard, P., Simonsen, E.B., Magnusson, S.P., Larsson, B. and Dyhre-Poulsen, P., 1998, A new concept for isokinetic hamstring: Quadriceps muscle strength ratio. *American Journal of Sports Medicine*, **26**, pp. 231–237.

Atkinson, G. and Batterham A., 2012, The use of ratios and percentage changes in sports medicine: time for a rethink?. *International Journal of Sports Medicine*, **33**, pp. 505–506.

Baltzopoulos, V. and Brodie, D., 1989, Isokinetic dynamometry: Applications and limitations. *Sports Medicine*, **8**, pp. 101–116.

Coelho-E-Silva, M.J., Vaz, V., Simões, F., Valente-Dos-Santos, J., Figueiredo, A., Pereira, V., Vaeyens, R., Philippaerts, R., Elferink-Gemser, M.T. and Malina R.M., 2012, Sport selection in under-17 male roller hockey. *Journal of Sports Sciences*, **30**, pp. 1793–1802.

Nevill, A.M., Ramsbottom, R. and Williams C., 1992, Scaling physiological measurements for individuals of different body size. *European Journal of Applied Physiology*, **65**, pp. 110–117.

Roche, A.F., Chumlea, C.W. and Thissen, D., 1988, *Assessing the Skeletal Maturity of the Hand-Wrist: Fels Method*, (Springfield, IL: CC Thomas).

Slaughter, M.H., Lohman, T.G., Boileau, R.A., Horswill, C.A., Stillman, R.J., Van Loan, M.D. and Bemben, D.A., 1988, Skinfold equations for estimation of body fatness in children and youth. *Human Biology*, **60**, pp. 709–723.

Winter, E.M. and Nevill A.M., 2001, Scaling: Adjusting for differences in body size. In *Kinanthropometry and Exercise Physiology Laboratory Manual: Tests, Procedures and Data*, 3rd ed., edited by Eston, R. and Reilly, T., (Oxon: Routledge), pp. 300–320.

Part V

Cardiovascular and Cardiorespiratory Fitness

CHAPTER NUMBER 17

ALLOMETRIC SCALING OF LEFT VENTRICULAR MASS IN RELATION TO BODY SIZE, FAT-FREE MASS AND MATURATION IN 13-YEAR-OLD BOYS

J. Castanheira[1], J. Valente-dos-Santos[2], J.P. Duarte[2], J.R. Pereira[2], R. Rebelo-Gonçalves[2], V. Severino[2], A. Machado-Rodrigues[2], V. Vaz[2], A.J. Figueiredo[2], M.J. Coelho-e-Silva[2], L.B. Sherar[4], M.T. Elferink-Gemser[5, 6], and R.M. Malina[7, 8]

[1]School of Health and Technology, Portugal; [2]University of Coimbra, Portugal; [3]Londrina State University, Brazil; [4]Loughborough University, UK; [5]University of Groningen, The Netherlands; [6]HAN University of Applied Sciences, The Netherlands; [7]University of Texas at Austin, USA; [8]Tarleton State University, USA

17.1 INTRODUCTION

A variety of methods have been used to normalize left ventricular mass (LVM) to body size, including dividing LVM by a body size variable such as stature or body surface area. However, body proportions change dramatically with growth and maturation, and the relationship between the LVM and stature differs depending on stage of development (Dewey *et al.*, 2008). Further, adjusting or scaling cardiac measurements to body surface area is influenced by body composition (Rowland and Roti, 2010), which in turn is related to growth and maturation. Ratio standards are routinely used to interpret physiological and morphological measurements of youth and adults contrasting in body size and composition descriptors. Allometric models are effective for partitioning the effects of body size and have been recommended as providing a "size-free" expression of physiological parameters (de Simone *et al.*, 1992). Dividing LVM by stature to a power of 2.7 (de Simone *et al.*, 1992) is the most widely accepted indexing method in older children and adolescents. Recent studies (e.g., Rowland and Roti, 2010), have shown that fat-free mass (FFM), a surrogate for metabolically active tissue, is most closely and positively related to LVM. The purpose of this study was to assess the influence of various body-size and body-composition indicators on LVM and, to explore the independent and combined effects of maturation, body-size and body-composition indicators on LVM, using proportional allometric modelling.

133

17.2 METHODS

A cross-sectional sample of 95 Caucasian boys (age 13.1 ± 0.2 years), from a school in the Midlands of Portugal, were enrolled in the study. The study was approved by the Scientific Committee of the University of Coimbra, and informed written consent was obtained from the parents of each boy.

Decimal age was computed from date of birth and date of testing. A single anthropometrist measured stature and body mass. Predicted mature (adult) stature was estimated using the Khamis–Roche protocol (Khamis and Roche, 1994). Current height was expressed as a percentage of predicted mature height and was used as an indicator of maturity status. Skinfolds were measured to the nearest mm using a Lange Caliper (Beta Technology, Ann Arbor, MI, USA). Percentage body fat was estimated from triceps and subscapular skinfold thicknesses using the protocol of Slaughter et al. (1988). Fat-free mass (kg) was derived.

A comprehensive resting echocardiography study was performed using a Vivid 3 ultrasound machine with a 1.5 to 3.6 MHz transducer (GE Vingmed Ultrasound, Horten, Norway). M-mode echocardiograms were derived from 2-dimensional images under direct visualization and were recorded at 100 mm/s. Left ventricular (LV) measurements were obtained in accordance with recommendations of the American Society of Echocardiography.

Data were expressed as means, standard deviations and ranges. The Kolmogorov-Smirnov test was used to confirm the Gaussian distribution of variables. Before the allometric analysis, correlation coefficients (Pearson) were calculated to examine the linearity of relationships between body size (stature and sitting stature), body mass, FFM and percentage of predicted mature stature with LVM.

An initial allometric model was adopted to examine the relationship between body descriptors and LVM ($y = a \cdot x^{k} \cdot \varepsilon$ [eq. 1]). Values of a and k were derived from linear regressions of the logarithmic regression transformations in the form of $\ln y = \ln a + k \cdot \ln x + \ln \varepsilon$ [eq. 2], where y was the dependent variable of LVM (ln LVM, i.e., natural logarithms), a was the scaling constant and k was the scaling exponent of the body size or body composition descriptor (i.e., ln stature, ln sitting stature, ln body mass or ln FFM). Subsequently, stepwise multiple linear regression on ln y based on proportional allometric models was used to fit the unknown parameters (Nevill and Holder, 1994). The models incorporated percentage of predicted mature stature as exponential term in addition to body descriptors (ln LVM = $k \cdot$ ln (body descriptor) + a + $b \cdot$ (% predicted mature stature) + ln ε [eq. 3]). Finally, different combinations of different body descriptors (e.g., stature and FFM) and the exponential term (i.e., % predicted mature stature) were simultaneously considered (ln LVM = $k_1 \cdot$ ln (body descriptor$_1$) + $k_2 \cdot$ log (body descriptor$_2$) + a + $b_1 \cdot$ (% predicted mature stature) + ln ε [Eq. 4]). Pearson's product-moment correlations were used to check the assumptions of scaled LVM independent of percentage of predicted mature stature, stature, sitting stature, body mass or FFM as well as homoscedasticity of residuals in the log-linear regressions (Nevill and Holder, 1994). A 2-tailed P value < 0.05 was considered statistically significant. Statistical analyses were performed using IBM SPSS version 19.0 software (SPSS Inc., IBM Company, NY, USA).

17.3 RESULTS

Chronological age, maturation, body size and composition and echocardiographic characteristics, of the boys, are summarized in Table 17.1. The exponents for stature, sitting stature, body mass and FFM from the independent allometric models of LVM are summarized in Table 17.2 (Models 1–4 derived from equation 2). The allometric models combining body descriptors with maturation (Table 17.2) explained 46% to 52% of variance in the LVM (Models 5–8 derived from equation 4).

Table 17.1 Descriptive statistics for the total sample ($n = 95$).

	Mean ± SD	Range	K-S	P
Chronological age (y)	13.1±0.2	12.8–13.4	0.52	NS
Predicted mature stature (%)	90.6±2.6	85.3–97.9	0.74	NS
Stature (cm)	159.5±9.3	136.4–187.6	0.55	NS
Sitting stature (cm)	82.5±4.8	68.2–96.2	0.55	NS
Body mass (kg)	51.5±11.6	32.6–86.8	0.92	NS
Fat-free mass (kg)	38.8±6.3	26.3–58.9	0.57	NS
Left ventricular internal dimension (mm) †	49.8±3.9	40.6–58.4	0.78	NS
Septal wall thickness (mm) †	6.9±0.6	5.8–9.3	2.08	<0.01
Posterior wall thickness (mm) †	6.6±0.4	5.1–8.7	2.31	<0.01
Left ventricular mass (g)	109.5±19.4	64.9–157.6	0.73	NS
Relative wall thickness	0.27±0.02	0.23–0.36	0.76	NS

†At end-diastole.

Table 17.2 Allometric modelling [eq. 2] and proportional multiplicative allometric modelling [eq. 4] of the LVM for body descriptors and for body descriptors and maturation, respectively ($n = 95$).

Eq.	Model †	Descriptors ‡	Exponents (95% CI)	Model Summary		
				R	R^2	Adj R^2
Eq. 2	1	Stature	1.99 (1.49 – 2.50)	0.63	0.40	0.39
	2	Sitting stature	2.15 (1.66 – 2.63)	0.67	0.45	0.45
	3	Body mass	0.58 (0.45 – 0.71)	0.68	0.46	0.45
	4	Fat-free mass	0.76 (0.59 – 0.94)	0.67	0.45	0.44
Eq. 4	5	Stature	0.89 (0.17 – 1.59)	0.71	0.49	0.48
		Body mass	0.40 (0.59 – 0.94)			
	6	Stature	0.80 (0.01 – 1.61)	0.69	0.47	0.46
		Fat-free mass	0.53 (0.24 – 0.82)			
	7	Sitting stature	1.22 (0.56 – 1.89)	0.73	0.53	0.52
		Body mass	0.34 (0.16 – 0.51)			
	8	Sitting stature	1.18 (0.15 – 2.21)	0.69	0.48	0.47
		Fat-free mass	0.39 (0.02 – 0.76)			

† Non-significant models are not presented; ‡ Non-significant predictors are not presented.

17.4 DISCUSSION

The present study investigated the influence of maturation and several indicators of body-size and composition on LVM in school boys using proportional allometric modelling procedures. Results of cross-sectional analyses were consistent with previous studies of adolescents in showing that stature, sitting stature, body mass and FFM were significant determinants of LVM (e.g., Valente-dos-Santos *et al.*, 2013). This study indicated no influence of percentage of predicted mature height, a non-invasive estimate of biological maturation, on LVM. The results for the allometric models suggest a lower exponent (i.e., 2.0, Table 17.2, [eq.2]), than the most widely accepted for normalizing LVM (i.e., 2.7) in older children and adolescents (de Simone *et al.*, 1992). The physiological basis for normalization LVM on stature alone is not particularly strong. LVM, like cardiac output, is determined primarily by the demands of metabolically active tissues or FFM (Rowland and Roti, 2010). The present study suggested that upper body length and body mass may be the best combination of body descriptors for normalizing LVM. The approach used in the present study offers a different statistical and biological approach to understanding LVM in pubescent boys.

17.5 ACKNOWLEDGMENT AND CONTRIBUTION

JVS who acted as second author [supported by *Fundação para a Ciência e a Tecnologia*: SFRH/BD/64648/2009] contributed as much as JC (the first author) and the database is part of PhD research project from JVS. JPD, JRP, RRG, VS, MJCS participated in the data collection. AMR and VV provided relevant contributions in the project design and management. AF is co-supervisor of JC. LBS contributed in the revision of the manuscript. MJCS is the research coordinator of the project and is co-supervisor of JC and JVS. MJCS, MEG and RMM are supervisors of JVS. MEG and RMM critically contributed in all phases of the project. All authors approved the final version.

17.6 REFERENCES

de Simone, G., Daniels, S.R., Devereux, R.B., Meyer, R.A., Roman, M.J., de Divitiis, O. and Alderman, M.H., 1992, Left ventricular mass and body size in normotensive children and adults: assessment of allometric relations and impact of overweight. *Journal of the American College of Cardiology*, **20**, pp. 1251–1260.

Dewey, F.E., Rosenthal, D., Murphy, D.J., Froelicher, V.F. and Ashley, E.A., 2008, Does size matter? Clinical applications of scaling cardiac size and function for body size. *Circulation*, **117**, pp. 2279–2287.

Khamis, H.J. and Roche, A.F., 1994, Predicting adult stature without using skeletal age: the Khamis-Roche method. *Pediatrics*, **94**, pp. 504–507.

Nevill, A. and Holder, R., 1994, Modelling maximum oxygen uptake: a case study in non-linear regression model formulation and comparison. *Journal of the Royal Statistical Society*, **43**, pp. 653–666.

Rowland, T. and Roti, M., 2010, Influence of sex on the "Athlete's Heart" in trained cyclists. *Journal of Science and Medicine in Sport*, **13**, pp. 475–478.

Slaughter, M.H., Lohman, T.G., Boileau, R.A., Horswill, C.A., Stillman, R.J., Van Loan, M.D. and Bemben, D.A., 1988, Skinfold equations for estimation of body fatness in children and youth. *Human Biology*, **60**, pp. 709–723.

Valente-dos-Santos, J., Coelho-e-Silva, M.J., Vaz, V., Figueiredo, A.J., Castanheira, J., Leite, N., Sherar, L.B., Baxter-Jones, A., Elferink-Gemser, M.T. and Malina, R.M., 2013, Ventricular mass in relation to body size, composition and skeletal age in adolescent athletes. *Clinical Journal of Sport Medicine*, **23**, pp. 293–299.

CARDIORESPIRATORY FITNESS AND ACADEMIC ACHIEVEMENT IN A LARGE COHORT OF BRITISH CHILDREN: DOES SELECTIVE ATTENTION MATTER?

D.M. Pindus, S. Bandelow, E. Hogervorst, S.J.H. Biddle, and L.B. Sherar

Loughborough University, UK

18.1 INTRODUCTION

British children have become progressively more unfit over the past decade (Sandercock *et al.*, 2010). Meanwhile, time dedicated to physical education in British schools is deemed insufficient to increase levels of cardio-respiratory fitness (CRF) in young people (Ofsted, 2013). Low levels of CRF have been associated with inferior academic performance (Van Dusen *et al.*, 2011) and cognitive function (Chaddock *et al.*, 2011) in children. Thus far, studies have focused on the independent associations between CRF and cognitive function, with the emphasis on cognitive control (Chaddock *et al.*, 2011), and CRF and academic achievement (Van Dusen *et al.*, 2011). The results from these studies indicate a positive and medium in magnitude association between CRF and children's scholastic performance. However, the role of cognitive function in the association between CRF and academic achievement has rarely been investigated. Specifically, selective attention has not been considered despite its likely instrumental role in scholastic performance across academic domains (Stevens and Bavelier, 2012). The current study aims to investigate the role of selective attention in the associations between CRF and academic performance in children from the Avon Longitudinal Study of Parents and Children (ALSPAC).

18.2 SUBJECTS AND METHODS

A sub-sample of 1978 (1160 females) cognitively healthy children from ALSPAC (1992 – present) at 9 and 11 years follow-ups were included in the analyses. Cognitive health was defined as the absence of mental disability based on the full scale IQ score greater than 69 on Wechsler Intelligence Scale for Children (WISC III), and no history of epilepsy or meningitis (parental report). CRF, selective attention and academic achievement were measured when children were on average 9.9 ($SD = 0.3$), and 11.8 ($SD = 0.2$) years old, respectively. Descriptive statistics for the sample are presented in Table 18.1. CRF was expressed as physical work capacity at a heart rate of 170 beats per minute (bpm) (PWC170) relative to body weight (kg). Fitness was assessed with a sub-maximal cycle ergometer test. Children were cycling at 55–65 revolutions per minute (rpm) for 3 minutes at each of the three workloads: 20, 40 and 60 Watts. The mean heart rates at the last minute of each stage were entered into linear regression equations to predict workload necessary to elicit a heart rate of 170 bpm. Weight was measured to the nearest 50g with a Tanita Body Fat Analyser (Model TBF 305). Selective attention was assessed with a Sky Search sub-test from the Test of Everyday Attention for Children (TEACh) (Robertson et al., 1996). Children were asked to identify identical spaceship pairs among distracters. Selective attention was expressed as time taken to complete the task (seconds) divided by the number of correctly identified pairs (targets), minus time taken to complete a basic motor speed task (sec). Total marks (out of 100) achieved on the national curriculum key stage 2 (K2) tests in English and mathematics were used as measures of academic achievement. Percent total body fat mass at the age of 11 years was assessed using Dual X-ray Absorptiometry (DXA) with a Lunar Prodigy narrow fan-beam densitometer (GE Healthcare, Bedford, UK). Biological maturation (at age 11 years) was expressed as years from predicted age at peak height velocity (APHV) estimated using the maturity off-set equation (Mirwald et al., 2002). Data were assessed for normality and screened for *outliers*. Selective attention scores were positively skewed and thus log transformed. First, relationships were explored using bivariate Pearson's rho product-moment correlations. Further, a multiple stepwise linear regression models were fit to the data. Data were assessed for multicollinearity. Statistical analyses were performed using IBM SPSS version 19.0 software (SPSS Inc., IBM Company, NY, USA).

18.3 RESULTS

Demographic, anthropometric, fitness and cognitive characteristics are summarized in Table 18.1. PWC170 adjusted for weight had a significant small positive association with average time (log transformed) taken to identify a target on the task of selective attention ($r = .09$, $p < .001$) but not with total marks achieved on the national curriculum test in mathematics or English (NS). Average time taken to identify a target on the selective attention task (log transformed) had a significant small negative association with total marks achieved on the national curriculum test in mathematics ($r = -.21$, $p < .001$) and English ($r = -.18$, $p < .001$). In the regression models, weight adjusted PWC170 was not associated with achievement in English ($\beta = .08$, $t(1408) = 2.9$), thus these analyses are not further presented. However, weight adjusted PWC170 was a significant predictor of marks achieved in the national curriculum test of mathematics (Table 18.2). Weight adjusted PWC170 and log transformed time on the selective attention task explained 5% of variance in children's marks on the national curriculum test of mathematics. Only log transformed time on the task of selective attention remained a significant predictor of achievement in mathematics after controlling for confounders. The results of the regression analyses are presented in Table 18.2.

Table 18.1 Descriptive statistics for the total sample ($n = 1977$).

	Mean	± SD	Range
Chronological age[1], (yrs)	11.8	0.19	11.3–12.9
Chronological age[2] (yrs)	9.9	0.26	9.3–11.5
Sex (% females)	58.6		
Gestational age (wks)	39.5	1.75	27 – 45
Birth weight (g)	3427.2	524.9	935–5080
BMI[1] (kg/m^2)	18.9	3.2	13.1–36.1
Total Body Fat mass[1], (%)	18.7	8.0	4.3–52.3
Years from PHV[1]	- 2.5	0.36	-3.51–-.91
Full Scale IQ (WISC-III)[3]	107.5	15.2	70–144
Maternal education[3] (%)			
None / CSE & Low GCSE	6.3		
Technical	7.0		
O-Level & High GSCE	33.6		
A-Level & Vocational	27.0		
University degree	20.5		
Time on Sky Search (sec)[1]	3.5	0.31	1.2–14.2
PWC170/kg (W/kg)[2]	1.9	0.4	0.68–3.2
Mathematics total marks (max. 100)[1]	72.6	18.2	10–100
English total marks (max.100)[1]	64.5	13.9	0–93

[1] measured at mean age of 11.8 years; [2] measured at mean age of 9.9 years; [3] measured when children were approx. 8.5 years.

18.4 DISCUSSION

The present study did not confirm the role of selective attention in the relationship between CRF and academic achievement in a large sample of British children. In contrast to previous studies (Van Dusen et al., 2011), our results suggest that CRF is weakly associated with academic achievement. This association was specific to achievement in mathematics. The discrepancy between the present study and that of Van Dusse et al., (2011) can partly be explained by the differences in the measurement of CRF. PWC170 is a relatively modest predictor of maximal oxygen consumption in contrast to FITNESSGRAM employed by Van Dussen et al. (2011) which is also linked to specific health outcomes in youth. Thus, in conjunction with a time lapse between the measurements of CRF and academic achievement in our study, a relatively modest sensitivity of PWC170 to detect health outcomes might have contributed to the observed small effects. Importantly, our models explained only one third of variance in academic achievement in mathematics. Since attainment in mathematics is influenced by a myriad of psychological, social and environmental factors (and genetic influence), it is possible that the effects of CRF (which is largely genetically determined), may be too specific to account for a larger portion of variance. In contrast, physical activity

(PA) behaviour has been shown to affect children's physical and psychosocial health. Thus, PA may be more strongly than CRF associated with academic achievement due to its broader impact on children's health and well being. Future studies should address the relative contribution of PA to academic achievement.

Table 18.2 Stepwise multiple regression model of academic achievement in mathematics regressed on PWC170 and selective attention after controlling for confounders ($n = 1418$).

	Predictors	B	$SE\ B$	β
Step 1	Constant	92.1[**]	3.8	
	Time on Sky Search (sec) †	-39.8	5.0	-.23[**]
	PWC170/kg (W/kg)	3.6	1.2	.08[**]
Step 2	Constant	115.5[**]	35.2	
	Time on Sky Search (sec) †	- 44.2	5.1	-.23[**]
	PWC170/kg (W/kg)	1.4	1.7	.03
	Chronological age (yrs)	-.08	2.8	-.00
	Sex	-4.331	1.0	-.12[**]
	Gestational age (wks)	-.131	.31	-.01
	Birth weight (g)	.00	.00	.06[*]
	Total Body Fat Mass (%)	-.10	.08	-.04
	Years from PHV	3.7	1.4	.07[*]
Step 3‡	Time on Sky Search (sec) †	-18.9	4.3	-.10[**]
	Sex	-2.9	.84	-.08[**]
	WISC-III Full Scale IQ	.65	.03	.55[**]
	Maternal Education	1.73	.35	.11[**]

† Log transformed; ‡ In Step 3 only significant predictors are presented; [**] $p \leq .001$, [*] $p < .05$. Note: For Step, 1 $R^2 = .05$, $F(2, 1415) = 34.6$, $p < .001$; for Step 2, $\Delta R^2 = .03$, $F(8, 1409) = 13.5$, $p < .001$; for Step 3, $\Delta R^2 = .33$, $F(10, 1407) = 93.8$, $p < .001$.

18.5 REFERENCES

Chaddock, L., Pontifex, M.B., Hillman, C.H. and Kramer, A.F., 2011, A review of the relation of aerobic fitness and physical activity to brain structure and function in children. *Journal of the International Neuropsychological Society*, **17**, pp. 975–985.

Mirwald, R.L.G., Baxter-Jones, A.D., Bailey, D.A. and Beunen, G.P., 2002, An assessment of maturity from anthropometric measurements. *Medicine and Science in Sports and Exercise*, **34**, pp. 689–694.

Ofsted, 2013, Beyond 2012 - outstanding physical education for all: Physical education in schools 2008 – 2012, (Manchester: OFSTED).

Sandercock, G., Voss, C., McConnell, D. and Rayner, P., 2010, Ten year secular declines in the cardiorespiratory fitness of affluent English children are largely independent of changes in body mass index. *Archives of Disease in Childhood*, **95**, pp. 46–47.

Stevens, C. and Bavelier, D., 2012, The role of selective attention on academic foundations: a cognitive neuroscience perspective. *Developmental Cognitive Neuroscience*, **2**, pp. S30–48.

Van Dusen, D.P., Kelder, S.H., Kohl, H.W., III, Ranjit, N. and Perry, C.L., 2011, Associations of physical fitness and academic performance among schoolchildren. *Journal of School Health*, **81**, pp. 733–740.

CHAPTER NUMBER 19

SOMATIC MATURITY AND CENTRAL OBESITY AS INDEPENDENT PREDICTORS OF CARDIORESPIRATORY FITNESS IN ADOLESCENTS

D.R.P. Silva[1], D. Ohara[1], C.M. Tomeleri[1], M.F. Souza[1], M.S. Carnelossi[1], R.A. Fernandes[2], M.J. Coelho-e-Silva[3], E.R.V. Ronque[1], and E.S. Cyrino[1]

[1] Londrina State University, Brazil; [2] University of São Paulo State, Brazil; [3] University of Coimbra, Portugal

19.1 INTRODUCTION

Cardiorespiratory fitness is recognized as an independent predictor of cardiovascular risk (Ekelund *et al.,* 2007). However due to changes occurring in society in recent decades, decreasing values of their indicators have been observed, especially in children and adolescents (Eisenmann, 2003). Among the main determinants of cardiorespiratory fitness is the level of adiposity, with consistently reported negative effects (Ornelas *et al.,* 2011). But in adolescence, a period characterized by significant changes, many analyses do not consider the maturity levels when testing the relationship between cardiorespiratory fitness and obesity. Additionally, the strong relationship observed between maturation and obesity confounds the interpretation of the results of some studies (Ortega *et al.,* 2007). In this context, our aim is to verify the independent relationship between somatic maturity and central obesity with cardiorespiratory fitness in adolescents.

19.2 METHOD

A school-based epidemiological survey was conducted with adolescents aged 10 to 16 years in the public schools of the urban area of Londrina/Brazil, in 2011. Located in Southern Brazil, Londrina has 515,707 inhabitants and a Human Development Index of 0.824. The sampling process was conducted in two stages. All public schools were listed by geographic region and two were randomly selected by region (10 schools). In these schools some classes were randomly selected and all students in those classes were invited to participate in the study. Two hundred and eighty-nine subjects of the 1,396 adolescents assessed, did not have complete data for the investigated variables. Thus, 1,107 adolescents were included in this study. Subjects were not taking any medication, were not being treated for any illness and returned the consent form signed by their parents or tutors. All procedures were approved by the Ethics Committee of the Londrina State University, Brazil.

The purchasing power (socioeconomic status) was obtained by "Brazil Criterion of Economic Classification" (ABEP 2006) which considers the education of household head and divides families into five groups, where "A" is the highest. The 20-m shuttle run test, held on indoor court and following the procedures suggested by Leger and Lambert (1982) was conducted to estimate cardiorespiratory fitness. The VO_{2peak} (ml/kg/min) was calculated using Léger *et al.'s* (1988) equation and was categorized according to the criteria proposed by Fitnessgram (2004). Waist circumference was measured by a single observer with an inelastic measuring tape (Sanny®). Both to measure and to categorize values the Katzmarzyk *et al.* (2004) recommendations were adopted.

The predicted age at peak height velocity was estimated as chronological age minus maturity offset, according to the suggestions of Mirwald *et al.* (2002). The adolescents' classification in Late, On time and Early was based on the standard deviation (±1SD) from predicted age at peak height velocity of the sample.

The Kolmogorov-Smirnov test analyzed the distribution of the numerical variables. Student t-test for independent samples was used to compare genders. Chi-square test assessed association among categorical variables. Additionally, multiple linear regression was used. All analyses were performed using SPSS 17.0 and statistical significance was set at $p < .05$.

19.3 RESULTS

The characteristics of the adolescents stratified by gender are presented in Table 19.1. Overall, significant differences were observed in age (boys older than girls) somatic maturity (higher frequency of girls and boys in early and late groups, respectively), waist circumference (higher prevalence of high waist circumference in girls) and VO_{2peak} (higher values in boys) between genders.

In the multivariable model we observed different results between genders (Table 19.2). In boys, somatic maturity (positive Std β) and waist circumference (negative Std β) were independently related with cardiorespiratory fitness. On the other hand, when the model was adjusted for chronological age in girls, only waist circumference was related to cardiorespiratory fitness (negative Std β).

Table 19.1 Characteristics of the sample by gender (n = 1,107).

	Boys (n = 504)		Girls (n = 603)	
	Mean / %	CI 95%	Mean / %	CI 95%
Age (y)*	13.1	12.9 13.2	12.8	12.6 12.9
Socioeconomic status (%)				
A/B	34.8	30.3 39.6	32.8	29.0 36.8
C/D/E	65.2	60.4 69.7	67.2	63.2 71.0
Somatic Maturity (%)*				
Early	6.8	4.9 9.3	20.0	17.1 23.3
On time	65.2	61.0 69.2	63.7	59.9 67.3
Late	28.0	24.3 32.0	16.3	13.6 19.4
Waist Circumference (%)*				
High	19.0	15.8 22.6	24.3	21.2 27.8
Normal	81.0	77.4 84.2	75.7	72.2 78.8
VO_{2peak} (mL/kg/min)*	42.1	41.7 42.5	38.2	37.9 38.5

Note. CI 95% = confidence interval of 95%; * p < .05 between genders.

Table 19.2 Linear multivariate model for predicting cardiorespiratory fitness in Brazilian adolescents (n = 1,107).

	Boys				Girls			
	Std β	t	p	R^2_{Adj}	Std β	t	P	R^2_{Adj}
$Age_{(y)}$	0.033	0.66	.510	0.18	-0.49	-11.84	< .001	0.40
$WC_{(cm)}$	-0.46	-9.50	<.001		-0.30	-8.14	< .001	
$SM_{(categories)}$	0.16	3.16	.002		0.04	0.91	.362	

Note. Dependent variable: VO_{2peak}; WC = Waist Circumference; MO = Somatic Maturity (1 = late, 2 = on time; 3 = early).

19.4 CONCLUSION

Based on the results, we conclude that somatic maturity and central obesity are independently related to cardiorespiratory fitness in boys. Among girls, the relationship between somatic maturity and cardiorespiratory fitness seems to be mediated by chronological age and central obesity.

19.5 ACKNOWLEDGEMENTS

Support: National Council of Scientific and Technological Brazil; Improving Coordination of Senior Staff Brazil.

19.6 REFERENCES

ABEP, 2006, Brazilian Association of Research Institute. *Brazilian criteria for economic classification.*
[http://www.abep.org/novo/index.htm], accessed on April 15, 2013.

Eisenmann J.C., 2003, Secular trends in variables associated with the metabolic syndrome of North American children and adolescents: a review and synthesis. *American Journal of Human Biology*, **15**, pp. 786 – 794.

Ekelund, U., Anderssen, S.A., Froberg, K., Sardinha, L.B., Andersen, L.B. and Brage,S., 2007, European youth heart study group. independent associations of physical activity and cardiorespiratory fitness with metabolic risk factors in children: The European youth heart study. *Diabetologia*, **50**, pp. 1832–1840.

Katzmarzyk, P.T., Srinivasan, S.R., Chen, W., Malina, R.M., Bouchard, C. and Berenson, G.S., 2004, Body mass index, waist circumference, and clustering of cardiovascular disease risk factors in a biracial sample of children and adolescents. *Pediatrics*,**114**, pp. 198–205.

Leger, L.A. and Lambert, J., 1982, A maximal multistage 20-m shuttle run test to predict $VO_{2máx}$. *European Journal of Applied Physiology and Occupational Physiology*, **49**, pp. 1–12.

Leger, L.A., Mercier, D., Gadoury, C. and Lambert, J., 1988, The multistage 20 metre shuttle run test for aerobic fitness. *Journal of Sports Science*, **6**, pp. 93–101.

Mirwald, R.L., Baxter-Jones, A.D., Bailey, D.A. and Beunen, G.P., 2002, An assessment of maturity from anthropometric measurements. *Medicine and Science in Sports & Exercise*, **34**, pp. 689–694.

Ornelas, R.T., Silva A.M., Minderico C.S. and Sardinha L.B., 2011, Changes in cardiorespiratory fitness predict changes in body composition from childhood to adolescence: findings from the European Youth Heart Study, *The Physician and Sportsmedicine*, **39**, pp. 78–86.

Ortega, F.B., Ruiz J.R., Mesa J.L., Gutiérrez A. and Sjöström M., 2007, Cardiovascular fitness in adolescents: the influence of sexual maturation status-the AVENA and EYHS studies. *American Journal of Human Biology*, **19**, pp. 801–808.

The Cooper Institute for Aerobics Research, 1999, *Fitnessgram: Test Administration Manual*, 2nd ed., edited by Meredith, M.D. and Welk, G.J. (Champaign: Human Kinetics), pp. 21–27.

ASSOCIATION BETWEEN SOMATIC MATURITY, PHYSICAL ACTIVITY AND BLOOD PRESSURE IN ADOLESCENTS

M.F. Souza[1], S.S. Kawagutti [1], M.C. Tadiotto[1], D. Ohara[1], D.R.P Silva[1], M.J. Coelho-e-Silva[3], E.S. Cyrino[1], R.A. Fernandes [2], and E.R.V. Ronque[1]

[1] State University of Londrina, Brazil
[2] State University of Paulista Júlio de Mesquita Filho, Brazil
[3] University of Coimbra, Portugal

20.1 INTRODUCTION

Hypertension is considered, singly, as an important risk factor for development of cardiovascular disease (Williams *et al.*, 2002). This fact becomes especially worrisome when high blood pressure (HBP) has already manifested itself in childhood and adolescence (Chiolero *et al.*, 2007). A period marked by numerous changes related to growth and development toward the mature state, which shows that children in the same chronological age may present variation in relation to the status in biological maturity. These differences may influence several morphological, physiological and behavioural transformations (Malina *et al.*, 2004), among which the relationship between HBP and biological maturity remains to be investigated. The aim of this study was to analyze the association between somatic maturity, physical activity and HBP in adolescents.

20.2 METHOD

The Scientific Commitee of the State University of Londrina reviewed and approved the procedure of this study. Adolescents and their parents were informed about the aim and design of the study. Signed informed consent was obtained before the start of data collection. A total of 1121 adolescents aged 10–17 years, enrolled in public schools in the urban area of Londrina, Brazil were included in the study. Height and weight were measured according to the standards described by Gordon *et al.* (1988) and BMI was calculated. The sitting height was measured using a bench of 50 cm attached to a stadiometer. The leg length was obtained by subtracting the sitting height from the height. As an indicator of somatic maturation, the age at peak height velocity (APHV) was used according to the recommendations of Mirwald *et al.* (2002). The adolescents were classified as early (boys: APHV <13,07; girls: APHV <11,70), on time (boys: 13,07 ≤APHV ≤15,04; girls: 11,70 ≤APHV ≤13,04) and late (boys: APHV> 15,04; girls: APHV> 13,04). The resting blood pressure was measured with an automatic device (OMRON–HEM-742), previously validated for this population (Christofaro *et al.*, 2009). For classification, the normative tables recommended by the National High Blood Pressure Education Program (2004) were adopted as well as being the 90th percentile the cutoff point for the HBP. The questionnaire proposed by Baecke *et al.* (1982) was used as a tool for assessment of physical activity (PA).

Descriptive statistics were used to characterize the sample. Binary logistic regression analysis was used to investigate the relationship between the main variables of the study, adjusted for PA (P <0.05). The analyses were performed in SPSS 20.

20.3 RESULTS

General characteristics of the sample are presented in Table 20.1. No significant association between HBP and somatic maturity status was observed in boys early [OR= 1.03 (0.56 - 1.92)] and late [OR= 0.52 (0.25-1.10)] and girls in early [OR= 0.78 (0.38 - 1.58)]. On the other hand, girls classified with late maturity were shown to have 65% less chance of having HBP than their peers with early maturity [0.35 (0.16 - 0.78)].

Table 20.1 General characteristics of the sample according to sex (n = 1121).

	Boys (489)	Girls (632)
Age (y)	13.02 (1.54)	12.81 (1.48)
Body Mass (Kg)	48.97 (14.01)	47.78 (11.73)
Stature (cm)	156.40 (11.86)	154.30 (8.54)
BMI (kg/m^2)	19.73 (3.94)	19.95 (4.05)

Table 20.2 Association between HBP and maturational stage in adolescents (n = 1121).

	PAE	
	Boys OR (IC95%)	Girls OR (IC95%)
On time	1	1
Late	0.52 (0.25 – 1.10)	0.35 (0.16 – 0.78)
Early	1.03 (0.56 – 1.92)	0.78 (0.38 – 1.58)

20.4 CONCLUSIONS

In summary, results from this study indicate that the relationship between HBP and biological maturity may occur regardless of the PA level, however, this ratio appears to be strongly influenced by characteristics inherent to sex, as observed in this study in which girls have the APHV later showed a lower prevalence of HBP.

20.5 REFERENCES

Baecke, J.A., Burema, J. and Frijters, J.E., 1982, A short questionnaire for the measurement of habitual physical activity in epidemiological studies. *American Journal of Clinical Nutrition* , **36**, pp.936–942.

Chiolero, A., Cachat, F., Burnier, M., Paccaud, F. and Bovet, P., 2007, Prevalence of hypertension in schoolchildren based on repeated measurements and association with overweight. *Journal of Hypertension*, **25**, pp.2209–2217.

Christofaro, D.G., Casonatto, J., Polito, M.D., Cardoso, J.R., Fernandes, R., Guariglia, D.A., Gerage, A.M. and Oliveira, A.R., 2009, Evaluation of the Omron MX3 Plus monitor for blood pressure measurement in adolescents. *European Journal of Pediatrics*, **168**, pp.1349–1354.

Gordon, C.C., Chumlea, W.C. and Roche, A.F., 1988, Stature, recumbent length, and weight. In *Anthropometric Standardization Reference Manual,* edited by Lohman, T.G., Roche, A.F., and Martorell, R., (Champaign: Human Kinetics Books), pp. 3–8.

Malina, R.M., Bouchard, C. and Bar-Or, O., 2004, *Growth, Maturation, and Physical Activity*, 2nd edition. (Champaign, IL: Human Kinetics).

Mirwald, R.L., Baxter-Jones, A.D., Bailey, D.A. and Beunen, G.P., 2002, An assessment of maturity from anthropometric measurements. *Medicine and Science in Sports and Exercise*, **34**, pp. 689–694.

National High Blood Pressure Education Program Working Group on High Blood Pressure in Children and Adolescents, 2004, The fourth report on the diagnosis, evaluation, and treatment of high blood pressure in children and adolescents. *Pediatrics,* **114** pp.555–576.

Williams, C.L., Hayman, I.L., Daniels, S.R., Robinson, T.N., Steinberger, J., Paridon, S. and Bazzarre, T., 2002, Cardiovascular Health in Childhood: A Statement for health professionals from (AHOY) of the Council on Cardiovascular Disease in the Young, American Heart the Committee on Atherosclerosis, Hypertension, and Obesity in the Young, *Circulation*, **106**, pp. 143–160.

MODELLING DEVELOPMENTAL CHANGES IN LEFT VENTRICULAR MASS USING MULTIPLICATIVE ALLOMETRIC AND ADDITIVE POLYNOMIAL MULTILEVEL MODELLING IN BOYS AGED 11–16 YEARS

J. Valente-dos-Santos[1], M.J. Coelho-e-Silva[1], J. Castanheira[2], E.R. Ronque[3], M.T. Elferink-Gemser[4, 5], and R.M. Malina[6, 7]

[1]University of Coimbra, PORTUGAL; [2]School of Health and Technology, Portugal; [3]Londrina State University, Brazil; [4]University of Groningen, The Netherlands; [5]HAN University of Applied Sciences, The Netherlands; [6]University of Texas at Austin, USA; [7]Tarleton State University USA

21.1 INTRODUCTION

Studies of developmental changes in left ventricular mass (LVM) among children and youth are still limited, and have not systematically considered the influence of habitual physical activity (PA) on LVM. Partitioning the relative contribution of PA to LVM from changes associated with growth and maturation requires longitudinal data and appropriate analytical techniques. To this end, multilevel modelling (Goldstein, 1995) is appropriate for the analysis of repeated measurements. It is also argued (Nevill *et al.*, 1998) that multiplicative rather than additive models would provide a superior fit and more plausible interpretation of such data. Accordingly, the current study was designed to identify the developmental predictors of LVM and to examine the contribution of multiplicative allometric structures as a relevant alternative to traditional multilevel model structures (i.e., additive polynomial models).

21.2 SUBJECTS AND METHODS

Boys in years 6, 7 and 8 from a school in the Midlands of Portugal (age 13.1±1.1 years) were invited to participate in a longitudinal study of LVM and PA; 136 boys volunteered for the study and of these 110 were randomly selected. The study was approved by the Scientific Committee of the University of Coimbra, and informed written consent was obtained from the parents of each boy. Subjects were tested at 6-month intervals over 2 years. A total of 429 observations (average 3.9 observations per subject) were available for each variable (Table 21.1).

Table 21.1 Number of subjects and number of measurements per age group.

Age	Number of measurements			
	2	3	4	Total
11 years	3	0	49	52
12 years	3	0	114	117
13 years	3	2	128	133
14 years	1	1	88	90
15 years	0	0	33	33
16 years	0	0	4	4
Total measurements	10	3	416	429
Number of subjects	5	1	104	110

Decimal age was computed from date of birth and date of testing. A single anthropometrist measured stature and body mass. Predicted mature (adult) stature was estimated using the Khamis–Roche protocol (Khamis and Roche, 1994) and was used as an indicator of maturity status.

ActiGraph GT1M accelerometers (ActiGraph™, LLC, Fort Walton Beach, FL) were used to estimate PA and sedentary time for 7 consecutive days. Non wear was defined as 60 min of consecutive zeros, allowing for 2 min of non-zero interruptions and 600 min of measured monitor wear was used as the criteria for a valid day. Subjects with at least one valid day of monitoring were retained for analysis. KineSoft programme (version 3.3.20; Loughborough, UK) was used to reduce the data in a file collected using a 15-second epoch.

A comprehensive resting echocardiography study was performed using a Vivid 3 ultrasound machine with a 1.5 to 3.6 MHz transducer (GE Vingmed Ultrasound, Horten, Norway). M-mode echocardiograms were derived from 2-dimensional images under direct visualization and were recorded at 100 mm/s. Left ventricular (LV) measurements were obtained in accordance with recommendations of the American Society of Echocardiography.

Means and standard deviations were calculated for all repeated measures. The multilevel regression analyses were performed using the MLwiN (version 2.02) software. First, an additive polynomial model was adopted, based on the models proposed by Goldstein (1995). Second, following the multiplicative model structure of Nevill *et al.* (1998), the model was linearized with a logarithmic transformation. The two model structures were compared based on the Akaike information criterion (Akaike, 1974): $-2 \times$ log likelihood $+ 2 \times$ number of parameters fitted. When the performance of competing models is assessed, the model that fits the data best is the one with the minimum Akaike information criterion (AIC) value.

21.3 RESULTS

Table 21.2 presents the characteristics of the study sample by moment of evaluation. Mean percentages of predicted mature stature (89.8±4.7%) tended to be greater than the longitudinal reference sample, suggesting that the participants were somewhat advanced in maturation. At baseline, the majority of participants (51.7%) were classified as 'on time' (or average) by the estimated maturity status. The proportion of participants classified as 'early' (36.6 %) was higher than those classified as 'late' (11.7 %). Boys had mean statures (157.9±11.4 cm) and mean body masses (51.1±12.5 kg) which approximated medians of US age-specific percentiles for boys. PA was monitored for an average of 5.1±1.5 days and 92.3% provided 3 or more days of valid recordings (> 600 min·day^{-1}). Mean daily accelerometer wear time was 801.7±69.0 min·day^{-1}. The registered amount of daily PA was 450.4±146.7 counts·min^{-1}. Among echocardiographic parameters, subjects showed an eccentric remodelling of LV structure within the reference range (i.e., $0.24 - 0.42$). Absolute LVM was also within normal limits.

Table 21.2 Characteristics of the study sample (mean ± SD) by wave cohort ($n = 429$).

	Moment 1 ($n = 110$)	Moment 2 ($n = 110$)	Moment 3 ($n = 105$)	Moment 4 ($n = 104$)
Chronological age (years)	12.34±0.97	12.87±0.97	13.36±0.96	13.88±0.97
Predicted mature stature (%)	87.1±4.1	89.1±4.2	90.8±4.3	92.8±4.2
Stature (cm)	152.9±10.4	156.4±10.7	159.3±11.0	163.2±11.0
Body mass (kg)	46.9±11.4	49.7±11.9	52.2±12.4	56.1±12.6
Total PA (counts·min^{-1})	480.2±121.1	519.5±164.0	472.7±116.3	423.0±129.5
AWT (min·d^{-1})	813.1±68.3	796.2±72.5	795.8±67.8	794.8±72.1
Time sedentary (min·d^{-1})	524.2 ± 64.0	506.5±74.0	560.5±63.5	547.2±61.4
MVPA (min·d^{-1})	66.8±20.6	73.0±26.4	48.9±18.0	58.4±22.1
Left ventricular mass (g)	98.3±18.6	104.3±19.7	109.7±21.8	116.2±21.6

Note: PA, physical activity. AWT, accelerometer wear time. MVPA, moderate-to-vigorous physical activity.

Results of the multilevel model analyses are summarized in Table 21.3. The predicted longitudinal scores for LVM in both multilevel regression analyses improved with stature ($P<0.01$), body mass ($P<0.01$), age ($P<0.01$) and maturity status ($P<0.05$).

Table 21.3 Multilevel regression analysis for LVM ($n = 429$).

Model 1: additive model structure		
Fixed explanatory variables	*P*	At final step
Constant	<0.01	− 67.851 ± 13.086
Stature	<0.01	0.588 ± 0.139
Body mass	<0.01	0.638 ± 0.115
Age	<0.01	3.642 ± 1.019
Age^2	NS	
Time sedentary	NS	
Moderate-to-vigorous PA	NS	
On time *vs* Late		0.018 ± 3.077
Early *vs* Late	<0.05	5.562 ± 2.749
Variance-covariance matrix		Age
Level 1 (within individuals)		
Constant	55.503 ± 4.856	
Level 2 (between individuals)		
Constant	413.466 ± 39.347	
Age	− 41.563 ± 6.253	4.467 ± 5.241
Log likelihood statistics = − 1581.15		
Model 2: multiplicative model structure		
Fixed explanatory variables	*P*	At final step
Constant	<0.01	− 1.137 ± 0.495
ln stature	<0.01	0.791 ± 0.214
ln body mass	<0.01	0.337 ± 0.059
Age	<0.01	0.034 ± 0.010
Age^2	NS	
Time sedentary	NS	
Moderate-to-vigorous PA	NS	
On time *vs* Late		− 0.004 ± 0.003
Early *vs* Late	<0.05	0.049 ± 0.018
Variance-covariance matrix	Constant	Age
Level 1 (within individuals)		
Constant	0.00511 ± 0.00045	
Level 2 (between individuals)		
Constant	0.00819 ± 0.00129	
Age	0.00004 ± 0.00565	0.00003 ± 0.00043
Log likelihood statistics = − 414.50		

Note: NS ($P>0.05$). Sedentary time and moderate-to-vigorous PA were adjusted for accelerometer wear time.

The multiplicative model required fewer parameters ($n=8$) than the additive model ($n=9$). The AIC criterion provided stronger support for the multiplicative model [AIC Model 2 = 845.0] compared to the additive model [AIC Model 1 = 3180.3].

Using the antilog function, the estimated curves for LVM derived from the multiplicative model structure (Model 2) were plotted in Figure 21.1. Figure 21.1 shows that the predicted LVM substantially increased from 11 to 16 yr (9.08 g / 38.7 %). Significant LVM differences were found among maturity groups from 11 to 16 yr [11 to 14 yr: 'early' maturers had, on average, more 15.73 g (11.5 %) and 27.87 g (20.3 %) of LVM than 'on time' and 'late' maturers, respectively ($P<0.05$). Also, 'on time' maturers had, on average, more 12.13 g (8.9 %) of LVM than 'late' maturers ($P<0.05$). 15 to 16 years: 'early' maturers had, on average, more 13.95 g (10.2 %) than 'on time' maturers ($P<0.05$)].

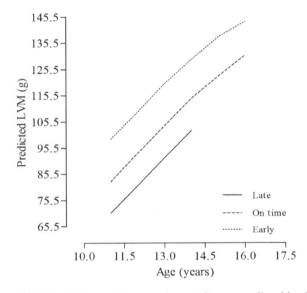

Figure 21.1 Predicted left ventricular mass, by maturity groups, aligned by chronological age. Data are predicted from the multiplicative model structure (Model 2) in Table 21.3.

21.4 DISCUSSION

The influence of body-size, age, estimated maturity status, PA and time sedentary on the developmental changes of LVM in school boys was evaluated using additive and multiplicative multilevel modelling procedures.

Results of the longitudinal analysis of data for boys spanning pre- to post-adolescence were consistent with previous studies of children and adolescents in showing that stature and body mass were significant determinants of LVM (Dai *et al.*, 2009). Consistent with a cross-sectional report showing a major influence of skeletal age on LVM of adolescent athletes (Valente-dos-Santos *et al.*, 2013), this study indicated a significant influence maturity status on LVM.

There were no significant longitudinal associations among PA or time sedentary and LVM. These results suggest that normal levels of PA do not independently predict LVM once LVM is adjusted for body size, body mass and age. It may be that stronger stimuli, i.e., more intense exercise training or elite levels of PA, are needed to substantially influence LVM in children. Nevertheless, it is important to consider that most children do not engage in highly structured training regimens such as those imposed in exercise training studies; therefore, the importance of considering the influence of habitual, free-living PA over a period of time (e.g., the adolescent growth spurt) is a novel and practical aspect of the present study.

On the basis of the AIC criterion, the multiplicative allometric model not only provided a superior fit to the LVM data compared with the additive polynomial model, but it also provided a simpler and more plausible interpretation of the data within and beyond the range of observations.

21.5 ACKNOWLEDGMENTS AND CONTRIBUTIONS

JVS is being supervised by MJCS, MEG and RMM. Data collected by JVS, ER, JC and MJCS. This output was designed by JVS and MJCS and analyses were done while JVS performed an outgoing mission in the University of Loughborough under the supervision of Lauren B Sherar. RMM, MEG substantially contributed in the interpretation of data and critically reviewed the chapter. All authors approved the final version. The authors acknowledged the contribution of Lauren B Sherar.

21.6 REFERENCES

Akaike, H., 1974, A new look at the statistical model identification. *IEEE Transactions on Automatic Control*. **19**, pp. 716–723.

Dai, S., Harrist, R.B., Rosenthal, G.L. and Labarthe, D.R., 2009, Effects of body size and body fatness on left ventricular mass in children and adolescents: Project HeartBeat. *American Journal of Preventive Medicine*, **37**, pp. S97–104.

Goldstein, H., 1995, *Multilevel Statistical Models*, 2nd ed., (London: Arnold).

Khamis, H.J. and Roche, A.F., 1994, Predicting adult stature without using skeletal age: the Khamis-Roche method. *Pediatrics*, **94**, pp. 504–507.

Nevill, A.M., Holder, R.L., Baxter-Jones, A., Round, J.M. and Jones, D.A., 1998, Modeling developmental changes in strength and aerobic power in children. *Journal of Applied Physiology*, **84**, pp. 963–970.

Valente-dos-Santos, J., Coelho-e-Silva, M.J., Vaz, V., Figueiredo, A.J., Castanheira, J., Leite, N., Sherar, L.B., Baxter-Jones, A., Elferink-Gemser, M.T. and Malina, R.M., 2013, Ventricular mass in relation to body size, composition and skeletal age in adolescent athletes. *Clinical Journal of Sport Medicine*, doi: 10.1097/JSM.0b013e318280ac63.

CHAPTER NUMBER 22

CRITERION-RELATED VALIDITY OF THE 20-M SHUTTLE RUN TEST IN BRAZILIAN ADOLESCENTS AGED 11– 13 YEARS

M.B. Batista[1], G. Blasquez[1], C.L.P. Romanzini[1], E.S. Cyrino[1], M.J. Coelho-e-Silva[2], M. Romanzini,[1] and E.R.V. Ronque[1]

[1]State University of Londrina, Brazil; [2]University of Coimbra, Portugal

22.1 INTRODUCTION

The assessment of cardiorespiratory fitness (CRF) has been considered an important factor in aspects related to public health, since high CRF levels can reduce the risk of morbidity and mortality due to various causes and from cardiovascular diseases in the adult population (Blair *et al.,* 1998). In the case of children and adolescents, this favourable aspect can also be observed, since youth with high values of cardiorespiratory indicators tend to have protection against the risk factors for cardiovascular diseases such as, obesity, high blood pressure, dyslipidaemia, and insulin resistance, among others (Eisenmann *et al.,* 2007).

With regard to the assessment of CRF, the peak oxygen uptake (VO_{2peak}) has been widely recognized as one of the best indexes to measure aerobic power during youth. In this sense, various field tests have been developed to estimate VO_{2peak} in children and adolescents. Among them, the 20-m shuttle run test (SR-20m) stands out (Léger *et al.,* 1988), which is a test widely used and recommended for battery tests to verify health-related CRF in youth, in addition to EUROFIT (1988) and FITNESSGRAM (1999). Additionally, it is noteworthy that the SR-20m test has some advantages such as: low cost, wide applicability, evaluation of various subjects simultaneously, a fact that contributes to epidemiologic studies, assessment in school and training environment (Ruiz *et al.,* 2009).

However, the increased use of the SR-20m test as an indicator of VO_{2peak} in children and adolescents is a fact that has aroused great interest in issues related to check its validity, since it is a field test that uses the indirect method to estimating CRF levels and therefore the measured values can present considerable measurement errors.

Thus, the aim of this study was to verify the validity of the SR-20m test in Brazilian adolescents based on the direct spirometry method.

22.2 METHOD

22.2.1 Sample

The sample consisted of 115 adolescents, 61 boys (12.25 ± 0.9 years) and 54 girls (12.06 ± 0.7 years) enrolled in a High School of Londrina, Paraná, Brazil. This study was approved by local ethic committees.

22.2.2 Procedures

Adolescents performed the SR-20m test and the VO_{2peak} was estimated using the original equation proposed by Léger *et al.* (1988).

Direct analysis of VO_2 (reference method) was performed in a laboratory with a portable gas analyzer (K4 b2, Cosmed) and a treadmill protocol specific to this sample. The test began with a 3 minute warm up exercise at speed of 6 km /h to 0% inclination, and subsequently, the inclination became 1% and the speed was increased by 1 km / h every minute, maintaining constant inclination successively until the completion of the test.

The criteria adopted for the end of the test were as follows: a) voluntary exhaustion of the subject, with request to finish the test, b) achieving maximal heart rate predicted for age (220 - age), c) respiratory exchange ratio higher than 1.1 detection of a plateau in the VO_2 curve, defined by an increase of less than 2 ml / kg / min in VO_2 with a change in the test stage. Therefore, when the subject expressed one or more of these criteria, the test was terminated and the highest VO_2 value obtained was considered as the VO_{2peak}, relatively represented ($mL.kg^{-1}.min^{-1}$).

22.2.3 Statistical Analysis

The validity of the SR-20m test, according to sex, was verified by analysis of variance for repeated measures, Pearson linear correlation coefficient and Bland and Altman (1986) analysis, which determined comparison, correlation and concordance between methods, respectively. The level of significance adopted was 5%.

22.3 RESULTS

The VO_{2peak} measured by the reference method was different ($P < 0.05$) from values estimated by the SR-20m test, for boys and girls (Table 22.1). The correlation coefficients found were classified as low for girls ($r = 0.49$) and moderate for boys ($r = 0.60$). Moreover, the method tested showed estimate bias, for boys and girls, with wide concordance limits between VO_{2peak} measured by the reference method and estimated by the SR-20m test (Table 22.2).

Furthermore, analysis was performed to identify trends in assessing by the techniques tested by means of a correlation between the mean and the difference between reference method and test investigated. In the present study, there was evidence of a trend in the individual variability to estimate VO_2 by the SR-20m test

160

for both sexes (P <0.001 – Table 22.2), demonstrating that the test tends to overestimate the result of young people with lower CRF levels and to underestimate the VO_2 of more fit adolescents.

Table 22.1 Comparison of relative VO_2 values (mL.kg^{-1}.min^{-1}) (mean ± standard deviation) measured by the reference method and estimated by the SR-20m field tests, according to sex.

Sex	Reference	SR-20m
Boys (n=61)	49.94 ± 9.5	41.58 ±4.2*
Girls (n=54)	42.18 ± 7.4	39.73 ±3.2*

Reference = VO_2 measured by the reference method, SR-20m = VO_2 estimated by the 20-m shuttle run test using the equation of Léger et al. (1988).
* = P <0.05.

Table 22.2. Correlation coefficient (r) and agreement (bias, limits and trends) between VO_2 measured by the reference method and estimated by SR-20m field test, according to sex.

SR-20m	r	Agreement		
		Bias	Limits	Trends
Boys (n=61)	0.60	8.36*	23.60; - 6.89	< 0.001
Girls (n=54)	0.49	2.45*	15.08; - 10.19	< 0.001

SR-20m= VO_2 estimated by the 20-m shuttle run test using the equation proposed by Léger et al. (1988).* = different from 0, P <0.05.

22.4 DISCUSSION

The correlation values between VO_2 measured by the reference method and estimated by the SR-20m test verified in this study varied from r = 0.49 to r = 0.60 for girls and boys, respectively. These values are considered lower than the correlation coefficient reported in the original study by Léger et al. (1988) (r = 0.71). However, results of this magnitude were also obtained in some more recent works such as Mahar et al. (2006) (r = 0.54) and Ruiz et al. (2009) (r = 0.58).

Moreover, the limits of agreement showed great range, and the best results found were for girls, demonstrating contrast in relation to results presented by correlation analysis. Such conflicting results for the validity of the equation of Léger et al. (1988) to estimate VO_2 in young individuals have been previously described in literature (Castro-Piñero et al., 2010).

In conclusion, the VO_{2peak} estimated by the SR-20m test was considered different from the direct spirometry method and therefore should be used with caution, especially when the results are individually analyzed.

22.5 REFERENCES

Blair, S.N., Wey, M. and Lee, C.D., 1998, Cardiorespiratory fitness determined by exercise heart rate as a predictor of mortality in the Aerobics Center Longitudinal Study. *Journal of Sports Sciences*, **16**, pp. S47–55.

Castro-Piñero, J., Artero, E.G., España-Romero, V., Ortega, F.B., Sjöström, M., Suni, J. and Ruiz J.R., 2010, Criterion-related validity of field-based fitness tests in youth: A systematic review. *British Journal of Sports Medicine*, **44**, pp. 934–943.

Cooper Institute for Aerobics Research. 1999, *FITNESSGRAM Test Administration Manual*, (Champaign: Human Kinetics).

Council of Europe Committee for the Development of Sport Eurofit. 1988, *Handbook for the EUROFIT Tests of Physical Fitness*, (Rome: Edigraf editoriale grafica).

Eisenmann, J.C., Welk, G.J., Ihmels, M. and Dollman, J., 2007, Fatness, fitness, and cardiovascular disease risk factors in children and adolescents. *Medicine and Science in Sports and Exercise*, **39**, pp. 1251–1256.

Léger, L.A., Mercier, D., Gadoury, C. and Lambert, J., 1988, The multistage 20-meter shuttle run test for aerobic fitness. *Journal of Sports Science*, **6**, pp. 93–101.

Mahar, M.T., Welk, G.J., Rowe, D.A., Crotts, D.J. and McIver, K.L., 2006, Development and validation of a regression model to estimate VO_2peak from PACER 20-m shuttle run performance. *Journal of Physical Activity and Health*, **3**, pp. S34–S46.

Ruiz, J.R., Silva, G., Oliveira, N., Ribeiro, J.C., Oliveira, J.F. and Mota, J., 2009, Criterion related validity of 20m shuttle run test in adolescents aged 13–19 years. *Journal of Sports Science*, **27**, pp. 899–906.

Part VI

Physical Fitness and Health

ANTHROPOMETRIC MODEL TO ESTIMATE BODY FAT IN BOYS USING A MULTICOMPARTMENTAL APPROACH

D.R.L. Machado[1], L.A. Gobbo[2], E.F. Puggina[1], E.L. Petroski[3], and V.J. Barbanti[1]

[1] School of Physical Education and Sport of Ribeirão Preto, University of São Paulo, Brazil; [2] Department of Physical Education, São Paulo State University, Presidente Prudente, Brazil; [3] Center of Sports, Center of Research in Kineanthropometrics & Human Performance, University of Santa Catarina, Brazil
[Financial Support: CNPq.]

23.1 INTRODUCTION

Dual Energy X-ray Absorptiometry (DXA) is an alternative method for body composition estimation in paediatric research with many clinical applications However research involving DXA in general population studies is expensive, precluding this method in large-scale use or non-clinical environments. The aim of this study was to develop equations for fat mass (FM) referenced in multi-component analysis by Dual Energy X-ray Absorptiometry (DXA).

23.2 METHODS

Body composition of 408 boys (8–18 years old) was assessed by DXA Scanner Lunar DPX-NT (GE Medical, Software Lunar DPX enCORE 2007 version 11.40.004, Madison, WI) according to the procedures recommended by the manufacturer. Fat mass (FM) was considered as the dependent variable by DXA (DXA_{FM}). Age (years), height (cm), body weight (kg), skinfold thickness (biceps, triceps, subscapular, midaxillar, iliac crest, vertical abdominal, thigh and medial calf), body circumferences (chest, relaxed arm, contracted arm, forearm, wrist, waist, gluteal, thigh and calf) and bone breadth (biacromial, biiliac, biepicondilar of humerus, bitrochanteric, biepiestiloidal of radius and ulna, femur biepicondilar and bimalleolar), were the independent variables. The measures were taken using conventional literature procedures (Lohman, 1986) with Sanny® equipment by the same evaluator. The consistency of measurements was assured, with absolute (TEM) and relative (%TEM) intra-evaluator technical error of measurement within acceptable limits. The study followed the guidelines and regulations governing human research, with parents or guardians consent, and the Ethics and Research School of Physical Education and Sport, University of São Paulo approved it.

An exploratory analysis showed absence of outliers and the Shapiro-Wilk test indicated the normality of data. Descriptive statistics were used to characterize the sample and Pearson correlations were performed to test the association between FM and independent variables. Stepwise regression was used to obtain the proposition of mathematic models (equations) to predict FM. Significance level was previously adopted ($p<0.05$) and SPSS 13.0 (SPSS, Chicago, EUA) statistical packages was used to perform the analysis.

23.3 RESULTS

Characteristics of the sample are presented in Table 23.1. Pearson correlations between independent and dependent variables showed association (r) between 0.27 to 0.93. Maintenance of low multicollinearity between the independent variables was considered. In the stepwise regression, eleven models were generated and indicated statistical significance ($p<0.05$), but just four revealed arbitrarily limited determination coefficient ($r^2>0.85$) to explain total variability (Table 23.2).

Table 23.1 Sample characteristics (mean, standard deviation, minimum and maximum).

(n=408)	Mean	SD	Minimum	Maximum
Age (yrs)	13.17	3.00	8	18
Height (cm)	158.06	17.67	120.3	196.8
Weight (kg)	50.28	17.41	20.6	119.4
%FM (%)	17.79	9.76	4.68	49.63
DXA$_{FM}$ (kg)	9.30	7.48	1.28	41.79

%FM= % of fat mass; DXA= Dual Energy X-ray Absorptiometry; FM=Fat Mass.

Table 23.2 Regression developments of predictive models for FM in boys.

Models	Independents variables				β	Adjusted r^2	SE
	Ab	W	Th	H			
1	0.578±0.01				-0.251±0.235	0.86	2.77
2	0.486±0.01	0.116±0.01			-4.537±0.335	0.92	2.20
3	0.310±0.02	0.147±0.01	0.237±0.02		-7.132±0.340	0.94	1.83
4	0.257±0.02	0.282±0.02	0.192±0.02	-0.127±0.01	-7.686±1.564	0.95	1.65

Ab=abdominal skinfold (mm), W=body weight (kg), Th=medial thigh skinfold (mm), H=height (cm).

Multicollinearity (calculated by dividing highest by the smallest eigenvalue) ranged from 0.191 (equation 1) to 0.250 (equation 4). As well, variance inflation factors (VIF) and tolerance of each model were calculated. Highest VIF and lowest tolerance were, respectively, 1.435 and 0.697 (equation 2), 4.446 and 0.225 (equation 3) and 10.450 and 0.096 (equation 4). For equation 1 (with one predictor only), tolerance and VIF value were 1. Comparison between the DXA_{FM} and predicted equations are shown in the Table 23.3.

Table 23.3 Mean and standard deviation in each age group for DXA_{FM} measured and predicted (equations 1 to 4) in boys.

	Measured	Predicted			
	DXA_{FM} (kg) Mean±Sd	Eq1 Mean±Sd	Eq2 Mean±Sd	Eq3 Mean±Sd	Eq4 Mean±Sd
8 (n=28)	6.08±4.44	8.25±5.94*	6.10±5.71	5.98±5.88	6.53±5.26
9 (n=32)	6.56±4.16	8.33±4.72*	6.38±4.55	6.50±4.65	6.89±4.50
10 (n=34)	7.01±4.47	8.23±5.39*	6.50±5.22	6.84±5.52	6.95±5.20
11 (n=40)	7.81±6.20	8.75±7.28*	7.28±7.07	7.14±6.90*	6.98±6.57*
12 (n=37)	8.41±6.52	8.10±6.50	7.49±6.45*	7.90±7.01*	7.63±6.98*
13 (n=39)	10.85±9.53	10.61±8.70	10.36±8.51	10.69±9.07	10.21±9.33*
14 (n=47)	10.28±9.43	9.74±8.54	10.30±8.40	10.17±8.54	9.83±8.69
15 (n=42)	11.08±8.15	10.61±7.10	11.88±6.98	11.73±7.13*	11.58±7.37
16 (n=39)	10.32±5.49	9.43±5.20*	11.0±5.14*	10.67±4.78	10.22±5.09
17 (n=40)	11.92±8.72	10.87±8.35*	12.64±8.35*	12.32±7.95	12.30±8.28
18 (n=30)	10.09±8.73	8.34±5.98*	10.49±6.39	10.52±6.84	10.60±7.49

DXA_{FM}=DXA fat mass; Eq1=equation1; Eq2=equation 2; Eq3=equation 3; Eq4=equation 4. *p<0.05.

23.4 DISCUSSION

The resulting four models in this study met the assumptions expected from regression analysis: a) strong correlation between independent and dependent variables; b) low multicollinearity among independent variables; and c) practical application of an equation. They were all developed for the whole sample, with all four predictive mean values significantly equal to the reference method (DXA). However, whenever analysed by age group, it could be noticed that each equation presented better statistical performance in one or more specific age groups, i.e., equation 1 was better fitted for subjects from 12 to 15 years old, and so on.

Proposals of multicomponent analysis of body composition normally are performed through molecular level, while anthropometric measurements are usually estimated from organ-tissue level. Although the use of these models facilitates clinical application (Kyle *et al.*, 2003), it does not always adopt valid assumptions, resulting in errors of equations of type II (Heymsfield *et al.*, 1997), for example: constant relation between FFM, FM and total body water (TBW) is problematic in paediatric populations. The changes in bone mineral content, TBW, protein and FFM during the growth process do not develop uniformly or proportionally. Thus, the use of multicomponent body composition methods in children and adolescents is indicated (Fields *et al.*, 2002); however, this practice is not common.

When well-founded models are proposed, they are restricted to pre-pubertal phases (Fomon *et al.*, 1982) or suggest the use of expensive and sophisticated procedures (Haschke, 1989). Quantification of children's FM in fields should favour the simplicity and practicality of the measures, the model should provide better accuracy with minimum error, respect for privacy of the child, low operating cost, and enable large-scale application.

The multicomponent anthropometric models presented in this study showed a high correlation in most of the comparisons between dependent and explanatory variables, and low estimation error, suggesting the preferred use of such models, than those on body density bases.

23.5 REFERENCES

Fields, D.A., Goran, M.I. and McCrory, M.A., 2002, Body-composition assessment via air-displacement plethysmography in adults and children: a review. *American Journal of Clinical Nutrition*, **75**, pp. 453–467.

Fomon, S.J., Haschke, F., Ziegler, E.E. and Nelson, S.E., 1982, Body composition of reference children from birth to age 10 years. *American Journal of Clinical Nutrition*, **35**, pp. 1169–1175.

Haschke, F., 1989, Body composition measurements in infants and children. In *Body Composition Measurements in Infants and Children - Report of the 98th Ross Conference on Pediatric Research*, edited by Klish, W.J. and Kretchmer, N. (Columbus, OH: Ross Laboratories), pp. 76–82.

Heymsfield, S.B., Wang, Z., Baumgartner, R.N. and Ross, R., 1997, Human body composition: advances in models and methods. *Annual Review of Nutrition*, **17**, pp. 527–558.

Kyle, U.G., Piccoli, A. and Pichard, C., 2003, Body composition measurements: interpretation finally made easy for clinical use. *Current Opinion in Clinical Nutrition and Metabolic Care*, **6**, pp. 387–393.

Lohman, T.G., 1986, Applicability of body composition techniques and constants for children and youths. *Exercise and Sport Sciences Reviews*, **14**, pp. 325–357.

IMPACT OF BEHAVIOUR DETERMINANTS ON OVERWEIGHT AND OBESITY AMONG BRAZILIAN SCHOOLCHILDREN: PARANA HEALTHY PROGRAM

D. Pinto-Guedes, D.J.Q. Martins, L.H.S. Martins, and E.R. Roman

State of Parana' Secretariat of Sport, Brazil

24.1 INTRODUCTION

The main causes of overweight and obesity are multifactorial and include genetic, biological and environmental factors, which impact on weight gain by acting through the mediators of energy intake, especially energy-dense food, and/or energy expenditure, especially daily physical activity. Despite the effect that genetic and biological factors can have, the rising prevalence among genetically stable population groups indicate that environmental factors must underlie the overweight and obesity epidemic (Krebs *et al.*, 2007). Current evidence suggests that the development and execution of intervention programmes related to prevention and management of overweight and obesity require the identification of obesogenic behaviour determinants (Bonsergent *et al.*, 2013). Studies available in the literature have shown the complex association between behaviour determinants and obesity (Ali *et al.*, 2011), but these studies were conducted in highly industrialized regions and whether these findings apply to other less developed societies remains to be determined. Therefore, the aim of this study was to identify the behaviour determinants that are most strongly associated with overweight and obesity in a representative sample of Brazilian schoolchildren assisted by the Parana Healthy Program.

24.2 METHODS

The Parana Healthy Program is an action of the State of Parana' Secretariat of Sport serving approximately 2 million schoolchildren. Its activities are focused on prevention and weight management through nutrition education and physical activity. The Parana is known as one of the most developed states in southern

Brazil. However, it has great socioeconomic diversity. With regard to the Human Development Index, 60% of the State's cities show values lower than 0.65 and 10% values great than 0.85, which represents a variation from 74% and 135% from the national average, respectively (UNDP, 2007). This study is part of a cross-sectional survey, which employed anthropometric indicators and social, environmental and behaviour determinants of the schoolchildren population from the State of Parana, Brazil. For selection of schoolchildren we used multistage sampling and a total of 5460 subjects (2946 girls and 2514 boys) aged 4 to 20 years were included in the study. Overweight and obesity were defined by body mass index (weight divided by the height squared – kg/m^2), based on sex-and-age-specific cut-off recommended by the *IOTF* (Cole *et al.*, 2000). Behaviour determinants were collected using a structured questionnaire. The data were collected between October and December of 2012. The prevalence of overweight and obesity were estimated for each stratum of schoolchildren classified according to behaviour determinants. The chi-square (χ^2) test was used to determine eventual differences between prevalence in each stratum. The impact of behaviour determinants on the prevalence of overweight and obesity were analysed using odds ratios (OR), established by binary logistic regression adjusted for sex, age and remaining independent variables included in the regression models. Only behaviour determinants that presented a level of significance ≤ 0.20 for the association with the prevalence of overweight and obesity in the chi-square test were included in the logistic regression model. All the analyses were performed for the whole sample considering the clustering effect.

24.3 RESULTS

In girls, prevalence of overweight and obesity were 18.9% and 8.2%, respectively, whereas the corresponding numbers in boys were 18.6% and 9.5%. Magnitude of the prevalence increases with age, these values being more pronounced among the boys. Chi-square (χ^2) analysis revealed that among the behaviour determinants analysed in this study, considering a level of significance ≤ 0.20, smoking, hours of sleeping and intake of milk showed no significant association with the prevalence of overweight and obesity. Notably, consuming alcohol, food consumption at school, transport to school, eating fruit/vegetables, sugar sweetened drinks, fast foods, moderate-to-vigorous physical activity and screen time were significantly associated with the prevalence of overweight and obesity among the schoolchildren. Table 24.1 shows ORs and their respective 95% confidence intervals for the prevalence of overweight of the schoolchildren selected in the study, according to behaviour determinants. The chance of overweight was higher in schoolchildren that engaged ≥ 4 hours/day screen time (OR = 2.41; 95% CI 1.72–3.28) and who did not eat five servings of fruit/vegetables daily (OR = 2.19; 95% CI 1.60–2.90). Other behaviour determinants that presented a significant odds of overweight were use of alcohol weekly, consuming foods sold in the school cafeteria, travelling by car to school, eating at fast food restaurants and drinking soft drinks. Risk to identify overweight in schoolchildren who reported moderate-to-vigorous physical activity daily was approximately two times lower than their sedentary peers (OR = 1.91; 95% CI 1.49-2.41).

Table 24.1 Multivariate analysis examining the odds ratios and their respective 95% confidence intervals (CIs) for the prevalence of overweight for schoolchildren from the State of Parana, Brazil, according to selected behavior determinants[1].

		Odds Ratios (95% CI)		p-value
Consuming alcohol				< 0.001
	No	Reference		
	Weekly	1.83	(1.41 – 2.34)	
Food consumption at school				0.027
	No	Reference		
	Bring from home	1.36	(0.95 – 1.86)	
	Refectory	1.88	(1.49 – 2.34)	
Transport to school				0.018
	Walking/bicycle	Reference		
	Public transport	1.25	(0.94 – 1.63)	
	Car	1.60	(1.24 – 2.07)	
Eating five servings fruit/vegetables daily				< 0.001
	Yes	Reference		
	No	2.19	(1.60 – 2.90)	
Sugar sweetened drinks				0.016
	Yes	Reference		
	No	0.71	(0.57 – 0.89)	
Eating at fast foods restaurants				0.017
	Yes	Reference		
	No	0.69	(0.54 – 0.89)	
Moderate-to-vigorous physical activity				0.001
	Daily	Reference		
	4–5 times/week	1.37	(0.98 – 1.82)	
	2–3 times/week	1.73	(1.38 – 2.14)	
	≤ 1 time/week	1.91	(1.49 – 2.41)	
Screen time (TV viewing/computer use)				< 0.001
	≤ 2 hours/day	Reference		
	2–4 hours/day	1.96	(1.50 – 2.63)	
	≥ 4 hours/day	2.41	(1.72 – 3.28)	

[1] Values adjusted for sex, age and remaining independent variables of the regression model.

24.4 DISCUSSION

Using the BMI scores we estimated the prevalence of overweight and obesity and the odds associated with behaviour determinants among schoolchildren in the State of Parana, Brazil. The results of this study revealed that, using the current method recommended by *IOFT* for age and sex, the joint prevalence of excess body weight (overweight + obesity) in the school population (27,6%) is higher than those reported in a study conducted from 2002–2003 in the young Brazilian population (20,3%) (IBGE, 2006). When comparing the results of the current study with the results of international studies, the prevalence of overweight and obesity was lower than that reported for young populations in North America (Ogden *et al.*, 2006), but similar to those reported in European countries (Janssen *et al.*, 2005).

Comparisons on overweight and obesity prevalence rates between studies must be done with caution, because of potential differences in the methodology, the cutoff points for weight status classification, and the study populations (sample size, maturation, and age). Even assuming these weaknesses, the current data revealed that although overweight and obesity prevalence were similar with estimates observed in other more industrialized areas, the proportion of schoolchildren who were overweight and obese was particularly worrying. Among all of the behaviour assessed, the primary determinants identified as potentially contributing to the incidence of overweight and obesity included eating habits (less frequent consumption of fruits/vegetables, eating at fast food restaurants and drinking soft drinks), school (go to school in motor vehicles and food consumption at school), use of alcohol weekly, less frequent moderate-to-vigorous physical activity and screen time spent per day, including TV viewing, video games, computer and internet use. The well documented adverse psychological, social and health consequences of overweight and obesity in young people and later in life, combined with the tracking of childhood overweight into adulthood, suggest the need to implement preventive programmes for the population studied. Preventive programmes taken should consider a multi-level intervention that includes the family, school and physical environment.

24.5 REFERENCES

Ali, M.M., Amialchuk, A. and Heiland, F.W., 2011, Weight-related behavior among adolescents: the role of peer effects. *Plos One*, **6**, e21179.

Bonsergent, E., Agrinier, N., Thilly, N., Tessier, S., Legrand, K., Lecomte, E., Aptel, E., Hercberg, S., Collin, J. F., Briançon, S. and the PRALIMAP Trial Group, 2013, Overweight and obesity prevention for adolescents a cluster randomized controlled trial in a school setting. *American Journal of Preventive Medicine*, **44**, pp. 30–39.

Cole, T.J., Bellizzi, M.C., Flegal, K.M. and Dietz, W.H., 2000, Establishing a standard definition for child overweight and obesity worldwide: international survey. *British Medical Journal*, **20**, pp. 1240–1243.

Instituto Brasileiro de Geografia e Estatística, 2006, *Pesquisa de Orçamentos Familiares – POF: Antropometria e Análise do Estado Nutricional de Crianças e Adolescentes no Brasil*, (Rio de Janeiro: IBGE).

Janssen, I., Katzmarzyk, P.T., Boyce, W.F., Verrecken, C., Mulvihill, C., Roberts, C., Currie, C. and Pickett, W., 2005, Comparison of overweight and obesity prevalence in school-aged youth from 34 countries and their relationships with physical activity and dietary patterns. *Obesity Review*, **6**, pp. 123–132.

Krebs, N.F., Himes, J.H., Jacobson, D., Nicklas, T.A., Guilday, P. and Styne D., 2007, Assessment of child and adolescent overweight and obesity. *Pediatrics*, **120**, pp. 193–228.

Ogden, C.L., Carroll, M.D., Curtin, L.R., McDowell, M.A., Tabak, C.J. and Flegal, K.M., 2006, Prevalence of overweight and obesity in the United States, 1999–2004. *Journal of the American Medical Association*, **295**, pp. 1549–1555.

United Nations Development Programme, 2007, *Human Development Report 2007/2008*, (New York: UNPD).

WEIGHT/HEIGHT$^{3.034}$ IS A NECESSARY TOOL IN RELATIVE BODY MASS ESTIMATION OF ADOLESCENTS

P.K. Prusov

Moscow scientific practical centre of medical rehabilitation and sports medicine,
Russia

25.1 INTRODUCTION

The relative body mass (RBM) is one of the major characteristics of physical development of the person and represents scientific interest for anthropometry, biomechanics, nutrition, sports and medicine. However the receipt of knowledge on determinants of its variability during growth and maturation in the adolescent period and development of algorithms on application of the given parameter in medicine and sports is limited to the presence of a suitable tool. The weight/height^2 index of body mass or body mass index (BMI), which has received the greatest dissemination, is considered basically for an epidemiological estimation of fatness independently of a person's age. Nevertheless, BMI correlations with height, individual distinctions on rates and phases of maturing in the teenage period cause additional anxiety of interpretation of BMI (Malina, 1999). We have proved theoretically the expediency of the development of an adolescent body mass index (ABMI) as RBM indicator on the basis of an experimental model of body weight change during growth in the pubertal period.

25.2 METHODS

The data from a prospective longitudinal study of physical development of 173 boys from 11 years till the completion of body height growth were analysed (Vitebsk, 1983–1992). Height, weight and level of pubertal maturation were measured with a frequency of up to four times a year and the general matrix made 2361 measurements of each parameter. Also two skinfolds subscapular and triceps and shoulder, forearm, hip, shin circumference and other anthropometrical parameters were measured. A level of biological maturation was defined on sexual attributes (SA), sum of pubis and axillary hair (P+Ax), % adult height (%Ah), age at peak height velocity (APHV). Individual data Ah, PHV and APHV were counted on a logistical model (Preece and Baines, 1978). The received results were repeatedly published in Russia since 1990. For establishment of the ABMI value for adaptable opportunities of organism to physical activities and development of separate testing algorithms alongside anthropometry, physical fitness, working capacity, sports successes were studied, questioning for an establishment of physical activity level was carried out. More than 550 young sportsmen and 450 schoolboys were investigated.

25.3 RESULTS

As a result of the statistical analysis it was established that the power function 3.034 most adequately reflects change of body weight during growth and maturation of adolescents (Prusov, 2000). For equivalence of the received values to percentage expression the calculation formula was presented in the form of ABMI $=M*10/H^{3.034}$ where ABMI-adolescent body mass index, M-weight, mg., H-height, cm. Average ABMI value was 100.1 ± 12.1 units, asymmetry coefficient was 1.04. Between values of ABMI and RBM calculated as observed weight/mean weight for height almost functional communication, r = 0.996 was defined. Correlation of ABMI with height 0.016 is not essential, and with the average value of skinfold thickness on the general matrix has made 0.76 whereas in different groups going in for sports was less and was in a range from 0.30–0.63. The percentile scales of ABMI estimation in view of a level of puberty allowing to spend individual monitoring of RBM during growth and maturing in the teenage period, Table 25.1, were developed.

Table 25.1 Dynamics and percentile scales of ABMI estimation during puberty of boys (P.K.Prusov, 2000).

(P+AX)*	M	S	Percentile						
			3	10	25	50	75	90	97
0	101	12.3	82	87	93	99	108	115	130
1	101.2	12.5	82	87	93	99	108	116	131
2	99.2	11.6	82	86	91	97	106	112	127
3	98.1	11.4	81	85	90	96	104	111	123
4	97.8	11.3	81	84	90	95	104	111	124
5	100.1	11.9	82	87	93	99	105	115	129
6	103.8	12.2	84	89	96	102	110	121	133
n=2361	100.1	12.1	82.5	86	92	98	106.5	113	127

*The estimation of a degree of pubis (P) and axillary (AX) hair-covering was spent by a technique recommended in Russia (Baranov and Kuchma, 1999). 1 point characterizes occurrence of initial attributes of hair-covering, whereas 0 means their absence.

Character of ABMI variability in view of phases and rates of biological maturing, value of parameters of physical development in the beginning of puberty is established (Prusov, 2005). In the beginning of puberty, in SA1 or (Tanner 2), or 86–88% AH ABMI compose about 101 units, then during maturing to moment SA4 or 94-95 %Ah ABMI steadily decreased. The lowest level "adolescent extension", about 98 units was registered in 0.5–1.0 years after the moment of

APHV. After this to the end of puberty and stop growth body height RBM is increased again up to 103–104 units. RBM decrease correlates positively with initial level of ABMI, % Fat, and PHV and negatively with APHV.

Longitudinal supervisions of young sportsmen have shown, that character of influence of physical activities on RBM dynamics depends on orientation of training process and its initial level in the beginning of puberty (Prusov, 2005). The young sportsmen having ABMI above an average level and more going in for kinds of sports on endurance (ski-race, run on average and long distances, sports walking, etc.), sports games have the tendency to decrease RBM. At deficiency of weight optimum loadings in kinds of sports with elements of a power orientation (struggle, weightlifting, athletic gymnastics, rowing, etc.) increase RBM during the growth. The statistical analysis of young sportsmen has shown essentially lower ABMI variability in separate kinds of sports in comparison with reference data that specifies value of an optimality of the given parameter for successful performance in concrete kinds of sports.

Also studying young sportsmen (Prusov, 2000) the dependence on RMB level of the maximal physical working capacity (PWCmx/kg) value at work on veloergometer and features of power supply of loading is established. The maximum PWCmx value was marked at having ABMI in a range below an average and an average level. The most corpulent were characterized by the minimum PWCmx values and productivity of cardiorespiratory systems. At having very low and low level of RBM the tendency to decrease PWCmx, the lowest profitability by power supply on 1 kg of a total body mass were marked. As a result it has been established that PWCmx in groups of young sportsmen with different RBM is defined not only by the maximal productivity of cardiorespiratory systems, but also somewhat by profitability of power supply of loading.

As RBM is a determinant for parameters of a fatty and muscular component (Prusov, 1998) in view of dependence of an average fatty fold and average muscular radius on ABMI and body height the mathematical models of calculation of its relative values are developed (Prusov, 2005). The given parameters as well as ABMI were important for development of some applied algorithms of physical training: allocation of hypokinesia group (Kuchma and Prusov, 2001); an individual estimation of physical fitness for 8 tests (Prusov, 2004); sports selection for some kinds of track and field athletics — high jumps, throwings, a sprinting and run on endurance (Prusov, 2005).

25.4 DISCUSSION

Thus on the basis of the analysis of longitudinal research it is established that height $^{3.034}$ most adequately reflects change of weight during growth and maturing of teenagers. It is shown that developed ABMI is a reliable and necessary tool of studying RBM variability during growth, adaptable opportunities to physical activities and development of practical algorithms for teenagers. Parameter RBM is very important not only for an epidemiological estimation of fatness but also for the decision of some scientific and practical questions in medicine and sports.

25.5 REFERENCES

Kuchma, V. and Prusov, P., 2001, Macro-morphological parameters in estimation of physical activity level of boys-teenagers. In *Materials of IX Congress of Pediatricians of Russia Children's Public Health Services of Russia: Strategy of Development*, (Moskow), pp. 477–478.

Prusov, P., 1998, Relative values of tissue body mass components depending on weight-height ratios at boys-teenagers. *Pediatrics*, **3**, pp. 40–42.

Prusov, P., 2000, New index for determination of weight-height ratio of boys-adolescents. *Pediatrics*, **2**, pp. 26–28.

Prusov, P., 2000, Physical working capacity and some features of power supply of young sportsmen depending on a weight-height ratio level. *Pediatrics*, **6**, pp. 61–65.

Prusov, P., 2004, Physical fitness of boys-teenagers (questions of individual estimation). *Magazine of the Russian association on sports medicine and rehabilitation of patients and invalids*, **1**, pp. 20–25.

Prusov, P., 2005, Features of Physical Development of Teenagers in a Control System of Health- Improving and Sports Process: Doctoral thesis of Medical Sciences, (Russia: Moscow scientific practical centre of medical rehabilitation and sports medicine, Russia).

SECULAR TREND OF NUTRITIONAL STATUS AND CARDIORESPIRATORY FITNESS IN CHILDREN

G. Blasquez[1, 2, 3], M.B. Batista[1], C.L.P. Romanzini[1], E.S. Cyrino[1], H. Serassuelo Jr[1], and E.R.V. Ronque[1]

[1]State University of Londrina, Brazil; [2]Paulista University, Brazil; [3]Rio Preto University Center, Brazil

26.1 INTRODUCTION

In recent decades, several studies have shown that inadequate cardiorespiratory fitness (CRF) levels have an inverse association with independent risk factors for chronic diseases and may lead to premature death in adults (Blair *et al.*, 1998; Lamonte *et al.*, 2005). In the case of children and adolescents, it was also observed that low CRF levels are strongly associated with the group of risk factors for cardiovascular disease such as high blood pressure, type-II diabetes, dyslipidaemia and body fat, regardless of sex and age (Andersen *et al.*, 2007). In addition, a worldwide increase in the overweight and obesity trend in children and adolescents has been observed, increasing the risk of morbidities that are associated with excess body weight and with the fact that this profile remains until adult age (Janssen *et al.*, 2005). Thus, the objective of this study was to investigate the secular trend of nutritional status and cardiorespiratory fitness indicators in Brazilian children between 2002 and 2010.

26.2 METHODS

In 2002, the sample consisted of 511 students, while in 2010, 303 subjects participated in the study. The samples had similar characteristics and the subjects analysed belonged to the age group between 7 and 10 years of both sexes. Data were collected in two private schools of the city of Londrina, Paraná, Brazil. All subjects and their parents were informed about the study proposal and signed an informed consent form. This study was approved by the local Research Ethics Committee.

Body mass (kg) and stature (cm) were measured and the body mass index (BMI) (kg/m^2) was calculated and used as nutritional status indicator. The cardiorespiratory fitness assessment was performed based on the 9-min run / walk test. All guidelines and procedures adopted during physical and motor assessments followed recommendations of the Physical Best (AAHPERD, 1988).

For the sample characterization, median values and interquartile intervals (Q1-Q3) were used, since the Shapiro-Wilk test indicated that the data were not normally distributed. To verify the secular trend in the variables analyzed, the Kruskal-Wallis test was applied, followed by Mann-Whitney U-test (P <0.05). Analysis of Covariance (ANCOVA) was used to compare studies, controlling variables: Age and Body Fat Percentage (F%), from dependent variables: Nutritional Status (BMI) and CRF (9min), respectively. To represent the percentage differences in dependent variables between studies, the delta percentage (Δ%) was used. The significance level adopted was 5%.

26.3 RESULTS

Table 26.1 shows the general characteristics of the sample expressed as median and interquartile interval, besides comparisons between 2010 and 2002, according to sex. Significant differences between studies were observed only in age for female sex, and in CRF indicator, both for males and females. The differences between 2010 and 2002 for nutritional status and cardiorespiratory fitness are shown in Table 26.2. Regardless of sex, no significant changes in the nutritional status (BMI) were observed in the period analysed (2002–2010). Moreover, the 9min test showed significant declines in 2010 compared to 2002 in both sexes (P <0.05).

Table 26.1 Descriptive characteristics of subjects, according to study and sex.

Variables	2002		2010	
	M (N=274)	F (N=237)	M (N=149)	F (N=154)
Age (y)	8.61 (1.80)	8.86 (1.85)	8.51 (2.04)	8.45 (5.03)[*]
BM (kg)	31.12 (11.86)	29.85 (10.33)	29.95 (10.40)	29.75 (9.95)
Stature (cm)	133.65 (12.60)	132.30 (11.70)	132.00 (13.90)	133.50 (14.00)
BMI (kg/m^2)	17.28 (4.30)	16.97 (3.37)	17.00 (3.63)	17.25 (3.86)
9min (m/min)	146.67 (31.70)	133.33 (25.00)	142.56 (31.3)	127.06 (19.00)[*]

Note: M= Male, F= Female, BM= body mass, BMI= body mass index; 9min= 9-minute run / walk test. * = P <0.05 (Kruskal-Wallis test, followed by the Mann-Whitney U-test, P <0.05).

26.4 DISCUSSION

This study found no secular trend in the nutritional status (BMI) indicator in the 8 year period, but negative secular trend for CRF was identified, regardless of sex. Some secular trend studies have also observed decline in performance on tests that estimate CRF, both for males and females in various countries from the decade of 1980 (Tomkinson and Olds, 2007; Ekblom et al., 2011). It was estimated that

178

there is an average decline of CRF each year in the order of 0.43%, and this fact can be explained at least in part by two factors: increase in body weight or reduction in the regular practice of physical activities (Tomkinson and Olds, 2007). Accordingly, since in the present study, excess body weight did not show significant changes in the nutritional status (BMI) indicator for both sexes between studies (2010–2002), it may be that the reduction in CRF in these subjects occurred due to the low practice of physical activities, although this variable was not controlled. Furthermore, some studies have shown that for physical activity to bring benefits to CRF levels, it must be conducted from moderate to vigorous intensities (Ortega *et al.*, 2008; Martinez-Gomez *et al.*, 2010), which may not be the reality of the regular practice of physical activities among individuals in this age group. Therefore, it could be concluded that there were no secular trends in nutritional status along the 8 year period; however, cardiorespiratory fitness is declining among children. In addition, further studies should be conducted to better understand the possible causes of these changes, especially longitudinal studies.

Table 26.2. Statistical significance of the secular trend analysis for variables nutritional status and cardiorespiratory fitness between studies (2002 and 2010), stratified by sex.

Sex	Variables	Co-variables	Difference (2002-2010)	ETA η^2	$\Delta\%$
M	BMI	- AG^I	ns ns	0.66	-1.93
M	9min	- $AG^I + F\%^I$	ns 0.007	0.24	-4.2
F	BMI	- AG^I	ns ns	0.03	1.32
F	9min	- $AG^I + F\%^I$	<0.001 <0.001	0.26	-5.2

- Kruskal-Wallis test, followed by the Mann-Whitney U-test, p <0.05, ns= not statistically significant, I= interaction between covariate and dependent variable. Note: M= Male, F= Female, AG= age; BMI= body mass index; F%= Fat Percentage; 9min= 9-minute run / walk test.

26.5 REFERENCES

American Alliance for Health, Physical Education, Recreation, and Dance. 1988, *American Alliance for Health, Physical Education, Recreation, and Dance*, (Reston, VA: Physical Best)

Anderssen, S.A., Cooper, A.R., Riddoch, C., Sardinha, L.B., Harro, M., Brage, S. and Andersen, L.B., 2007, Low cardiorespiratory fitness is a strong predictor for clustering of cardiovascular disease risk factors in children independent of country, age and sex. *European Journal of Cardiovascular Prevention and Rehabilitation,* **14**, pp. 526–531

Blair, S.N., Wey, M. and Lee, C.D., 1998, Cardiorespiratory fitness determined by exercise heart rate as a predictor of mortality in the aerobics center longitudinal study. *Journal of Sports Sciences*,16, pp.S47–S55.

Ekblom, O.B., Bak, E.A.M.E. and Ekblom, B.T., 2011, Cross-sectional trends in cardiovascular fitness in Swedish 16-year-olds between 1987 and 2007. *Acta Pædiatrica,* 100, pp. 565–569.

Janssen I., Katzmarzyk, P.T., Srinivasan, S.R., Chen, W., Malina, R.M., Bouchard, C. and Berenson G.S., 2005, Utility of childhood BMI in the prediction of adulthood disease: comparison of national and international references. *Obesity Research,* 13, pp. 1106–15.

Lamonte, M.J., Barlow, C.E., Jurca, R., Kampert, J.B., Church, T.S. and Blair, S.N. 2005, Cardiorespiratory fitness is inversely associated with the incidence of metabolic syndrome: a prospective study of men and women. *Circulation,* 112, pp.505–512.

Martinez-Gomez, D., Ruiz, J.R., Ortega, F.B., Casajús, J.A., Veiga, O.L., Widhalm, K., Manios, Y., Béghin, L., González-Gross, M., Kafatos, A., España-Romero, V., Molnar, D., Moreno, L.A., Marcos, A., Castillo M.J., Sjöström M. and HELENA Study Group, 2010, Recommended levels and intensities of physical activity to avoid low-cardiorespiratory fitness in european adolescents: The Helena Study. *American Journal of Human Biology*, 22, pp.750–756.

Ortega, F.B., Ruiz, J.R., Hurtig-Wennlöf, A. and Sjöström, M. 2008, Physically active adolescents are more likely to have a healthier cardiovascular fitness level independently of their adiposity status. The European Youth Heart Study. *Revista Española de Cardiolía*, 61, pp.123–129.

Tomkinson, G.R. and Olds, T.S., 2007, Secular changes in pediatric aerobic fitness test performance: the global picture. *Medicine and Sport Science*, 50, pp. 46–66.

MULTIVARIATE ASSOCIATION BETWEEN HEALTH-RELATED QUALITY OF LIFE AND PHYSICAL FITNESS IN FEMALE STUDENTS

G.E. Furtado, M.J. Coelho-e-Silva, A.J. Figueiredo, and J.P. Ferreira

University of Coimbra, Portugal

27.1 INTRODUCTION

Concerns about the state of global health have contributed to a progressive operational update of the concept of health-related physical activity (PA) in paediatric populations. In addition to the value of a complete classification of the several organic system markers and cardiometabolic profile, importance is given to various mental health indicators associated to psychological well-being (WHO, 1995). For this reason studies that associate health-related quality of life (HRQoL) and physical fitness indicators (PhF) have received more attention in the last years (Cumming et al., 2011). There is consensus that the components of PhF are solid indicators of health status in children and adolescents (Malina, 1995). Currently, there is a lot of alarming evidence to support the involvement of low levels of PA and consequently a decrease in general health, that is associated with an increase in obesity (Smart et al., 2012). Likewise, it is important to emphasize that there is little evidence between low levels of physical fitness and overweight in female adolescents associated to global self-esteem, body image and perception of feelings of satisfaction and well-being (Frost and McKelvie, 2005). The purpose of this study was to examine the associations between HRQoL and PhF indicators in adolescent females.

27.2 METHODS

Participants: Participants were 233 female secondary school students (M = 14.9, SD = 0.6) from Azores Islands, Portugal aged 14–15.9 years. This study was approved by the ethics committee of the University of Coimbra and the Direction of Regional Sports by Government of the Azores Islands. **Field Protocol:** Data collection was conducted during regular physical education classes with the agreement and cooperation of physical educators. Participants completed the Portuguese language version of a series of self-reported psychological questionnaires to assess HRQoL followed by the administration of a test battery to assess PhF indicators. Chronological age in decimals was calculated as the difference between date of birth and date of measurement. Height, weight, percentage of fat mass and body mass index were measured using standardized procedures (Malina, 1995). **Health-related quality of life:** i) *The Satisfaction With Life Scale (SWLS)* is a unidimensional instrument that evaluates individual satisfaction with life in general. The original instrument has demonstrated adequate levels of internal consistency of .87 (Diener *et al.*, 1985), and the Portuguese version presented a Cronbach alpha value of .78 (Marques *et al.*, 2007). In the present study, SWLS revealed a good level of internal consistency with a Cronbach alpha value of .81. ii) *The Children and Youth Physical Self-Perception Profile (CY-PSPP)* is a multidimensional questionnaire that assesses physical self-perceptions in six dimensions (sport competence, physical condition, body attractiveness, physical strength, physical self-worth and global self-worth). In the original validation study Whitehead and Corbin (1997) reported Cronbach alpha values ranging between .86 and .90. The Portuguese version, adapted by Bernardo and Matos (2003), reported Cronbach alpha values ranging between .66 and .85. In the present study Cronbach alpha values ranged from 87. to .88. iii) *The Perceived Stress Scale (PSS)* is a unidimensional instrument developed to quantify the stress level that each individual experiences subjectively, in daily life (Cohen *et al.*, 1983). The Portuguese version of the PSS was translated by Mota-Cardoso *et al.* (2002) and reported Cronbach alpha values of .86 indicating a good internal consistency. In the present study, *PSS* revealed a Cronbach alpha value of .71. For data analysis extension limitations associated to the present short article we will present only data from two of the six dimensions of the CY-PSPP: The *Physical Self-Worth (PSW)* hypothesized as a general or global measure of happiness, pride, satisfaction and confidence in the physical self, and perceived to be a super-ordinated representation of all perceptions in the four physical self sub-domains and *Global Self-Worth (GSW)* as an overall measure of self-esteem. **Physical Fitness Test assessment:** A specific test battery based on the FITNESSGRAM was used to collect data about the youth level of PhF (Plowman, 2008). The battery included: (a) anthropometric assessment: height, weight, body mass index (BMI), triceps and biceps skinfold for percentage of body fat (%BF); (b) strength assessment: The medicine ball forward (MBF), "Softball throwing", hand grip test (HGT) and the standing broad jump test (SBJ); (c) endurance/speed assessment: Sit-Ups in 60 seconds (St-Up), 25 metres endurance shuttle run test (25M-SR) and multi-stages 20 m shuttle run test (PACER). **Statistical analyses:** Descriptive statistics were calculated for age, HRQoL and PhF indicators. The canonical correlation analysis was used to examine the relationships between the two dimensions.

27.3 RESULTS

Table 27.1 shows mean and standard deviation values for chronological age (M = 14.9, SD = 0.6 years), the four dimensions of the HRQoL and the PhF variables, based on anthropometrics, strength and endurance/speed indicators assessment. The multivariate statistic was used to examine the relationship between the

HRQoL and PhF variables. A significant canonical correlation (Eigenvalue = 0.131, Wilks Lambda = 0.762, F = 1-206, p<0.05, r^c=0.340) was extracted from the relationship between the two sets of variables. The variables of the X-side (PhF) explained 15.7% of the variance and the variables of the Y-side (HRQoL) explained 2.2% (rc = 0.340, rc^2 = 0.112). This first canonical correlation explained 46.1% of the total variance. Figure 27.1 shows that the canonical variates emerged from %BF (+0.789), 25M-SR (-0.537), SLJT (-0.492) and that the linear combination of variables were SWLS (-0.532) and PSS (-0.407). The pair of the linear functions correspond to an inverse and positive relationship between BMI (+0.382), %BF (+0.789), HGT (+0.081) and all other variables form both sides. The direct and negative relationships can be observed in the other PhF variables (X-side) and in the four variables that represent the HRQoL (Y-side).

Table 27.1 Descriptive statistics of the health-related quality of life and physical fitness

	Min	max	M	DP
Chronological age (y)	14.0	15.9	14.9	.6
Height (cm)	148.2	179.8	160.3	5.6
Weight (Kg)	36.7	101.4	57.7	10.7
Skinfold triceps (mm)	5	37	18.1	6.0
Skinfold biceps (mm)	5	51	15.2	8.6
Body Mass Index (kg.m^{-2})	16.40	40.11	22.41	3.95
Body Fat mass (%)	11.6	67.4	27.5	8.8
Standing long jump (cm)	67	206	139.4	22.6
2-kg medicine ball throw (m)	2.21	9.05	4.78	1.00
Softball throwing (m)	8.66	39.20	16.76	5.09
Handgrip strength (kg)	14.0	42.5	28.2	5.2
25-m dash (s)	4.17	6.74	5.16	.46
60-s situps (rep)	12	60	31.5	8.9
PACER, aerocbic endurance (m)	240	1240	450	194
Satisfaction With Life	5	35	23.32	6.06
Perceived Stress	25	59	43.21	5.68
Physical Self-Worth	1.00	3.83	2.36	.55
Global Self-Worth	1.00	3.83	2.64	.55

27.4 DISCUSSION

The purpose of this study was to examine the associations between health-related quality of life and physical fitness assessment tests in female adolescents. The results of the study support the hypothesis that it is possible to find a direct and negative relationship between HRQoL and PhF in females expect for BMI, %BF and HGT, which have a direct relationship between specific dimensions of HRQoL and athletic related fitness tests. Previous studies have reported direct relationships between physical fitness and psychological variables in adolescent females (Cumming et al., 2011; Frost and McKelvie, 2005) and similar results occur in the present study. Additionally, a moderated and inverse association was found with

%BF. The canonical correlation indicates, in general, significant but no substantial canonical correlation among HRQoL and PhF dimensions in our sample of Azorean female youth. Future research will examine sex differences, variation by contrasting maturity status and also between sport participants and non-participants in organized sports.

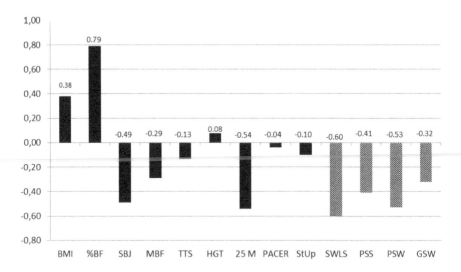

Figure 27.1 Correlations of Physical fitness and Health-related quality of life items with their respective canonical correlation [X-side = PhF: i) anthropometric: mass index (BMI), percentage of body fat mass (%BF); ii) strength: The medicine ball forward (MBF), "Throwing the softball", Hand grip test (HGT), Standing broad jump test (SBJ); iii) endurance/speed: Sit-Up in 60 seconds (St-Up), 25 meters endurance shuttle run (25M-SR), multistage 20 m shuttle run test (PACER); Y-side = HRQoL: i) Satisfaction With life (SWLS); ii) Physical self-Worth (PSW), iii) Global Self-worth (GSW), iv) Perceived Stress (PSS).]

27.5 ACKNOWLEDGMENT AND CONTRIBUTION

MJCS designed the 2008 edition of the Azores Growth Study. JPF coordinated the the psychological domain. GF is being supervised by MJS, AF and JPF. Data were collected by students from the 3rd edition of the Master Programme in Youth Sports.

27.6 REFERENCES

Bernardo, R.P. and Matos, M.G., 2003, Adaptação Portuguesa do Physical Perception Profile for Children and Youth e do Perceived Importance Profile for Children and Youth. *Análise Psicológica*, **2**, pp. 127–144.

Cohen, S, Kamarck, T. and Mermelstein, R., 1983, A global measure of perceived stress. *Journal of Health and Social Behavior*, **24**, pp. 385–395.

Cumming, S.P., Standage, M., Loney, T., Gammon, C., Neville, H., Sherar, L.B. and Malina R.M., 2011, The mediating role of physical self-concept on relations between biological maturity status and physical activity in adolescent females. *Journal of Adolescence*, **34** pp. 465–473.

Diener, E., Emmons, R.A., Larsen, R.J. and Griffin, S., 1985, The Satisfaction With Life Scale. *Journal of Personality Assessment*, **49**, pp. 71–75.

Frost, J. and Mckelvie, S., 2005, The relationship of self-esteem and body satisfaction to exercise activity for male and female elementary school, high school, and university students. *Athletic Insight – The on line Journal of Sport Psychology*, **4**, pp. 36–49.

Malina, R.M., Beunen, G.P., Classens, A.L., Lefevre, J., Vanden Eynde, B.V., Renson, R., Vanreusel, B. and Simons J., 1995, Fatness and physical fitness of girls 7 to 17 years. *Obesity Research*, **3**, pp. 221–231.

Marques, S.C, Pais-Ribeiro, J.L. and Lopez, S.J., 2007, Validation of a Portuguese Version of the Students' Life Satisfaction Scale. *Applied Research in Quality of Life*, **2**, pp. 83–94.

Mota-Cardoso, R., Araújo, A., Carreira-Ramos, R., Gonçalves, G. and Ramos, M., 2002, *O stress nos Portugueses. Estudo do Instituto de Prevenção do Stress e Saúde Ocupacional*, (Porto: Porto Editora).

Plowman, S.A., 2008, Muscular Strength, Endurance, and Flexibility Assessments. In *FITNESSGRAM/ACTIVITYGRAM: Reference Guide* edited by Welk, G. and Meredith, M., (Dallas, TX: The Cooper Institute), pp. 1–40.

Smart, J.E., Cumming, S.P., Sherar, L.B., Standage, M., Neville, H. and Malina, R.M., 2012, Maturity associated variance in physical activity and health-related quality of life in adolescent females: a mediated effects. *Journal of Physical Activity and Health*, **9**, pp. 86–95.

Whitehead, J.R. and Corbin, C.B., 1997, Self-esteem in children and young: The role of sport and physical education. In, *The Physical Self*, edited by K. R. Fox, (Champaign, IL: Human Kinetics), pp. 175–204.

WHOQOL Group, 1995, The World Health Organization quality of life assessment (WHOQOL): Position paper from the World Health Organization. *Social Science and Medicine*, **10**, pp. 1403–1409.

Part VII

Physical Activity and Sedentary Behaviour

THE EFFECTS OF A 6-WEEK RESISTANCE TRAINING PROGRAMME IN CHILDREN WITH JIA: A PILOT STUDY

C.V. Oort[1], S. Tupper[2], A. Rosenberg[3], J. Farthing[1], and A. Baxter-Jones[1]

[1]College of Kinesiology, University of Saskatchewan, Canada; [2]School of Physical Therapy, University of Saskatchewan, Canada; [3]Department of Pediatrics, Royal University Hospital, Canada

28.1 INTRODUCTION

Juvenile idiopathic arthritis (JIA) is the most common rheumatic disease in children and due to its enigmatic nature it is very difficult to treat (Weiss and Ilowite, 2007). JIA is also the most common cause of chronic pain in adolescents (Schanberg and Sandstrom, 1999). Participating in regular physical activity is necessary for children and adolescents to grow properly and attain optimal musculoskeletal health (Mackelvie *et al.*, 2003). Establishing physical activity patterns and proper musculoskeletal health at an early age may set the foundation for adult health, helping to prevent numerous chronic diseases. JIA patients are known to be less physically active during the growing years, compromising their musculoskeletal health (Giannini and Protas, 1993). Through a mechanism labeled exercise induced hypoalgesia, resistance training in healthy populations decreases sensitivity to pain for a short period after exercise training (Cote and Hoeger-Bement, 2010). However, it is yet to be understood whether similar benefits would be achieved in children with JIA.

Chronic pain is a dynamic variable and of major concern in children with JIA because it may significantly affect an individual's health related quality of life, including their ability to participate in physical activity (Hunfeld *et al.*, 2001). Furthermore, chronic pain is a complex and multidimensional (intensity, affect, and interference) health problem that requires careful assessment. In order to properly assess chronic pain researchers need to understand all aspects contributing to and affecting that pain (Cohen *et al.*, 2008). Real time data capture (RTDC) is a concurrent pain measurement tool where patients report chronic pain via pain diaries (Stinson, 2009). This method relies on current levels of pain as opposed to recall, avoiding recall bias, and can be performed in a naturalistic environment. Compliance can also be improved through the use of RTDC devices, both by informing patients that the responses are time-stamped and that data points can be entered through a simple screen tap, reducing response times (Stinson *et al.,* 2006). As well, researchers are able to formulate within-subject comparisons and attain more accurate treatment response measures by used RTDC assessment approaches (Stinson, 2009).

Previous studies assessing exercise training programmes in children with JIA have found inconsistent results. Takken *et al.* (2003) observed no significant difference in functional ability, joint status, health-related quality of life, or physical fitness between a 20 sessions, 1 hour per week, aquatic training group compared to controls. Similarly, in a pilot study Singh-Grewal *et al.* (2006) reported no significant differences between a pre and post 12 week aerobic fitness training programme in functional ability, VO_{2peak} or leg anaerobic capacity. Pain intensity was also measured during each exercise session for this study using a visual analog scale (VAS). No pain was reported in 50.4% of the exercise sessions. One subject with severe polyarticular arthritis needed modification to the training protocol due to pain severity. Epps *et al.* (2005) compared a 2 month land-based exercise programme to a mixed aquatic/land-based programme, finding that both groups increased in strength and aerobic capacity to similar amounts. The common denominator in all these studies was that there were no adverse effects of the exercise; however, none of these studies measured the multidimensional aspects of pain concurrently. Therefore, the main purpose of this study was to pilot the effects of a 6 week resistance training programme on concurrent measures of pain in children with JIA. It was hypothesized that 6 weeks of resistance training would significantly improve pain scores in children with JIA. Secondary aims were to assess changes in muscle thickness and strength, inflammation and functional ability.

28.2 METHODS

Five (two males, and five females) with clinically diagnosed JIA (age range 8 to 18 years) have been recruited so far from an outpatients clinic at the Royal University Hospital, Saskatoon, Canada. All procedures were approved by the University of Saskatchewan's Research Ethics Board and written informed guardian consent attained as well as verbal assent from the child.

The training programme consisted of a 6 week home-based video guided resistance training programme, performed three times per week. The training programme consisted of seven exercises (squats, lunges, step-ups, planks, seated rows, bicep curls/shoulder presses, and push-ups) that were repeated three times each, using body weight and/or a resistance band, during a 40 minute guided video session. Each session involved a 10 minute full body warm-up, followed by 20 minutes of resistance exercises and ended with a 10 minute cool-down with stretching exercises. To accommodate joint pain or swelling in certain locations of the body, modified exercises were also demonstrated in the exercise video that would allow for alternative movements to be performed. The exercise programme varied slightly every second week in order to keep participant interest and increase intensity.

Pain data were reported once a day on non-exercise days (at the end of day) and three times a day on exercise days (before exercise, after exercise, and at the end of day). Before beginning the exercise programme participants answered the pain questionnaire once a day for one week to estimate typical pain. Perceptions of pain were monitored using an application-based tablet device. Participants were instructed to answer each question on the app's questionnaire (PinGo©). The RTDC of pain asked participants to report the pain location (body diagram), intensity (VAS), affect (pain faces scale), and interference (VAS). Additionally, the application measured self-reported stiffness (VAS), mood (VAS), fatigue (VAS), rate of perceived exertion from exercise (Borg scale), and the ability to perform individual exercises. Based on competition of the after-exercise questionnaire the study used the information to assess adherence to the training programme.

Secondary outcome measures were measured pre and post the exercise training programme. Measures included inflammation (at any joint), muscle thickness (vastus lateralis and biceps brachii of the dominant limb), muscle strength (knee extension and elbow flexion of the dominant limb), and functional ability. Inflammation and muscle thickness were measured via ultrasound (Doppler and B-mode, respectively). Muscle strength was determined via Biodex dynamometer and functional ability via a Childhood Health Assessment Questionnaire (CHAQ). An exit questionnaire was also given to participants to understand their perceptions of the exercise programme as well as the PinGo app. Finally, baseline physical activity was measured via accelerometers (Actigraph GT3X) 1 week prior to each participant beginning the exercise programme, coinciding with the initial week of once a day pain measurements.

To test for changes in reported pain over the 6 week duration of the resistance exercise programme repeated measures analysis of variance (ANOVA) were conducted. Comparisons at weeks one (baseline), four and seven of the exercise programme for the three dimensions of pain (intensity, affect, and interference) were assessed. If there was a significant main effect of time, paired samples t-tests were then used to determine where the effect occurred. Independent Paired samples t-tests were used to assess for differences between the first and last week's after-exercise stiffness and rating of perceived exertion (RPE) scores, as well as muscle thickness, muscle strength, and functional ability. An alpha of $p<0.05$ was considered significant for all analyses. All analyses were performed using IBM Statistical Package for the Social Sciences 20.0 for Windows (IBM SPSS, Champaign, IL, USA).

28.3 RESULTS

All participants completed the baseline and post-training measurements and completed the pain diary throughout the training programme. The mean amount of exercise sessions completed was 12.4 ± 3.8 out of a possible 18. Median age was 13.7 years (females=14.6; males=12.3). Median height was 154.7cm (females=161.6 cm; males= 144.35cm) at baseline and 154.83cm (females=161.2cm; males=145.3cm) at post-testing. This puts the females at the 50th percentile and the males between the 15th and 25th percentile for height according to WHO growth reference tables (2007). Median weight was 49.1kg (females=58.9kg; males=34.4kg) at baseline and 49.02kg (females=58.9kg; males=34.2kg) at post-testing. At post-training, average body mass index (BMI) was 22.7 and 16.2 for females and males, respectively. This puts the females between the 75th and 85th percentile and the males between the 15th and 25th percentile for BMI according to WHO BMI reference tables for females and males (2007). Two participants had seronegative polyarticular JIA, one had seronegative arthritis, and 2 had oligoarticular JIA. No significant differences were observed for within-subjects variables of pain intensity, pain affect, or pain interference (p>0.05). Paired samples t-tests also showed no significant differences between the first and last week's self-reported, after exercise scores of stiffness or RPE. Pre and post scores of muscle thickness, muscle strength, and functional ability showed no significant change (p>0.05)

28.4 DISCUSSION

The results of this pilot study suggest that resistance training had no significant effects on pain scores in children with JIA over a six week exercise training period. It is important to note that greater emphasis is now put on patient-centred outcomes, as opposed to the traditional foci of inflammation. The novelty of this study is that it is the first study to incorporate a resistance training specific exercise programme in a population of children with JIA that incorporates an assessment of pain perception. Additionally, pain was measured concomitantly as the child was participating in the training programme. A Cochrane Review of randomized control trials (RCT) of exercise programmes in JIA patients showed no significant decreases in self-reported pain (Takken *et al.*, 2008). That being said, all of those studies measured pain retrospectively, while limiting their outcome to pain intensity.

Secondary outcome variables also did not show significant differences over time. Concurrently self-reported stiffness and RPE are unique to this study in that they were self-reported throughout the training period. Stiffness, as measured through joint range of motion previously showed no significant improvement in any RCT for JIA patients (Takken *et al.*, 2008). RPE scales have been used in this population and correlate well with heart rate, giving a good representation of how hard the individual is working (Singh-Grewal *et al.*, 2006). Muscle thickness is unique to this study, while muscle strength has been examined after a 2-month training programme with small increases occurring, although none being statistically significant (Epps *et al.,* 2005). Finally, the CHAQ is the most widely used health status measure in children with JIA (Singh *et al.,* 1994). This functional ability measure also showed no significant differences in a previous Cochrane Review (Takken *et al.,* 2008). The CHAQ score ranges from 0 to 3, 0 being no disability and three being unable to do. All participants were at 0.13 of a disability index score, being very close to the lowest possible score and giving reason to postulate a floor effect.

Because this is a pilot study, measuring adherence to the home-based exercise program was also a goal. In the 6 weeks, three times a week programme each participant should have completed 18 exercise sessions. The mean amount of exercise sessions completed was 12.4 (69%). Singh-Grewal *et al.* (2006) reported that only 56% completed training sessions in their experimental group, with an average of two training sessions being completed per week as opposed to the desired three. As with many studies, a major limitation to this study is adherence. A home-based exercise programme, although potentially more externally valid, may suffer from compliance. One common denominator with other exercise research in JIA is that no adverse outcomes have been reported (Takken *et al.,* 2008).

Resistance training in children with JIA is a type of exercise that has not been previously investigated for safety or therapeutic benefit. Pain is a barrier to physical activity and youth with JIA show reduced levels of physical activity. The hope is that larger studies can be suitably designed and health professionals may be able to give resistance training recommendations for JIA patients. Upon completion of this study, the results will be used to identify sample size that would be required to determine a definitive research study to answer the questions related to pain control and improvements in health status.

28.5 REFERENCES

Cohen, L., Lemanek, K., Blount, R., Dahlquist, L., Lim, C., Palermo, T., McKenna, K. and Weiss, K., 2008, Evidence-based assessment of pediatric pain. *Journal of Pediatric Psychology,* **33**, pp. 939–955

Cote, J. and Hoeger-Bement, M., 2010, Update on the relation between pain and movement: Consequences for clinical practice. *Clinical Journal of Pain,* **26**, pp. 754–762.

Epps, H., Ginnelly, L., Utley, M., Southwood, T., Gallivan, S., Sculpher, M. and Woo, P., 2005, Is hydrotherapy cost-effective? A randomised controlled trial of combined hydrotherapy programmes compared with physiotherapy land techniques in children with juvenile idiopathic arthritis. *Health Technology Assessment,* **9**, pp. 1–59.

Giannini, M.J. and Protas, E.J., 1993, Comparison of peak isometric knee extensor torque in children with and without juvenile rheumatoid arthritis. *Arthritis Care and Research,* **6**, pp. 82–88.

Hunfeld, J., Perquin, C., Duivenvoorden, H., Hazebroek-Kampschreur, A., Passchier, J., Lisette W., van Suijlekom-Smit, A. and van der Wouden, J., 2001,

Chronic pain and its impact of quality of life in adolescents and their families. *Journal of Pediatric Psychology*, **26**, pp. 145–153.

Mackelvie, K. Khan, K., Petit, M., Janssen, P. and McKay, H., 2003, A school-based exercise intervention elicits substantial bone health benefits: A 2-year randomized controlled trial in girls. *Pediatrics*, **112**, pp. 447–452.

Schanberg, L. and Sandstrom, M., 1999, Causes of pain in children with arthritis. *Rheumatic Disease Clinics of North America*, **25**, pp. 31–53.

Singh-Grewal, Wright, D., Bar-Or, O. and Feldman, B., 2006, Pilot study of fitness training and exercise testing in polyarticular childhood arthritis. *Arthritis and Rheumatism*, **55**, pp. 364–372.

Singh D, Athreya B, Fries J. and Goldsmith D., 1994, Measurement of health status in children with juvenile rheumatoid arthritis. *Arthritis and Rheumatism*, **37**, pp. 1761–1769.

Stinson, J. 2009. Improving the assessment of pediatric chronic pain: Harnessing the potential of electronic diaries. *Pain Research and Management*, **14**, pp. 59–64.

Stinson, J. Petroz, G., Tait, G., Feldman, B., Streiner, D., McGrath, P. and Stevens, B., 2006, e-Ouch: Usability Testing of an Electronic Chronic Pain Diary for Adolescents With Arthritis. *Clinical Journal of Pain*, **22**(3), pp. 295–305.

Takken, T., van der Net, J., Kuis J. and Helders, P., 2003, Aquatic fitness training for children with juvenile idiopathic arthritis. *Pediatric Rheumatism*, **42**, pp. 1408–1414.

Takken, T., Van Brussel, M., Engelbert, R., van der Net, J., Kuis, W. and Helders, P., 2008, Exercise therapy in juvenile idiopathic arthritis (Review). *The Cochrane Collaboration*, Review, pp. 1–21.

World Health Organization, 2007, *BMI-for-age BOYS,* (Geneva: World Health Organization).

World Health Organization, 2007, *BMI-for-age GIRLS,* (Geneva: World Health Organization).

World Health Organization, 2007, *Height-for-age BOYS*, (Geneva: World Health Organization).

World Health Organization, 2007, *Height-for-age GIRLS*, (Geneva: World Health Organization).

NATURE NINJAS: PILOTING A NATURE-BASED PHYSICAL ACTIVITY AND YOUTH DEVELOPMENT INTERVENTION IN ELEMENTARY SCHOOL CHILDREN

K.A. Pfeiffer, D.R. Gould, C. Vogt, E. Oregon, E. Martin, C. Gammon, and M. Maienbrook

Michigan State University, USA and Flint (Michigan) Community Schools, USA; Supported by the Michigan State University College of Education and the Crim Fitness Foundation

29.1 INTRODUCTION

Physically active individuals have been documented as being at lower risk for deleterious medical conditions and having lower rates of chronic disease than those who are inactive (Physical Activity Guidelines Advisory Committee, 2008). National surveys report a low prevalence of meeting physical activity guidelines in United States children and adolescents (~40%; Troiano *et al.,* 2008). In addition, low income, minority populations in the U.S. are less physically active than their white counterparts (Flegal *et al.,* 2010, Sallis *et al.,* 2000). Thus, it is important to design innovative, effective interventions to increase physical activity (PA) in low income, minority populations.

Time spent outside is positively correlated with PA in children and adolescents (Sallis *et al.,* 2000), yet it has not been well-examined as an intervention strategy. Research has shown that exposure to natural settings enhances health-related factors (Mowen et al., 2008). Thus, simply having nature experiences is likely to improve health, but being in nature is also likely to increase PA, which also improves health. Children who live in urban environments are likely to experience difficulty finding safe outdoor spaces, and learning character-developing traits such as responsibility and respect could be particularly useful in navigating those environments. Creating an intervention for adolescents that provides a combination of nature experiences, PA, and positive youth development could positively enhance physical and psychological health-related characteristics. The purpose of this study was to conduct an exploratory study examining physical, psychological, and process outcomes of a nature-based PA pilot intervention in a racially diverse sample of children from a low socioeconomic status, urban community.

29.2 METHODS

Participants were 26, 5th and 6th grade students (14 boys and 12 girls; mean age 10.5 ± 0.6 yrs; 58% African American; 81% receiving free/reduced price lunch), from one classroom at a school whose population was predominantly minority (~46% African American) and low income (~88% eligible for free/reduced price lunch). Prior to beginning the project, participants provided assent and parents/guardians provided informed consent. The study was approved by the Michigan State University Biomedical Institutional Review Board.

The intervention was designed using Attention Restoration Theory (Kaplan, 1995). The school physical education (PE) teacher delivered all sessions during the 5-week intervention. Sessions were held during (4–5 days/week, 30–45 min.) and after school (1–2 days/week, 60–90 min.) and included nature-awareness and nature-based PA. Students hiked for 2 weeks and cycled, fished, and learned archery for 1 week each. Sessions also featured instruction in positive youth development ("life skills": participation, self-direction, respect, caring, and teamwork/leadership). Students also spent 1 day at an outdoor nature camp.

All measures were assessed pre- and post-intervention. PA was assessed using self-report (Physical Activity Questionnaire for Children (PAQ-C); Crocker *et al.,* 1997). Height and weight were assessed according to standardized procedures, and body mass index (BMI) was calculated ($kg \cdot m^{-2}$). BMI percentiles were also calculated according to the Centers for Disease Control and Prevention (CDC) growth charts. Cardiorespiratory fitness was assessed using a shuttle run (PACER, Fitnessgram). Four domains of self-efficacy (Leisure time and extracurricular, Self-regulated learning, Social, Self-assertive from Multidimensional Scales of Perceived Self-Efficacy; Bandura, 1990) and connection with nature were assessed using surveys. All measures were taken by trained staff. The PE teacher recorded number and content of sessions delivered and attendance, and three investigators conducted post-intervention focus groups. Participant responses were not audio recorded; investigators recorded responses to questions on-site.

Descriptive statistics were calculated, and pre- to post-intervention differences were examined using paired t-tests. Sex differences were examined using repeated measures ANOVA. Descriptive statistics were used to examine program characteristics. Focus group data were coded according to standardized procedures.

29.3 RESULTS

Pre- and post-intervention values for outcome variables are listed in Table 29.1. Mean BMI approximated the 78th percentile, with 62% of the sample classified as overweight or obese. There were no sex differences for any outcome variables

196

except PACER score (boys scored higher; F $(1,20)=4.846$, $p<0.05$). Additionally, there were no significant ($p<0.05$) differences in pre- and post-intervention values for any of the outcome variables. The PE teacher delivered 12 in-school sessions, with average attendance of 24.4 students/session and five after-school sessions, with average attendance of 16.6 students/session. Students reported overwhelming satisfaction with the programme; the most popular activities were camouflage hiking and the outdoor camp. Their main source of dissatisfaction was that the programme did not last longer. Participants also noted that they learned to face their fears and try new things.

Table 29.1 Pre- and post-intervention values for outcome variables.

	Pre-intervention	Post-intervention
BMI (kg·m^{-2})	21.7 ± 4.2	22.2 ± 4.0
PAQ-C	2.9 ± 0.8	2.8 ± 0.9
PACER (laps)	26.7 ± 19.4	24.7 ± 16.3
Leisure	5.1 ± 1.1	4.9 ± 1.3
Self-regulated	5.8 ± 1.0	5.6 ± 1.2
Social	5.9 ± 1.2	5.9 ± 1.1
Self-assertive	5.7 ± 1.1	5.5 ± 1.3
Connect nature	4.7 ± 0.7	4.6 ± 0.9

PAQ-C is score on PAQ instrument (1–5); Leisure, self-regulated, social, and self-assertive are self-efficacy subscale scores (1–7); Connect nature is connection to nature score (1–6); All scales 1=low.

29.4 CONCLUSION

Although the research team was interested in examining pre- and post-intervention differences in this exploratory study, a major purpose of the investigation was to examine feasibility and acceptability of the intervention. Several sources of information, including lack of differences in the outcome measures and commentary from participants, indicated that a higher intervention dose was necessary for future study. This is not surprising given that recent literature reviews have indicated high quality studies typically implement PA interventions that are at least 3 months in duration (Kriemler *et al.*, 2011). Regardless, the research team learned valuable lessons regarding how to conduct this type of intervention in this population, including participant impressions and suitability of measures used.

29.5 REFERENCES

Bandura, A., 1990, *Multidimensional Scales of Perceived Self-Efficacy*, (Stanford, CA: Stanford University).

Crocker P.R., Bailey D.A., Faulkner R.A., Kowalski K.C. and McGrath R., 1997, Measuring general levels of physical activity: preliminary evidence for the Physical Activity Questionnaire for Older Children. *Medicine and Science in Sports and Exercise,* **29**, pp. 1344–49.

Flegal K.M., Ogden C.L., Yanovski J.A., Freedman D.S., Shepherd J.A. Graubard B.I. and Borrud L.G., 2010, High adiposity and high body mass index-for-age in US children and adolescents overall and by race-ethnic group. *American Journal of Clinical Nutrition,* **91**, pp. 1020–1026.

Kaplan, S., 1995, The restorative benefits of nature: toward an integrative framework, *Journal of Environmental Psychology,* **15**, pp. 169–182.

Kriemler, S., Meyer, U., Martin, E., van Sluijs, E.M.F., Andersen, L.B. and Martin, B.W., 2011, Effect of school-based interventions on physical activity and fitness in children and adolescents: a review of reviews and systematic update, *British Journal of Sports Medicine,* **45**, pp. 923–930.

Mowen, A., Kaczynski, A. and Cohen, D. A., 2008, The potential of parks and recreation in addressing physical activity and fitness. *President's Council on Physical Fitness and Sports,* **9**, pp. 1–6.

Physical Activity Guidelines Advisory Committee, 2008, *Physical Activity Guidelines Advisory Committee Report,* (Washington, DC: U.S. Department of Health and Human Services).

Sallis J.F., Prochaska J.J. and Taylor W.C., 2000, A review of correlates of physical activity of children and adolescents. *Medicine and Science in Sports and Exercise,* **32**, pp. 963–975.

Troiano R.P., Berrigan D., Dodd K.W., Masse L.C., Tilert T. and McDowell M., 2008, Physical activity in the United States measured by accelerometer. *Medicine and Science in Sports and Exercise,* **40**, pp. 181–188.

CHAPTER NUMBER 30

THE IMPACT OF SOCIAL COMPETENCE AND MOTOR PERFORMANCE ON PHYSICAL ACTIVITY

B. Martin, and J. Hay

Brock University, Canada

30.1 INTRODUCTION

Social competence (SC) is defined as the perception of one's ability to engage in social interactions (Lee *et al.*, 2010). Children who fail to develop adequate SC often feel they are incapable of making appropriate choices to better their health (WHO, 2009). This is problematic as many adult lifestyle choices, such as physical activity (PA) participation, are established in childhood (Daniels *et al.*, 2008). A socially competent child is more likely to become involved in regular PA and maintain an active lifestyle (Rovniak *et al.*, 2002). Another factor that directly influences a child's PA levels is motor performance (MP) as children with lower MP have a well-established activity deficit (Cairney *et al.*, 2009). This activity deficit is persistent over time especially in those with developmental coordination disorder (DCD); a chronic and normally permanent condition found in children characterized by significant motor impairment (Cairney *et al.*, 2009). Children with DCD also demonstrate poor SC (Dewey *et al.*, 2002). However, it is unclear whether the relationship between physical inactivity and motor incompetence is moderated by SC. Gender is also at play here with social norms being more influential for boys PA participation as opposed to girls. The objective of this study is to identify the risk of low PA in children with poor MP and to determine the potential moderating role of self-perceived SC.

30.2 METHODS

Data were obtained from the winter term (2007) of the Physical Health Activity Study Team (PHAST) which followed students in the District School Board of Niagara Ontario. Eighty three % (83) of schools participated with parental consent obtained from 1958 of 2278 children (50.15% males; mean age=11.91 years).

PA is the outcome variable and was determined using the Participation Questionnaire (PQ) which measures a child's frequency and nature of PA (Hay, 1992). The PQ displays strong construct validity with a test-retest reliability of 0.81 for this age (Hay, 1992). MP is a predictor variable and children were screened using the short form of Bruininks-Oseretsky Test of Motor Proficiency (BOTMP-SF). The BOTMP-SF has been validated against the full test with correlations between 0.90 and 0.91 for children ages 8 to 14 years (Cairney *et al.*, 2010). SC is the moderating variable and the well-established Harter Self-Perception Scale was employed (Harter, 1982). Children completed the Harter scale and the PQ in the classroom, while the BOTMP-SF was administered in the schools' gymnasia. Confounders considered were age, gender, BMI, and SES.

All statistical analyses were completed using Statistical Analysis Software 9.3. Demographics and key variable means of the sample population are provided in Table 30.1. Pearson correlation matrices were used to detect collinearity. Simple linear regression (SLR) was performed to determine the direction of each relationship. All analyses were run separately by gender due to social norms differences (Cairney *et al.*, 2009). Comparative tests determined if any differences existed between MP quartiles or SC groups for PA. Multiple regression models were run on PA to show the relationships of the key variables, as well as the effect of potential confounders. Logistic regressions were then performed with Z scores used as PA and SC cut offs, with a z score of less than 0 being 'low'. BOTMP-SF quartiles were used for MP cut offs, with 1st and 2nd quartiles as a 'low MP' level.

30.3 RESULTS

Only motor performance was significantly different between genders. For males, a one-way ANOVA (F=18.11; p<.0001) revealed significant differences in PQ score between all MP levels apart from between the 1st and 2nd quartiles. For females, significant differences in PQ score were present except between the 2nd with 3rd MP quartiles (F=15.30; p<.0001). Using t test results, all t values were significant (p<.0001) with PA being higher in those with high SC in both males (t= -8.51) and females (t= -9.69).

Table 30.1 Descriptive Characteristics Means (SD) by Males and Females.

	Males (n=982)	Females (n=976)
Age (years)[†]	11.92 (0.35)	11.90 (0.34)†
BMI (kg/m^2)[£]	19.95 (3.94)	20.14 (4.11)
PQ Total	17.47 (7.39)	16.88 (6.73)
BOTMP Rank*	71.55 (28.98)	62.39 (30.49)
Social Competence	19.69 (3.86)	19.56 (3.99)
College Education (%)	31.93	33.82

*Statistically different means between genders (p<0.05); [£]5 males and 4 females did not have a BMI reading; [†]1 female did not record age.

Both MP and SC remained as independent predictors of PA in the multiple regression models after adjusting for age, BMI, and SES. When parental education, a proxy for SES, was added to the model, the adjusted R^2 increased in the male model (+0.0053) but not in the female model (-0.0167).

The first set of odds ratios took MP and SC as separate exposures on PA participation. Based solely on MP quartiles as the exposure, males are at risk of low participation in PA in the lower MP quartiles. After adjusting for age, BMI and SES the third quartile was no longer at significant risk. In contrast, results for females — before adjustment — were similar although females in the 2nd MP quartile were not at increased risk of low PA relative to the 4th MP quartile. These results remained after adjustment after adjusting for age, BMI, and SES. With only low SC as the exposure, there is an increased risk of low participation in PA compared to children from both genders with high SC which remains after adjusting for age, BMI, and SES. This is a significant finding as this is the central concept of this analysis. This can therefore be distributed through different MP scenarios to determine the moderating effect of SC on PA.

The second set of odds ratios (Table 30.2) dichotomizes SC (z scores) and MP (1st and 2nd quartiles as 'low') leaving four groups with children with both high MP and high SC as the reference group.

Table 30.2 Odds ratios on low participation in physical activity by gender.

	MALES: Unadjusted	MALES: Adjusted[£]	FEMALES: Unadjusted	FEMALES: Adjusted[£]
Low SC/Low MP	5.47*	5.29*	3.36*	2.60*
High SC/Low MP	2.63*	2.92*	3.38*	3.64*
Low SC/High MP	1.87*	1.86*	1.47*	1.31
High SC/High MP	1.00	1.00	1.00	1.00

*confidence interval does not include 1·[£]adjusted for age, BMI and SES.

The results of odds ratios for low PA determined with both MP and SC as exposures, make it apparent that high SC is protective against low MP's effect on PA for boys in the lower MP quartiles. This protective effect was not as clear in females, with the risk of low PA in females being similar for those with low MP regardless of SC level with increased risk removed in those with low SC and high MP after adjusting for age, BMI and SES. It appears that by improving either of MP or SC in children, their risk of low participation in PA is lessened and that improved SC may moderate the negative effect of low MP particularly for boys.

30.4 DISCUSSION

It is clear that SC has an important role in regard to MP and PA. The ANOVA and t test results demonstrate that the higher your MP and the more socially competent you are, participation in PA was higher. Multiple regression models demonstrate that MP and SC are independent contributors to PA participation in both genders. The result adding parental education into the male model reflects the role that a more educated parent would be more aware of the social worth and benefits of promoting PA in early years (Cairney *et al.*, 2009). The impact of SC was evident in the odds ratios, distinguishing that low MP and low SC negatively affect one's participation in PA. Therefore, being socially competent was uncovered as a facilitator of PA in younger years, where we adapt our healthy lifestyle choices. Since social competence is far more amenable to change than motor performance this aspect of a child's makeup should receive significant attention in the development of physical activity promotion programmes.

We cannot conclude causation with a cross sectional study. There was no information on ethnicity or pubertal stage. The ethnicity was homogeneous and the age suggests most if not all at the same Tanner Stage. Self-report bias may exist with the use of questionnaires. However, both have been validated against higher measurement tools. The categorization of key components in our study eliminates their continuous nature. However, MP quartiles are commonly used, and z scores maintain a continuous nature by using measures of central tendency to categorize. Social competence plays an independent role in children's physical activity and moderates the detrimental effects of motor incompetence.

30.5 REFERENCES

Cairney, J., Hay, J., Veldhuizen, S. and Faught, B.E., 2010, Trajectories of cardiorespiratory fitness with and without developmental coordination disorder: a longitudinal analysis. *British Journal of Sports Medicine,* **45**, pp. 1196-1201.

Cairney, J., Hay, J.A., Veldhuizen, S., Missiuna, C. and Faught, B.E., 2009, Developmental coordination disorder, sex, and activity deficit over time: a longitudinal analysis of participation trajectories in children with and without coordination difficulties. *Developmental Medicine and Child Neurology*, **52**, pp. E67-72.

Daniels, S.R., Greer, F.R. and Committee of Nutrition 2008, Lipid screening and cardiovascular health in childhood. *Pediatrics,* **122**, pp. 198-208.

Dewey, D., Kaplan, B.J., Crawford, S.G. and Wilson, B.M., 2002, Developmental coordination disorder: Associated problems in attention, learning, and psychosocial adjustment. *Human Movement Science,* **21**, pp. 905-918.

Early Childhood Development, 2009, In World Health Organization. Retrieved from http://www.who.int/mediacentre/factsheets/fs332/en/.

Harter, S., 1982, The Perceived Competence Scale for Children. *Child Development,* **53**, pp. 87-97.

Hay, J. A., 1992, Adequacy in and predilection for activity. *Clinical Journal of Sport Medicine*, **2**, pp. 192-201.

Lee, A., Hankin, B.L. and Mermelstein, R.J., 2010, Perceived social competence, negative social interactions and negative cognitive style predict depressive symptoms during adolescence. *Journal of Clinical Child and Adolescent Psychology,* **39**, pp. 603-615.

Rovniak, L.S., Anderson, E.S., Winett, R.A. and Stephens, R.S., 2002, Social cognitive determinants of physical activity in young adults: A prospective structural equation analysis. *Annals of Behavioural Medicine*, **24**, pp. 149-156.

ASSOCIATION BETWEEN BONE MINERAL DENSITY AND PHYSICAL ACTIVITY IN 12-TO-14-YEAR-OLD UNDERWEIGHT BOYS

D. Vaitkeviciute, E. Lätt, J. Mäestu, M. Saar, P. Purge, T. Jürimäe, K. Maasalu, and J. Jürimäe

University of Tartu, Estonia

31.1 INTRODUCTION

Optimising peak bone mineral parameters during adolescence is an important factor for the prevention of osteoporosis in later years. The pubertal growth spurt is the period of rapid acceleration in the growth velocity of almost all skeletal tissue. Usually studies have examined differences in bone mineral density (BMD) between underweight adolescents attributed to diseases such as anorexia nervosa and their normal weight peers (Castro *et al.*, 2002; Misra *et al.*, 2008). Vigorous physical activity has been related to BMD in adolescent boys (Garcia-Marco *et al.*, 2011). However, most studies of physical activity (PA) and bone mineral parameters in adolescents have been carried out on elite sporting populations, while normally active underweight adolescent boys have not been widely studied. The aim of this study was to investigate the relationship between BMD, body composition and PA parameters in underweight boys during pubertal growth spurt and to compare the results with normal weight boys.

31.2 METHODS

Participants were 145 boys between the ages of 12 and 14 years and they were divided into underweight (BMI ≤ 15.84 kg/m^2) and normal weight (BMI $\geq 15.85 - 21.91$ kg/m^2) groups. The cut-off points for BMI were set according to Cole *et al.* (2007). Pubertal development was assessed according to Tanner (1962) and years from peak height velocity (APHV) were calculated (Mirwald *et al.*, 2002). Bone age was assessed with an X-ray of the left hand and wrist, and determined according to the method of Greulich and Pyle (1959). Bone mineral and body composition parameters were measured by DPX-IQ densitometer (Lunar Corporation, Madison, WI, USA) for whole body (WB), lumbar spine (LS) and femoral neck (FN). A uniaxial accelerometer (Actigraph GT1M; Monrovia, USA) was used to assess PA for 7 days. At least 3 days of recording with the minimum of 8 hours recording per day was set as an inclusive criterion. Total PA (TPA) was calculated as the total number of counts divided by total daily registered time (counts/min). Moderate-to-vigorous PA (MVPA; >3 METs) was calculated as the sum of moderate and vigorous PA. Standard statistical methods were used to calculate the means and standard deviations ($\pm$ SD). Normality of parameters was controlled by a Shapiro-Wilks test. An unpaired, two-tailed t-test was used to compare the differences between groups. Pearson correlation coefficients and multiple regression analyses controlled for body mass and pubertal stage were applied to examine relationships of FFM, FM, TPA and MVPA with BMD parameters. The level of significance was set at $p < 0.05$.

31.3 RESULTS

Underweight and normal weight adolescent boys significantly differed by anthropometric, body composition, maturity and BMD parameters (Table 31.1). WB, FN and LS BMD values were positively correlated with TPA and MVPA in the underweight group (Table 31.2).

Table 31.1 Comparison between the measured parameters of underweight and normal weight.

	Underweight (n = 17)	Normal weight (n = 128)
Age (y)	12.9 ± 0.6	13.0 ± 0.7
Bone age (y)	11.9 ± 0.9	$12.8 \pm 1.3*$
Pubertal stage (1/2/3/4/5)	(0/4/10/3/0)	(0/13/60/43/12)
APHV (y)	-1.4 ± 0.7	$-0.7 \pm 0.8*$
Height (cm)	154.1 ± 6.2	$161.9 \pm 9.5*$
Body mass (kg)	36.1 ± 3.2	$49.4 \pm 7.5*$
BMI (kg/m^2)	15.2 ± 0.7	$18.7 \pm 1.5*$
Fat mass (kg)	4.7 ± 1.4	$8.8 \pm 3.5*$
Fat free mass (kg)	29.4 ± 3.2	$38.3 \pm 7.3*$
BMD$_{WB}$ (g/cm^2)	0.913 ± 0.045	$1.007 \pm 0.068*$
BMD$_{FN}$ (g/cm^2)	0.839 ± 0.093	$0.939 \pm 0.106*$
BMD$_{LS}$ (g/cm^2)	0.761 ± 0.069	$0.886 \pm 0.111*$
TPA (counts/min)	491.8 ± 187.3	486.9 ± 159.3
MVPA (min/day)	62.7 ± 32.2	58.7 ± 26.1

* Significantly different from underweight group ($p < 0.05$).

In normal weight boys only BMD$_{FN}$ was positively related to measured PA parameters. FM was negatively correlated with BMD$_{FN}$ in underweight group, whereas all BMD parameters were positively correlated with FFM. In addition, BMD$_{FN}$ and BMD$_{LS}$ values were negatively correlated with FM in normal weight group (Table 31.2). Stepwise multiple regression analysis indicated that MVPA ($R^2 = 0.336$) and FM ($R^2 = 0.289$) were the best predictors ($p < 0.05$) of BMD_{FN} in underweight boys, while FFM was the most important predictor ($p < 0.05$) for BMD_{LS} ($R^2 = 0.494$) and BMD_{FN} ($R^2 = 0.341$) in normal weight boys.

Table 31.2 Correlations between BMD, body composition and physical activity controlled for body mass and pubertal stage in underweight (U) and normal weight (N) pubertal boys.

		FM (kg)	FFM (kg)	TPA (counts/min)	MVPA (min/day)
BMD_{WB} (g/cm^2)	U	.114	-.160	.530[*]	.567[*]
	N	-.007	.589[*]	.115	.105
BMD_{FN} (g/cm^2)	U	-.577[*]	.200	.546[*]	.580[*]
	N	-.188[*]	584[*]	.293[*]	.272[*]
BMD_{LS} (g/cm^2)	U	-.126	-.022	.496[*]	.545[*]
	N	-.229[*]	.703[*]	.003	-.007

[*] Correlations are significant at the 0.05 level.

31.4 DISCUSSION

The major factor for thinness in adolescents is due to malnutrition, but thin adolescents are not undernourished necessarily. Underweight adolescent boys are largely under studied compared with underweight girls or overweight and obese adolescents. Our current study mainly focused on healthy underweight boys during the pubertal growth spurt.

Both groups of adolescents in our study satisfied the recommendation of Physical Activity Guidelines for children and adolescents to spend 60 min in MVPA per day (DHHS). However, stepwise multiple regression analysis showed that this amount of PA was not related to any of the BMD parameters in the normal weight group. In contrast, MVPA had an influence on BMD_{FN} in underweight boys. Underweight boys had significantly lower FFM compared with normal weight boys. According to Misra et al. (2008), one of the best predictors of BMD in underweights is FFM, but we did not find any associations between FFM and BMD parameters in underweight group. However, in the normal weight group, FFM was the main factor that had a positive association with BMD_{LS} and BMD_{FN} values similarly to other results (Pietrobelli et al., 2002).

The difference between constitutionally thin and anorexic (AN) adolescents in body composition and BMD was reported by Galusca et al., (2008) who stated that constitutionally thin subjects had higher percentage of FM than AN subjects but similar BMD_{LS} and BMD_{FN}, and these values were lower in comparison with normal weight controls. BMI is known as an important predictor of low BMD, emphasizing that body weight recovery is critical (Misra et al., 2008). It has been shown that the decline in bone mineral mass still continues despite the recovery of normal weight in adolescents with AN (Castro *et al.*, 2002).

Our study supports the findings of Artero *et al.* (2010) that there is a need for PA programmes that are specially designed for improving health-related fitness in underweights and the main aim of this programme should be to increase FFM in underweight adolescents. This was also indicated by our study that showed significant contribution of FFM to BMD_{FN} in normal weight subjects but no such relation was found in underweight boys. In conclusion, underweight boys have lower BMD compared with normal weight peers during pubertal growth spurt and PA should be kept as one of the major factors that increase BMD through increasing FFM in underweight adolescents.

31.5 REFERENCES

Artero, E.G., Espana-Romero, V., Ortega, F.B., Jimenez-Pavon, D., Ruiz, J.R., Vicente-Rodríguez, G., Bueno, M., Marcos, A., Gómez-Martínez, S., Urzanqui, A., González-Gross, M., Moreno, L.A., Gutiérrez, A. and Castillo, M.J., 2010, Health-related fitness in adolescents: underweight, and not only overweight, as an influencing factor. The AVENA study. *Scandinavian Journal of Medicine and Science in Sports*, **20**, pp. 418–427.

Castro, J., Toro, J., Lazaro, L., Pons, F. and Halperin, I., 2002, Bone mineral density in male adolescents with anorexia nervosa. *Journal of the American Academy of Child and Adolescent Psychiatry*, **41**, pp. 613–618.

Cole, T.J., Flegal, K.M., Nicholls, D. and Jackson, A.A., 2007, Body mass index cut offs to define thinness in children and adolescents: international survey. *British Medical Journal*, **335**, pp. 194–201.

Galusca, B., Zouch, M., Germain, N., Bossu, C., Frere, D., Lang, F., Lafage-Proust, M.H., Thomas, T., Vico, L. and Estour, B., 2008, Constitutional thinness: unusual human phenotype of low bone quality. *The Journal of Clinical Endocrinology and Metabolism*, **93**, pp. 110–117.

Garcia-Marco, L., Moreno, L.A., Ortega, F.B., Leon, F., Sioen, I., Kafatos, A., Martinez-Gomez, D. Widhalm, K., Castillo, M.J., Vicente-Rodríguez, G. and HELENA Study Group, 2011, Levels of physical activity that predicts optimal bone mass in adolescents: The HELENA Study. *American Journal of Preventive Medicine*, **40**, pp. 599–607.

Greulich, W.W. and Pyle, S.I., 1959, *Radiographic Atlas of Skeletal Development of Hand and Wrist,* 2nd ed., (California: Stanford University Press).

Mirwald, R.L., Baxter-Jones, A.D., Bailey, D.A. and Beunen, G.P., 2002, An assessment of maturity from anthropometric measurements. *Medicine and Science in Sports and Exercise*, **34**, pp. 689–694.

Misra, M., Katzman, D.K., Cord, J., Manning, S.J., Mendes, N., Herzog, D.B., Miller, K.K. and Klibanski, A., 2008, Bone metabolism in adolescent boys with anorexia nervosa. *Journal of Clinical Endocrinology and Metabolism*, **93**, pp. 3029–3036.

Pietrobelli, A., Faith, M.S., Wang, J., Brambilla, P., Chiumello, G. and Heymsfield, S.B., 2002, Association of lean tissue and fat mass with bone mineral content in children and adolescents. *Obesity Research*, **10**, pp. 56–60.

Tanner, J., 1962, *Growth at Adolescence*, 2nd ed., (Oxford: Blackwell Scientific Publications).

OBJECTIVELY ASSESSED PHYSICAL ACTIVITY AND GUIDELINE COMPLIANCE: THE MIDLANDS ADOLESCENT LIFESTYLE STUDY

M.J. Coelho-e-Silva[1], I. Rego[1], J.P. Rodrigues[1], E.S. Cyrino[2], and A.M. Machado-Rodrigues[1]

[1]University of Coimbra, Portugal; [2]Londrina State University, Brazil

32.1 INTRODUCTION

Adolescence is characterized by an increasing amount of sedentary behaviours and acquisition of unhealthy dietary behaviours, all of which increase the risk of obesity. The need to promote regular involvement in physical activity (PA) in young people is recognized by public health authorities throughout the world as an important health-related strategy in part because children and adolescents with overweight and obesity have a higher risk of co-morbidities (Strong *et al.*, 2005). Evidence relating to PA and health emphasizes that adolescents should spend at least 60 min in moderate to vigorous physical activity (MVPA) each day, to promote a broad range of health improvements (Strong *et al.*, 2005). However, data derived from objective measurements of PA such as accelerometry in adolescents to determine the prevalence reaching that PA guideline varies across countries and also within a specific country. Given that the youth from Southern European countries have the highest prevalence of overweight and obesity in Europe (Sardinha *et al.*, 2010) and the apparent decline of physical activity and the high level of sedentariness among adolescents still require complementary research in different cultural contexts, the main purpose of this study was to assess the proportion of adolescents in a Midlands Portuguese sample that met the guidelines of 60 min of MVPA on week days and at the weekend.

32.2 METHODS

The *Midlands Adolescent Lifestyle Study* (MALS) was a school-based study conducted in Midlands of Portugal which was part of a cross-sectional survey of the prevalence of overweight/obesity in Portugal (Sardinha *et al.*, 2010). The sample comprised 580 youth aged 11 to 18 years, 253 males and 327 females. The research was approved by the Scientific Committee of the University of Coimbra.

Informed consent was provided by parents and pupils. Height and weight were measured with participants in t-shirt and shorts, and without shoes.

The *GT1M Actigraph* accelerometer was used and placed over the hip. The sampling period was set at 1 minute as in other studies of adolescents (Troiano *et al.*, 2008). Participants who did not complete a minimum of 600 min of accelerometer data per day (after removing sequences of 20 or more consecutive zero counts) were excluded from subsequent analyses. MVPA was estimated for 5 consecutive days (3 week days and both weekend days). The threshold of MVPA was determined using age-specific regression equations published in Trost and colleagues (Trost *et al.*, 2002). These criteria have been used in epidemiological studies of youth (Troiano *et al.*, 2008).

Percentage of youth engaged in 60 min of continuous MVPA each day was calculated to determine how many participants met recommended physical activity guidelines.

32.3 RESULTS

Percentages of active adolescents who met the international PA guideline (≥ 60 min of MVPA per day, ≥ 5 days/week) for week and weekend days are presented in graphs 1 and 2. On week days, over 86% of the males and 64% of the females met that international PA guideline at the 13–14 year-old; corresponding values for 17–18 year-old age group were 5% and 3%, respectively – (Figure 32.1).

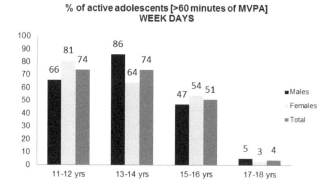

Figure 32.1. Prevalence of adolescents who achieve 60 minutes of moderate-to-vigorous physical activity per day, by sex and age group on week days.

At the weekend (Figure 32.2), over half of 11–12 year-old youth from both sexes met the PA guideline; however, just about 8% of 17–18 year-old participants fulfilled the 60 min of MVPA on a daily basis – (Figure 32.2). Compliance with this PA guideline decreased markedly with age in both male and female youth, particularly from 13–14 years to 17–18 years on week days and from 11–12 years to 17–18 years at the weekend.

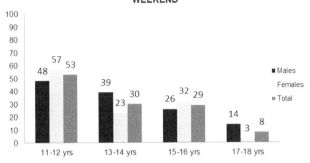

Figure 32.2. Prevalence of adolescents who achieve 60 minutes of moderate-to-vigorous physical activity per day, by sex and age group at the weekend.

32.4. DISCUSSION

The current survey was conducted in five out of six districts from Portuguese Midlands and describes the PA guideline compliance among adolescents aged 11–18 years. The main finding revealed that compliance with this PA guideline decreased markedly with age in both male and female youth. The findings also support the notion that males and females dramatically decreased their PA at the weekend. To our knowledge, this is the first quantification of PA using objective measures to evaluate compliance with guidelines in Portuguese youth from the Midlands.

Previous studies from different geographic contexts have reported worrying rates of the compliance with PA guidelines, especially in late adolescence. For example, in the USA, only 42% of children and an alarming 6–8% of adolescents achieved the recommended levels of PA objectively assessed (Troiano *et al.,* 2008). In contrast, based on accelerometry data, among 9-year-olds, 75.2% of the girls and 90.5% of the boys met the Norwegian PA guidelines of 60 min of moderate-intensity physical activity every day (Kolle *et al.,* 2010); the corresponding value among the 15-year-olds was 49.9% among females and 54.1% among male adolescents. Recently, in Portugal, and according to the recommendations of, 36% of participants age 10–11 years (boys = 51.6%, girls = 22.5%) and 4% age 16–17 years (boys = 7.9%, girls = 1.2%) were considered sufficiently active, achieving at least 60 min/day of MVPA (Baptista *et al.,* 2012). Accurate estimates of how many males and females can be classified as inactive according to the current recommendations are clouded by methodological inconsistencies, such as the selected epoch, the number of measured days, the number of hours representing a single day, among others. Limitations of the study should be recognized. The study is cross-sectional in design. In addition, the PA assessment was limited to the number of accelerometers available. In spite of all data collection being done in the springtime, youth were measured over several months. In summary, the present study examined the PA guidelines compliance of adolescents from Portuguese Midlands. The findings indicate the majority of the females failed to meet the current guideline of 60 min of continuous MVPA per day. The prevalence of inactivity increased at the weekend for both sexes.

32.5 ACKNOWLEDGMENT AND CONTRIBUTIONS

Data collection was obtained by students: (i) supervised by MJCS (Aristides Machado-Rodrigues, Ana Simões, Joana Amaral, Arlindo Araújo, José M. Gonçalves, Vítor Coelho, Nuno Dias); (ii) co-supervised by MJCS and AMR (José Alfredo Proença, Juliana Cordeiro, Vanessa Nunes, Paulo Francisco); (iii) co-supervised by MJCS and IR (Carlos Santos). JPR organized the full database. ESC critically reviewed the final document. All authors approved the final version.

32.6. REFERENCES

Baptista, F., Santos, D., Silva, A.M., Mota J., Santos, R., Vale, S., Pereira, J.P., Raimundo, A.M., Moreira H. and Sardinha L.B., 2012, Prevalence of the Portuguese population attaining sufficient physical activity. *Medicine and Science in Sports and Exercise,* 7, pp. 369–374.

Sardinha, L.B., Santos, R., Vale, S., Silva, A.M., Ferreira J.P., Raimundo A.M., Moreira, H., Baptista, F. and Mota, J., 2010, Prevalence of overweight and obesity among Portuguese youth: A study in a representative sample of 10-18-year-old children and adolescents. *International Journal of Pediatric Obesity,* pp. 1–5.

Strong, W.B., Malina R.M., Blimkie, C.J., Daniels, S.R., Dishman, R.K., Gutin, B., Hergenroeder, A.C., Must, A., Nixon, P.A., Pivarnik, J.M., Rowland, T., Trost, S. and Trudeau, F., 2005, Evidence based physical activity for school-age youth. *Journal of Pediatrics*, 146, pp. 732–733.

Troiano, R.P., Berrigan, D., Dodd, K.W., Masse, L.C., Tilert, T. and McDowell, M., 2008, Physical activity in the United States measured by accelerometer. *Medicine and Science in Sports and Exercise,* 40, pp. 181–188.

Trost, S.G., Pate, R.R., Sallis, J.F., Freedson, P.S., Taylor, W. C., Dowda, M. and Sirard, J., 2002, Age and gender differences in objectively measured physical activity in youth. *Medicine and Science in Sports and Exercise,* 34, pp. 350–355.

PHYSICAL ACTIVITY INTENSITY OF THE WII DANCE GAME FOR CHILDREN 6—9 YEARS OF AGE

C.L.P. Romanzini, M.B. Batista , G. Blasquez, T.H. Volpato, E.S. Cyrino, M. Romanzini, and E.R.V. Ronque

Londrina State University, Brazil

33.1 INTRODUCTION

Technological advances have enabled new forms of physical activity by means of "exergames" (EXGs), which are "a combination of physical exercise with games" (Sinclair *et al.*, 2007). This new form of physical activity can be considered a technology with great potential for encouraging the practice of physical activities, especially among children and adolescents (Biddiss and Irwin, 2010). A very successful game that uses dance is the Dance Dance Revolution (DDR), which combines music, rhythm and physical exercises (Höysniemi, 2006). Epstein (2007) observed that the use of DDR motivates children to be more active, when compared with the interactive bicycle game. More recently, the Just Dance game has been spread among Nintendo Wii players, which consists of reproducing the movements shown on screen using a controller with a motion sensor that is picked up by the console (Nintendo, 2009). Some studies have shown that in the short term, the use of active videogames increased the levels of physical activity in children, thereby increasing their energy expenditure (Mhurchu *et al.*, 2008; Bailey and McInnis, 2011) and that the use of active videogames provided energy expenditure similar to other physical activities such as: fast walking, jumping, running and climbing stairs (Maddison *et al.*, 2007). Accordingly, the aim of this study was to determine what is the physical activity intensity that the Just Dance Kids game offers to children 6–9 years old.

33.2. METHOD

Study participants were six children, all girls, aged 6–9 years, practitioners of jazz in a School of Dance in the city of Londrina / PR / Brazil. To participate in the study, after authorization provided by the School of Dance, parents also provided consent for children to participate by signing an Informed Consent Form. The study was approved by the local Ethics Committee on Human Research. The Just Dance Kids game for Nintendo Wii was used in two alternate sessions during 1 week, each session lasting 40 min. Data collection occurred on October 2012 and was performed by a single researcher. To assess the level of physical activity intensity, GT3X ActiGraph accelerometers were used and the data were recorded in units of counts.15seg^{-1}. Before data collection, participants were submitted to a process of familiarization with the game, since it occurred through different choreographic sequence for each song. For each session of activities, a sequence of different songs was selected. Each period of physical activity related to units of counts.15seg^{-1} was classified according to cutoffs proposed by Evenson *et al.* (2008), which are defined as: sedentary (0–25 counts.15seg^{-1}), light (26–573 counts.15seg^{-1}), moderate (574–1002 counts.15seg^{-1}) and vigorous (greater than or equal to 1003 counts.15seg^{-1}).

For data analysis, the IBM SPSS Statistics 20.0 software for Windows was used and firstly, the data normality was verified through the Kolgomorov Smirnov test. Since data were not normally distributed and the number of subjects in the sample was small, nonparametric procedures were used by applying the Wilcoxon signed rank test for comparing the values of physical activity intensity corresponding to the magnitude vector for both physical activity sessions. The significance level adopted was p <0.05.

33.3 RESULTS

The physical activity intensity values through dance game for Nintendo Wii in both physical activity sessions with children are shown in magnitude vector (counts.15seg^{-1}) in Table 33.1. The physical activity sessions conducted with children through the use of the Just Dance Kids dance game were characterized in different physical activity intensity levels. The first session had mostly vigorous intensity (40.1%), followed by light (38.1%), moderate (18.3%) and sedentary (3.5%), while the second session had predominantly light intensity (55.1%), followed by moderate (22.3%), vigorous (20.1%) and sedentary (2.6%). The comparison between the means of both physical activity sessions showed significant difference (P <0.001).

Table 33.1 Physical activity intensity in the Just Dance Kids dance game during sessions.

	Mean and SD	Intensity	P
Session 01	932.06 ± 748.85	Vigorous	P<0.001
Session 02	638.44 ± 522.73	Light	

33.4 DISCUSSION

After the application of two physical activity sessions with the use of the Just Dance Kids dance game for Nintendo Wii with children aged 6–9 years, it was observed that the performance of 40 min of physical activity using this game, divided into two sessions of 20 min was sufficient to promote physical activity levels from light to vigorous intensity. However, it was observed that the physical activity levels of sessions were different. This may have occurred because the game allows the choice of different types of dance. The activity offered by exergames of intermittent nature performed for short periods of time can provide physical activity from light to moderate intensity (Maddison *et al.,* 2007; Maddison *et al.,* 2009; Biddiss and Irwin, 2010), and can also achieve vigorous intensities (Bailey and McInnis, 2001). In this sense, it is suggested that the Just Dance Kids dance game, performed through the use of exergames is potentially important to increase the physical activity intensity of children, making it a viable alternative for interventions with this population. However, the songs that will compose the physical activity session must be selected with caution, since they can influence the session intensity.

33.5 REFERENCES

Bailey, B.W. and Mcinnis, K., 2011, Energy cost of exergaming: A comparison of the energy cost of 6 forms of exergaming. *Archives of Pediatrics and Adolescent Medicine*, **165**, pp. 597–602.

Biddiss, E. and Irwin, J., 2010, Active video games to promote physical activity in children and youth: A systematic review. *Archives of Pediatrics and Adolescent Medicine*, **164**, pp. 664–672.

Epstein, L.H., Beecher, M.D., Graf, J.L. and Roemmich, J.N. 2007, Choice of interactive dance and bicycle games in overweight and nonoverweight youth, *Annals of Behavioral Medicine*, **33**, pp. 124–131.

Evenson, K.R., Catellier, D.J., Gill, K., Ondrak, K.S. and McMurray R.G., 2008, Calibration of two objective measures of physical activity for children. *Journal of Sports Sciences*, **26**, pp. 1557–65.

Höysniemi, J., 2006, International Survey on the Dance Revolution Game. *Computers in Entertainment*, **4**, pp. 1–30.

Maddison, R., Maddison, R., Mhurchu, C.N., Jull, A., Jiang Y., Prapavessis, H. and Rodgers, A., 2007, Energy expended playing video console games: An opportunity to increase children's physical activity? *Pediatric Exercise Science*, **19**, pp. 334–343.

Maddison, R., Foley, L., Mhurchu, C.N., Jull, A., Jiang, Y., Prapavessis, H., Rodgers, A., Vander Hoorn, S., Hohepa, M. and Schaaf D., 2009, Feasibility, design and conduct of a pragmatic randomized controlled trial to reduce overweight and obesity in children: The electronic games to aid motivation to exercise (eGAME) study. *BMC Public Health*, **146**, pp. 1–9.

Mhurchu, C.N., Maddison, R., Jiang, Y., Jull, A., Prapavessis, H. and Rodgers, A., 2008, Couch potatoes to jumping beans : A pilot study of the effect of active video games on physical activity in children. *International Journal of Behavioral Nutrition and Physical Activity*, **5**, pp. 1–5.

Sinclair, J., Hingston, P. and Masek, M., 2007, Considerations for the design of exergames. In *Proceedings of the 5th International Conference on Computer graphics and interactive techniques in Australia and Southeast*, Perth, edited by Rohl, A., (Perth: Australia), pp. 289–296.

CHAPTER NUMBER 34

VALIDITY OF ACCELEROMETER REGRESSION MODELS TO ESTIMATE METs IN ADOLESCENTS

D. Ohara[1], M.F. Souza[1], M. Romanzini[1], D.R.P. Silva[1], A.C. Dourado[1], E.R.V. Ronque[1], F. Adami[2], and E.S. Cyrino[1]
[1] Londrina State University, Brazil; [2] Faculty of Medicine of the ABC, Brazil

34.1 INTRODUCTION

Physical activity has been measured with self-report instruments such as questionnaires and interviews, mainly in large-scale research. In children and adolescents, these instruments must be used with care, because of their inability to accurately recall intensity, frequency and duration of the activities (Sirard and Pate, 2001). However, gold-standard methods such as doubly labeled water and indirect calorimetry are expensive and unfeasible in large-scale epidemiological studies. Therefore, advancements in technology have increased in both number and type of objective physical activity measurement devices including accelerometers. Accelerometers are lightweight electronic devices, able to measure and store accelerations in one to three axis. Nevertheless, the accelerometer output value, typically called "counts", still remains without a biological meaning. Thereby, different cut-points of physical activity intensity and predictive energy expenditure equations have been published. We examined the validity of two METs regression models of ActiGraph, the most widely used accelerometer (De Vries *et al.*, 2009).

34.2 METHODS

Seventy-nine adolescents aged 10–15 years (40 boys and 39 girls) enrolled from 5th to 8th grades from a public school of Londrina (Southern Brazil) and participated in the study. A comprehensive verbal description of the nature and purpose of the study was provided to the participants and their parents or tutors. Written informed consent was obtained from the adolescents' parent or legal guardian and all participants gave verbal consent. This study was approved by the local ethical committees and all procedures were in accordance with those outlined by the Declaration of Helsinki. Oxygen uptake and accelerometer data were collected by Cosmed K4b2 (Cosmed, Rome, Italy) portable metabolic system and ActiGraph (MTI Health Services, Fort Walton Beach, FL) model GT3X accelerometer, respectively. The subjects used the accelerometer and the portable metabolic unit at rest and during 11 activities at different intensities. The rest period and sedentary activities were conducted in an air-conditioning laboratory and the other physical activities were held in a ventilated gymnasium. The rest period lasted 20 min and all other activities were performed for 5 min. Subjects rested for 5 min between each activity. MET score was computed by dividing VO_2 (ml.kg.$^{-1}$min^{-1}) recorded in each activity by the VO_2 (ml.kg^{-1}.min^{-1}) value obtained at rest. Two regression models were examined: Freedson *et al.* (1997) (1.1) and Treuth *et al.* (2004) (1.2). Root mean squared error (RMSE), bias with 95%CI and analysis of variance (ANOVA) for repeated measures (comparisons between measured and predicted MET values for activities) were used. Statistical significance was set at $P<0.05$. All analyses were conducted using IBM SPSS Statistics 20.0 and GraphPad Prism 5 for Windows.

$$METs = 2.757 + (0.0015 \times cpm)-(0.08957 \times age)-(0.000038 \times cpm \times age) \quad (1.1)$$
$$METs = 2.01 + (0.000856 \times cpm) \quad (1.2)$$

where age = years and cpm = counts per minute.

34.3 RESULTS

The general characteristics of the sample are presented in Table 34.1. No significant difference was found between boys and girls for all variables. The RMSE between measured and predicted MET values were greater for the Freedson equation (1.7) than the Treuth model (1.5). Both Freedson and Treuth regression models overestimated MET values for all activities (Bias 0.54, 95% CI -2.8,3.9) and (Bias 0.54, 95% CI -2.5,3.6) respectively. Significant differences ($P<0.05$) were found between both regression models vs. measured MET values (Figure 34.1), but did not between models ($P>0.05$).

Table 34.1 General characteristics of the sample (n=79).

	All subjects (n=79)	Boys (n=40)	Girls (n=39)
Age (years)	12.5 (1.3)	12.6 (1.3)	12.5 (1.4)
Body Mass (kg)	48.5 (10.7)	48.8 (10.7)	48.3 (10.7)
Height (cm)	156.3 (8.8)	157.1 (9.3)	155.5 (8.2)
BMI (kg/m^2)	19.7 (3.2)	19.6 (3.1)	19.8 (3.4)

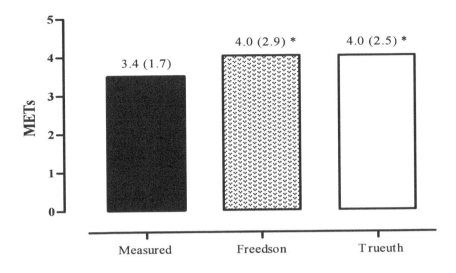

Figure 34.1 Comparison between measured and estimated METs values for all activities. *$P<0.05$ vs. Measured.

34.4 CONCLUSION

Our results suggest that the regression models analyzed in this study are inadequate to estimate the MET values in adolescents aged 10–15 years. Despite the Treuth model being developed only with girls, no significant differences were found when compared with the Freedson model which includes both sexes.

34.5 REFERENCES

De Vries S.I., Van Hirtum, H.W., Bakker, I., Hopman-Rock, M., Hirasing, R.A. and Van Mechelen, W., 2009, Validity and reproducibility of motion sensors in youth: a systematic update. *Medicine and Science in Sports and Exercise*, **41**, pp. 818–827.

Freedson, P., Sirard, J., Debold, E.,Pate, R.R., Dowda, M., Trost, S. and Sallis, J., 1997, Calibration of the Computer Science and Application Inc. (CSA). *Medicine and Science in Sports and Exercise*, **29**, pp. S45.

Sirard, J.R. and Pate, R.R., 2001, Physical activity assessment in children and adolescents. *Sports Medicine*, **31**, pp. 439–454.

Treuth, M.S., Schmitz, K., Catellier, D.J., McMurray, R.G., Murray, D.M., Almeida, M.J., Going, S., Norman, J.E. and Pate, R.R., 2004, Defining accelerometer thresholds for activity intensities in adolescent girls. *Medicine and Science in Sports and Exercise*, **36**, 1259–1266.

EFFECTS OF A 1-YEAR TRAINING PROGRAMME ON THE SKELETON OF DOWN SYNDROME CHILDREN

M Gavris[1,3], B. Ferry[1,4], S. Serbanoiu[2], I. Hantiu[3], K. Kiss[2], G. Lucaciu[3], C. Tifrea[2] and D. Courteix[1]

[1] Clermont Université, Université Blaise Pascal, EA 3533, Laboratoire des Adaptations Métaboliques à l'Exercice en Conditions Physiologiques et Pathologiques, Clermont-Ferrand, France; [2] Centre de Recherche Interdisciplinaire "Dr. Alexandru Partheniu", UNEFS Bucarest, Romania; [3] Research Center on Human Performance, Oradea University, Romania; [4] Université Limoges, Faculté des Sciences et Techniques, STAPS, Limoges, France

35.1 INTRODUCTION

Down syndrome (DS) is a genetic disability caused by the presence of all or part of an extra 21st chromosome (Lejeune *et al.,* 1959) which may be responsible for skeletal abnormalities, short stature and other mechanisms of premature aging (Roth *et al.,* 1996). Such disease is able to generate physiological and physical developmental disorders (Thibaut *et al.,* 2006). In recent years the life expectancy of this population has grown over 60 years (Bittles and Glasson, 2004). Osteoporosis has been identified in individuals with DS. Lower levels of bone mineral content (BMC) have been observed not only in adults (Angelopoulou *et al.,* 1999; Baptista *et al.,* 2005; Sakadamis *et al.,* 2002; Sepulveda *et al.,* 1995) but also in children and adolescents with Down syndrome (Gonzalez-Aguero *et al.,* 2010) compared with the general population. So bone fragility, and related fractures are expected to increase, being one of the main factors contributing to both premature morbidity and mortality in this population (Chaney and Eyman, 2000). Thyroid impairment, abnormalities of sexual development, musculoskeletal troubles as well as poor calcium and vitamin D intakes may contribute to the development of osteoporosis. Moreover, both paediatric and adult cohorts display a lower level of physical fitness (Fernhall *et al.,* 1996) than individuals without Down syndrome. The purpose of this study was to assess the effects of a 1-year training programme based upon impact activities on the skeleton of DS children.

35.2 METHOD

A group of 24 men and 18 women with Down syndrome, aged between 13 to 19 years participated in this study. Subjects were divided into two groups, non-exercising group (CTL, n=22, 14 males and 8 females) and exercising group (AP, n=20, 10 males and 10 females). They were selected from different schools and specialized institutions in Oradea and Bucharest, Romania. Parents and children were informed about the objectives and procedures. Written informed consent was obtained from all parents or subjects. All measurements were performed at baseline and after 1 year.

35.2.1 Anthropometric Measurements

Body height and body mass were measured. Skinfold thickness was assessed at bicipital, tricipital, subscapular and suprailiac regions of interest.

35.2.2 Bone Measurements

Bone mineral density at the lumbar spine and predominant hip was measured with dual-energy X-ray absorptiometry (Hologic QDR Explorer). Ultrasound bone attenuation (BUA) and speed of sound (SOS) were measured using an Achilles Insight device.

35.2.3 Training Programme

The subjects assigned in AP group participated in a programme of extra-curricular physical activities, sessions of 60 min two times a week, over 12 months. These training sessions were aimed at developing general physical abilities. Each child received a support person, students from the Faculty of Physical Education and Sport Oradea_who helped and encouraged. Each session had a content of 15 min warm-up, 60 min of moderate activity to vigorous exercises with gravitational impact (plyometric jumps, bodybuilding exercises, games and various tasks including: racing speed, slalom, jumps, obstacles, gymnastic routines, all in the form of dynamic games).

35.2.4 Statistical Analyses

All values were expressed as mean and standard deviation (SD). The Gaussian distribution of the variables was assessed using the Shapiro-Wilk test. Comparisons between groups were made using a one-way ANOVA (CTL / AP) with repeated measures (baseline / 1 year). In case of non Gaussian distribution, data were Ln-transformed. All analyses were conducted using SPSS software (PASW version 20).

35.3 RESULTS

The control and AP groups had increased their body mass (+ 0.55 ± 0.21 kg) and their body height (+0.9 ± 0.2 cm). The sum of skinfolds thickness did not change for CTL whereas it decreased significantly in EXE, suggesting a fat mass loss. As shown in Table 35.1, all the bone parameters had increased in both groups. It was noticeable that the AP group displayed higher increases for Neck, Total Hip and

Lumbar spine BMD's compared with CTL. There was no difference regarding the quantitative ultrasound parameters.

Table 35.1 Bone data at baseline and after intervention in CTL and AP groups. Significance is specified for interaction, time effect (duration of intervention) and group effect.

	DS-CTL		DS-AP		Inter action	Time effect	Group effect
	Baseline	End of intervention	Baseline	End of intervention			
BUA(dB/MHZ)	47.59±16.31	50.57±15.09	47.52±18.17	48.83±17.11	NS	.001	NS
SOS(m/s)	1579.5±15.4	1582±13.8	1580±17.1	1589±19.5	NS	.001	NS
Hip_BMC (g)	21.64±6.9	22.11±6.9	19.0±6.7	22.14±6.1	.001	.001	.001
LS_BMC (g)	43.48±10.5	46.00±8.8	42.46±8.6	46.03±7.1	NS	.002	NS
FN_BMD (g/cm²)	0.838±0.134	0.853±0.135	0.834±0.10	0.874±0.10	.008	.001	.002
Hip_BMD (g/cm²)	0.901±0.122	0.913±0.114	0.847±0.09	0.889±0.10	.008	.001	.017
LS_BMD (g/cm²)	0.925±0.128	0.938±0.127	0.875±0.157	0.924±0.154	.005	.001	.004
Troch_BMD (g/cm²)	0.69±0.121	0.74±0.104	0.674±0.07	0.757±0.08	NS	.001	NS

35.4 DISCUSSION AND CONCLUSION

The main result of the present study points out the responsiveness of the skeleton of Down syndrome subjects to mechanical constraints induced by physical exercise. One year of specific training had increased all the bone parameters in the two groups of subjects. This was due to a growth effect in this range of age (13 to 19 years). In addition, the trained group had increased Hip BMC and BMD, and Femoral Neck and Lumbar spine BMD more than the controls. Down syndrome disease seems to not disturb the response of bone tissue to a physical stress. The hip and lumbar spine sites were both improved by the practice, suggesting that axial and appendicular skeleton may respond to such stimulations. The lack of difference in improvement of bone quantitative ultrasound between groups can be explained by the less sensitivity of this measure, and the fact that the two groups were not different as regards the genetic disease. A previous study showed that patients with mental retardation have a marked reduction in BUA and SOS measurements at the heel, compared with age-matched control subjects (Aspray *et al.*, 1998). We did not compare our sample with healthy subjects, the purpose of the study being rather a study between DS subjects. Another study performed in subjects with genetic disorders and healthy controls, using quantitative ultrasound at hand phalanges (Halaba *et al.*, 2006) reported that, despite comparable improvement in measured ultrasound parameter in patients and controls observed over the study duration, the difference between them remained stable. The present results confirm that regular physical activity must be practiced in order to maintain bone integrity, especially in individuals with fracture risk. The benefit of physical activity was obtained after a 1-year period of specific training, suggesting that a long programme must be performed to reach this objective. In conclusion one can propose that an active lifestyle should be instituted as well as a programme of physical exercise characterized by impact loading, in order to improve the bone mass and therefore avoid the development of osteoporosis in individuals with Down syndrome.

35.5 REFERENCES

Angelopoulou, N., Souftas, V., Sakadamis, A., and Mandroukas, K. 1999. Bone mineral density in adults with Down's syndrome. *European Radiology,* **9**, pp. 648–651.

Aspray, T. J., Francis, R. M., Thompson, A., Quilliam, S. J., Rawlings, D. J., and Tyrer, S. P. 1998. Comparison of ultrasound measurements at the heel between adults with mental retardation and control subjects. *Bone,* **22**, pp. 665–668.

Baptista, F., Varela, A., and Sardinha, L. B. 2005. Bone mineral mass in males and females with and without Down syndrome. *Osteoporos Int,* **16**, pp. 380–388.

Bittles, A. H., and Glasson, E. J. 2004. Clinical, social, and ethical implications of changing life expectancy in Down syndrome. *Developmental Medicine Child Neurology,* **46**, pp. 282–286.

Chaney, R. H., and Eyman, R. K. 2000. Patterns in mortality over 60 years among persons with mental retardation in a residential facility. *Mental Retardation,* **38**, pp. 289–293.

Fernhall, B., Pitetti, K. H., Rimmer, J. H., McCubbin, J. A., Rintala, P., Millar, A. L., et al. 1996. Cardiorespiratory capacity of individuals with mental retardation including Down syndrome. *Medicine and Science in Sports and Exercise,* **28**, pp. 366–371.

Gonzalez-Aguero, A., Vicente-Rodriguez, G., Moreno, L. A., & Casajus, J. A. 2010. Bone mass in male and female children and adolescents with Down syndrome. *Osteoporosis International,* **22**, pp. 22.

Halaba, Z., Pyrkosz, A., Adamczyk, P., Drozdzowska, B., and Pluskiewicz, W. 2006. Longitudinal changes in ultrasound measurements: a parallel study in subjects with genetic disorders and healthy controls. *Ultrasound Medicine Biology,* **32**, 409–413.

Lejeune, J., Turpin, R., and Gautier, M. 1959. [Mongolism; a chromosomal disease (trisomy)]. *Bulletin Academic National Medicine,* **143**, pp. 256–265.

Roth, G. M., Sun, B., Greensite, F. S., Lott, I. T., & Dietrich, R. B. 1996. Premature aging in persons with Down syndrome: MR findings. *American Journal Neuroradiology,* **17**, pp. 1283–1289.

Sakadamis, A., Angelopoulou, N., Matziari, C., Papameletiou, V., and Souftas, V. 2002. Bone mass, gonadal function and biochemical assessment in young men with trisomy 21. *European Journal of Obstetric Gynecology Reproductive Biology,* **100**, pp. 208–212.

Sepulveda, D., Allison, D. B., Gomez, J. E., Kreibich, K., Brown, R. A., Pierson, R. N., Jr., *et al.* 1995. Low spinal and pelvic bone mineral density among individuals with Down syndrome. *American Journal of Mental Retardation,* **100**, pp. 109–114.

Thibaut, J. P., Elbouz, M., and Comblain, A. 2006. Apprentissage, mémorisation, et généralisation de nouveaux noms chez l'enfant trisomique 21. Une comparaison avec l'enfant en développement normal. *Psychologie Française,* **51**, pp. 413–426.

CHAPTER NUMBER 36

AGREEMENT OF PHYSICAL ACTIVITY ASSESSED BY OBJECTIVE AND SELF-REPORTED MEASURES: VARIATION BY WEIGHT STATUS

A.M. Machado-Rodrigues[1], J. Mota[2], and M.J. Coelho-e-Silva[1]

[1] University of Coimbra, Portugal; [2] Faculty of Sport, University of Porto, Portugal

36.1 INTRODUCTION

Physical activity (PA) in adolescence may contribute to the development of healthy adult lifestyles, helping reduce chronic disease incidence. However, research in PA associated with health outcomes is normally assessed by self-reported measures, which inevitably leads to misclassification. Therefore, adequate and comprehensive PA assessment techniques are needed to evaluate relationships between PA and indicators of health status, fitness and behaviour. PA tends to decrease, on average, with age. This decline in PA with age may be influenced by differences between overweight and normal-weight adolescents to recall information. Overweight and obese adults tend to overestimate involvement in PA compared to normal weight adults (Lee *et al.*, 1993). Differences between actual and reported involvement PA in normal weight and obese/overweight youth are less well documented, though McMurray *et al.* (2008) reported that overweight and obese girls aged 11–14 years were also more likely to overestimate involvement in moderate-to-vigorous PA. The purpose of this study was to evaluate the concordance between self-reported and objective estimates of activity energy expenditure (AEE) among female adolescents by weight status (normal weight and overweight/obese).

36.2 METHODS

The present study was part of a cross-sectional research which was approved by the *Portuguese Commission for Data Protection* and it is available elsewhere (Machado-Rodrigues *et al.*, 2012). The sample comprised 265 girls (13–16 years of age). Informed consent were provided by parents and pupils. ***Anthropometry:***

Height and weight were measured with participants in t-shirt and shorts, and without shoes. The body mass index (BMI) was calculated and adolescents were grouped into two groups: normal weight (NW) and overweight/obese (OW/OB) based in age- and gender-specific cut-offs (Cole *et al.*, 2000). ***Three-day diary:*** The diary protocol (Bouchard *et al.*, 1983) was used and participants were required to rate the intensity of the primary activity performed in each 15-min period using a numeric code ranging from one to nine. Energy expenditure (EE) was subsequently estimated from equivalents of the original version. ***Accelerometry:*** The *GT1M Actigraph* accelerometer was used and placed over the hip. The sampling period was set at 1 minute as in other studies of adolescents. Participants who did not complete a minimum of 600 min of accelerometer data per day (after removing sequences of 20 or more consecutive zero counts) were excluded from subsequent analyses. ***Data Reduction:*** The accelerometer was used for three consecutive days, the same days that the diary protocol was completed. The diary (Bouchard *et al.*, 1983) assumes a standard energy equivalent for all activity codes, including code 1 which represents resting activities (resting EE, REE). AEE was derived by subtracting REE ($0.26 \text{ kcal kg}^{-1} 15 \text{ min}^{-1}$) from daily energy expenditure (DEE). For accelerometry, average counts per minute were converted to AEE using the equation proposed by Trost (Trost *et al.*, 1998). Activity counts were strongly correlated with indirect calorimetry EE ($r=0.86$). ***Statistical Analysis:*** Partial correlations between methods controlling for body mass were calculated by weight status. Fisher's r to z transformation procedure was used to determine the variability in magnitude of correlations. According to Nevill and Atkinson (1997), and assuming a relation exists between the measurement differences (errors) and the mean, an analysis was conducted to determine the ratio limits of agreement using natural log transformed measurements. SPSS 15.0 was used for all the analyses.

36.3 RESULTS

Partial correlations between the diary and accelerometry, controlling for body mass, ranged between 0.39 and 0.42 (Table 36.1). The 3-day diary markedly underestimates AEE in overweight/obese. Table 36.2 summarises the mean of the log transformed measurement, and their mean differences, and the "limits of agreement". By observing the agreement ratios, the worst agreement was found on normal weight female group; although the bias ratio is not great, given as 0.94, the agreement ratio ($*/\div 1.73$) implies that 95% of ratios will lie between 173% of the mean bias (Table 36.2).

Table 36.1 Partial correlations (controlling for body mass) between estimates of activity energy expenditure by the diary and accelerometry, bias and its limits of agreement between two AEE estimates by weight status.

Weight status	# observed days	Partial		Bias	Agreement [1]		Trend
		r	p		Limits		
					Lower	Upper	
Nw	495	0.42	p<0.01	-0.11	-1.25	1.02	-0.05
Ow/Ob	156	0.39	p<0.01	-0.74	-2.36	0.89	0.07
		Δr=0.03	n.s.				

Nw (normal-weight); Ow/Ob (overweight + obese participants); [1] Diary – Accelerometry; ** (p<0.01).

Table 36.2 The log transformed (ln) measurement means and differences, the "ratio limits of agreement", together with the correlation between the absolute differences and the mean (log transformed) by weight status.

Weight status	# of days	Log transformed measurements			Ratio limits	Correlation *(abs(diff) v mean)*
		Mean 1 Diary	Mean 2 Accelerometry	Difference (SD)		
Nw	495	0.673	0.772	-0.065(0.28)	0.94(*/÷1.73)	-0.11**
Ow/Ob	156	0.975	1.230	-0.259(0.25)	0.77(*/÷1.64)	0.03

Nw (normal-weight); Ow/Ob (overweight + obese participants); ** (p<0.01).

36.4 DISCUSSION

This study examined the agreement of AEE derived from a 3-day diary and accelerometry relative to weight status in female adolescents. Bias ranged between -0.11 and -0.74. Since self-reported PA is prone to misreporting and the correlations between the 3-day diary and accelerometer were no more than moderate, results should be interpreted with caution. At higher intensity levels of AEE, overweight adolescents tended to overestimate PA, while the opposite tendency was observed among normal weight youth (Table 36.2). Previous research suggested that overweight and obese adolescents provided less accurate self-assessments of PA (McMurray *et al.*, 2008; Slootmaker *et al.*, 2009). American girls classified as overweight and obese, for example, had 17.7% and 19.4% fewer minutes of MVPA based on a self-instrument compared to normal weight girls (McMurray *et al.*, 2008). In contrast, European adolescents 12 to 18 years self-reported more time on moderate and vigorous PA compared to objective accelerometry data, and results significantly differed in all subgroups (i.e. gender, weight status, and education) (Slootmaker *et al.*, 2009). The current study suggests that the overweight/obese participants underestimated their AEE. Accordingly, further investigation is needed to examine the agreement between self-reported and objective measures at high intensity levels of PA. The results of the present study showed a moderate relationship between AEE assessed by accelerometry and a 3-day diary. The diary markedly underestimated AEE in overweight youth.

36.5 ACKNOWLEDGMENT AND CONTRIBUTION

The first author was supported by *Fundação para a Ciência e a Tecnologia*: [SFRH/BD/38988/2007]. AMR was supervised by JM and MJCS and obtained the PhD in December 2011. All authors approved the final version. The contributions of Robert M Malina, Joey C Einsemnann, Sean Cumming, Chris Riddoch, Lauren Sherar, Gaston Beunen, Enio Ronque, Edilson Cyrino, Cristina Padez, Rute Santos and António Figueiredo in the *Midlands Adolescent Lifestyle Study* (MALS) were appreciated.

36.6 REFERENCES

Bouchard, C., Tremblay, A., Leblanc, C., Lortie, G., Savard, R. and Theriault, G., 1983, A method to assess energy expenditure in children and adults. *American Journal of Clinical Nutrition*, **37**, pp. 461–467.

Cole, T.J., Bellizzi, M.C., Flegal, K.M. and Dietz, W.H., 2000, Establishing a standard definition for child overweight and obesity worldwide: International survey. *British Medical Journal*, **320**, pp. 1240–1243.

Lee, I.M., Cook, N.R. and Henneckens, C.H., 1993, Actual versus self-reported intake and exercise in obesity. *New England Journal of Medicine*, **328**, pp. 1494–1496.

Machado Rodrigues, A.M., Mota, J., Cumming, S.P., Eisenmann, J.C., Malina, R.M. and Coelho-e-Silva M.J., 2012, Concurrent validation of estimated activity energy expenditure using a 3-day diary and accelerometry in adolescents. *Scandinavian Journal of Medicine and Science in Sports*.

McMurray, R.G., Ward, D.S., Elder, J.P., Lyttle, L.A., Strikmiller, P.K. and Baggett, C.D., 2008, Do overweight girls over report physical activity? *American Journal of Health Behavior*, **32**, pp 538–546.

Nevill, A.M., and Atkinson, G., 1997. Assessing agreement between measurements recorded on a ratio scale in sports medicine and sports science. *British Journal of Sports Medicine*, **31**, pp. 314–318.

Slootmaker, S.M., Schuit, A.J., Chinapaw, M.J., Seidell, J.C., and van Mechelen, W., 2009, Disagreement in physical activity assessed by accelerometer and self-report in subgroups of age, gender, education and weight status. *International Journal of Behavioral Nutrition and Physical Activity*, **6**, pp.17.

Trost, S.G., Ward, D.S., Moorehead, S.M., Watson, P.D., Riner, W., and Burke, J. R., 1998. Validity of the computer science and applications (CSA) activity monitor in children. *Medicine and Science in Sports and Exercise*, **30**, pp. 629–633.

Part VIII

Sport Participation and The Young Athlete

DROP-OUT IN BRAZILIAN YOUTH TENNIS PLAYERS: A COMPARATIVE STUDY

F. de Oliveira Matos[1], R. Assis Garcia[1], D. Martin Samulski[1], and S. Soares da Silva[2]

[1]Federal University of Minas Gerais, Brazil; [2]Federal University of Rio Grande do Norte, Brazil

37.1 INTRODUCTION

In the late 90s and early 2000s, with the emergence of the phenomenon "Guga" (Gustavo Kuerten), the Brazilian tennis player who was three-time Roland Garros champion, when he finished the year ranked number one by the Association of Tennis Professionals (ATP). At this time, tennis became more popular in Brazil, with an exponential increase in the number of practitioners in the country, including children, young people and adults. However, the practice of tennis at a high level requires dedication, physical and psychological preparation. At this time, there is a concern regarding competitive pressures placed by the coach, family and the competition environment on junior players. Thus, one of the major problems involving children and competition is burnout. According to Smith (1986), burnout is a psychological, emotional and physical withdrawal from a formerly pursued and enjoyable sport as a result of excessive stress over time. Burnout, a negative effect of stress from training and competition, impairs the quality of life of the athletes, causing the abandonment of the sport and abbreviating careers (Gould *et al.,* 1996). Since this phenomenon can be deleterious to the athlete's career, researchers and coaches should investigate the possible reasons that lead young people to abandon competitive tennis practice. Thus, the main purpose of this study is to compare gender and age to increase knowledge of the topic in a Brazilian sample. Also, we hope that our results will support coaches in the development of training programmes and competitions that encourage young people to maintain involvement in sports like tennis.

37.2 METHODS

Data collection for this study was approved by the Ethics Committee in Research of the Federal University of Minas Gerais (ETIC 650/08) and all procedures were in accordance with the Declaration of Helsinki. The sample included 71 tennis players (30 girls), age 12–18 years (15.36 ± 1.64 years) and sport practice between 3 and 9 years (5.98 ± 1.47 years), who were involved in competition at national level in their respective age groups, 14 (N = 22), 16 (N = 28) and 18 (N = 21) years, according to the Brazilian Tennis Confederation. The athletes and parents were informed about the aim and design of the study, and signed informed consent was obtained prior to data collection.

The reasons for drop-out were determined with the subscale of the Motivos de Início, Manutenção, Troca e Abandono Esportivo, MIMCA-BR (Carmo *et al.*, 2008). The instrument consists of 10 items that address the possible reasons for the abandonment of the sport. The answers are given on a Likert scale of 5 points (totally agree) 1(totally disagree). This instrument has shown good internal consistency in several studies. Cronbach's alpha range between .82 and .94 (Lucas, Alonso and Izquierdo, 2003; Carmo *et al.*, 2008).

Description of variables was made through median, minimum and maximum values. For the interpretation of data we used a Mann-Whitney test to compare gender and Kruskal-Wallis for age. Data were analyzed with SPSS for Windows (version 15.0) and we adopted a significance level of $p<.05$.

37.3 RESULTS

Initial data screening showed that all variables did not meet assumptions of normality. Thus there were no statistical significance between gender and age, ($p>.05$). However, "injuries that preclude them from training" was the main reason given for the possible drop-out of tennis (median 4) (Vide graph 37.1).

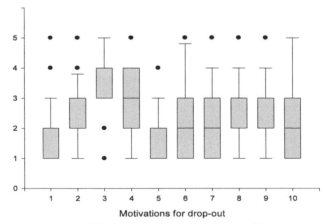

Graph 37.1 Motives for drop-out tennis competition.

Tables 37.1 and 37.2 show the median, minimum and maximum values found in the subscale of drop-out comparing gender and age.

Table 37.1 Descriptive scores for drop-out according gender.

Itens	Minimum		Maximum		Median	
	Male	Female	Male	Female	Male	Female
A1	1	1	5	4	1	1
A2	1	1	4	5	3	3
A3	2	1	5	5	4	3,5
A4	1	1	5	5	3	2,5
A5	1	1	4	4	1	1
A6	1	1	5	5	2	2
A7	1	1	5	5	2	2
A8	1	1	5	5	3	3
A9	1	1	5	5	3	2
A10	1	1	5	5	2	2

Table 37.2 Descriptive scores for drop-out according age.

Itens	Minimum			Maximum			Median		
	14	16	18	14	16	18	14	16	18
A1	1	1	1	5	4	4	1	1	1
A2	1	1	1	5	5	5	3	3	3
A3	1	2	1	5	5	5	4	4	4
A4	1	1	1	5	5	5	3,5	3	2
A5	1	1	1	4	4	3	1	1	1
A6	1	1	1	5	5	5	2	2,5	2
A7	1	1	1	5	5	4	2	3	2
A8	1	1	1	5	5	5	2,5	3	3
A9	1	1	1	5	5	5	2	3	3
A10	1	1	1	5	5	5	3	2	2

According to the results, "injury" had great prominence in relation to other possible reasons for the drop-out of the tennis competitions. This finding is also presented in other studies that have investigated possible reasons for drop-out of Brazilians and Spaniards (Rodriguez, Alonso and Lucas, 1999), and in retrospective studies such as that of Bara Filho and García (2008) in Spanish athletes, and Samulski et al. (2009) who identified the reasons for retirement in elite sports in Brazil. According to Gould et al. (1996), by the fact that high demands of training and competitions during adolescence make young players reach higher levels of physical and psychological stress, which can increase susceptibility to injury and drop-out of competitive tennis, shortening promising careers.

37.4 CONCLUSION

The results showed that the main reason for the dropout of competitive tennis by young Brazilian athletes are injuries that preclude the involvement in sports. Researchers have not found statistical differences between gender and between ages. Thus, there should be more attention from coaches in the preparation and control of training programmes in order to prevent injuries and possible shortening of promising careers.

37.5 REFERENCES

Bara Filho, M.G. and Garcia, F.G., 2008, Motivos do abandono no esporte competitivo: Um estudo retrospectivo. *Revista Brasileira de Educação Física e Esportes*, **22**, pp. 293–300.

Carmo, J., Matos, F.O., Bara Filho, M., Miranda, R., Ribas, P., Alonso, J.L.N. and Lucas, J.M., 2008, Validação preliminar de Questionário de Início, Manutenção, Mudança e Abandono (MIMCA) no Esporte para a língua Portuguesa. *Revista Conexões*, **6**, pp. 540–551.

Gould, D., Tuffey, S., Udry, E. and Loehr, J., 1996, Burnout in competitive junior tennis players: II Qualitative analysis. *The Sport Psychologist,* **10**, pp. 341–366.

Lucas, J.M-A., Alonso, J.L.N. and Izquierdo, J.G.N., 2003, La Evolución motivacional como criterio discriminante de los deportes. *Revista Latinoamericana de Psicología,* **35**, pp. 1–23.

Rodríguez, G.M., Alonso, J.L.N. and Lucas, J.M.A., 1999, *Motivos, motivación y deporte,* (Salamanca: Tesitex).

Samulski, D.M., Moraes, L.C.C.A., Ferreira, R.M., Marques, M.P., Silva, L.A., Lôbo, I.L.B., Matos, F.O., Santiago, M.L.M. and Ferreira, C.H.S., 2009, Análise das transições das carreiras de ex-atletas de alto nível. *Motriz,* **15**, pp. 310–317.

Smith, R., 1986, Toward a cognitive-affective model of athletic burnout. *Journal of Sport Psychology,* **8**, pp. 36–50.

SYSTEMATIZED LEARNING ASSESSMENT IN SWIMMING PRACTICE

A. Custódio-Marques[1], O. Andries-Júnior[1], R. Carvalho de Moraes[1], M. Vinicius Machado[2], E.S. Cyrino[3], and E. Colantonio[4]

[1]State University of Campinas, Brazil; [2]Oswaldo Cruz Institute, Brazil; [3]State University of Londrina, Brazil; [4]Federal University of São Paulo, Brazil.

38.1 INTRODUCTION

Intensive studies regarding swimming specific analyses of physiological and biomechanical variables are performance-oriented (Gatti *et al.,* 2004). Although it can be understood that motor aspects in the initial formation process are important in order to obtain technical efficiency entailing less energy expenditure when performing work and therefore improving performance (Oliveira, 2011). The systematized learning assessment contributes to the evolution (Xavier Filho and Manoel, 2002) and criteria for monitoring must be established to have an analysis standard regarding qualitative variables. Therefore, the objective of this study is to compare the effect upon a content package divided into specific and systematized modules to 6–17 year old children spread throughout provinces with distinct socioeconomic indices located in Pará and Espírito Santo, Brazil.

38.2 METHODS

The sample is composed of 183 male volunteers and 144 female volunteers, aged 6–17 years, from a social sportive formation project developed in the North region (Pará – PA) and Southwest region (Espírito Santo – ES). The module content is described in the swimming learning – Cycle I (Table 38.1). All procedures were approved by the Ethics Committee where such research is linked to the respective institution and also to the authors and study.

Divided modules presented in Table 38.1 compound learning processes belonging to Cycle I, where each content is measured through three criteria to be object of observation transformation in quantitative values. Thus, it was established concepts to such quantifications and they are divided and presented according to the following: a) it performs completely the task (R=3 points): volunteer performs completely proposed activity; b) has difficulty in performing activity (RD=1 point): volunteer partially performs proposed activity. Such criteria have been established due to partial activity performance; c) volunteer doesn´t perform activity (NR=0 point): volunteer doesn´t perform proposed activity and demonstrates a lot of difficulty when it comes to motor perception settle. All assessment patterns were previously established based on theory postulates in the learning process on swimming (Corazza *et al.*, 2006; Freudnheim *et al.*, 2005; Catteau and Garoff, 1990; Aplmer, 1990). It has been previously taken into account the minimum learning value where all were able to perform activities and get started with the AML process. It was composed of three weekly sessions lasting 45 minutes each session. Volunteers were submitted to a systematized process composed of 72 classes, having the same pattern, where all received the same content in class. Assessments were performed in two steps, after 12 weeks (36 classes) in order to control it and at the end of the learning process (72 classes). Volunteers were submitted to qualitative evaluation process considering modules´ content. Assessments were performed by two professionals, capable and trained with more than 2 years experience of carrying out the test. Upon doubts, a third evaluator took part in the process.

The normality of the data was analysed using a Kolmogorov-Smirnov test. Data are described using the median (Md) calculation of respective content modules, for boys and girls and in the states of Pará and Espírito Santo (PA *vs.* ES). The Mann-Whitney test, with a significance value of $p<0.05$, was used to compare modules (AML, PP, NC_r, NC) between boys and girls, as well as, the cumulative calculation regarding module learning between the states of PA *vs.* ES.

Table 38.1 Modules that compound Cycle I regarding swimming learning.

Modules	Content	Total Score
Adjustment to liquid base (AML)	Breathtaking control, ventral fluctuation, ventral slide, backbone fluctuation and slide besides changes in the prone position.	18 points
Leg range propulsion (PP)	Legs range propulsion regarding crawl and backstroke swimming style (with implements), legs range propulsion regarding crawl and backstroke swimming style (without implements), resources displacement (dog paddle swimming style), front breathtaking, side breath in.	21 points
Front-crawl swimming style (NC_r)	Stroke support during displacement, completion of strokes during pathway, recovery of strokes (elbow positioning), continuous legs range propulsion, synchronized swimming (arms + breathtaking), synchronized swimming itself, somersault.	21 points
Backstroke swimming style (NC)	Aligned body (water level), arms extension during aerial swimming style step, propulsive completion of arms during water phase, swimming style coordination, and somersault.	15 points
		75 points

38.3 RESULTS

The analysis demonstrated volunteers reached maximum score in the AML module, where it occurred variation in median values between sports programme participants in Southwest Pará region (PA) *vs.* metropolitan area in the state of Espírito Santo (ES), showing that volunteers from PA presented better results for PP, NC_r and NC in both genres. It has been possible to verify a representative statistical difference for AML, PP, NC_r and NC in both genders between PA *vs.* ES (table 38.2) and the total accumulate regarding learning process, supporting findings in isolated modules (Figure 38.1)

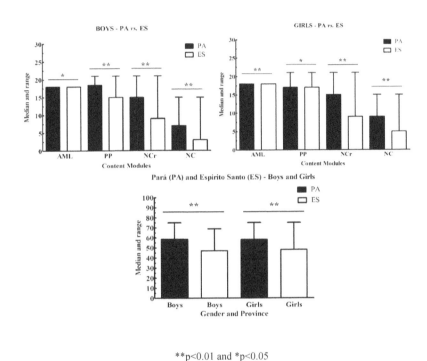

**p<0.01 and *p<0.05

Figure 38.1 Median (Md) and Mann-Whitney test regarding all modules (AML, PP, NC_r and NC) developed between Pará (PA) and Espírito Santo (ES) provinces driven to boys and girls individuals.

38.4 CONCLUSION

With results in hand we are able to conclude that, volunteers from the Southwest region at PA with a lower socio-economic index achieved better results from a systematized programme lasting 24 weeks. This may be associated with motor experiences acquired on a daily basis from activities but also external ones to the swimming programme and learning linked to specific existing opportunities in the region. The smaller variation found between median calculations in such regions may be associated with such suppositions.

Table 38.2 Median (Md) and Amplitude (Am) of developed modules during 72 classes between the provinces of Pará (PA) and Espírito Santo (ES) driven to boys and girls individuals.

	Boys				Girls			
	PA (n=102)		ES (n=81)		PA (n=71)		ES (n=72)	
	Md	Am	Md	Am	Md	Am	Md	Am
AML	18.00^{*}	10 – 18	18.00	08 – 18	18.00^{**}	10 – 18	18.00	08 – 18
PP	18.50^{**}	07 – 21	15.00	00 – 21	17.00^{*}	07 – 21	17.00	06 - 21
NC_r	15.00^{**}	00 – 21	9.00	00 – 21	15.00^{**}	00 – 21	9.00	00 – 21
NC	7.00^{**}	00 – 15	3.00	00 – 15	9.00^{**}	00 – 15	5.00	00 – 15

$**p<0.01$ and $*p<0.05$ – PA vs. ES

38.5 REFERENCES

Catteu, R. and Garoff, G., 1990. *O ensino da natação*, (São Paulo: Editora Manole).

Corazza, S.T., Pereira, E.F., Villis, J.M.C. and Katzer, J.I., 2006. Criação e validação de um teste para medir o desempenho motor do nado crawl. *Revista Brasileira de Cineantropometria e Desempenho Humano*, **8**, pp. 73–78.

Freudenheim, A.M., Basso, L., Xavier Filho, E., Madureira, F., Silva, C.G.S. and Manoel, E.J, 2005. Organização temporal da braçada do nado crawl: iniciantes *vs* avançados. *Revista Brasileira de Ciência e Movimento*, **13**, pp. 75–84.

Gatti, R., Oliveira, G., Erichsen, A.O., Iberes, S. and Melo, L., 2004. Respostas fisiológicas e biomecânicas de nadadores em diferentes intensidades de nado. *Revista Brasileira de Cineantropometria e Desempenho Humano*, **6**, pp. 26–35.

Mansoldo, A.C., 1986, *Estudo Comparativo da Eficiência do Aprendizado da Natação (Estilo Crawl) Entre crianças de três a oito anos de idade*. Dissertação do Título de Mestre em Educação Física (São Paulo: USP).

Oliveira, F.S., 2011. Avaliação da aprendizagem nas aulas de natação. *Revista Digital EFDeportes.com*, **16**, pp. 162. [http://www.efdeportes.com/efd162/a-avaliacao-da-aprendizagem-de-natacao.htm] accessed on December 25, 2012.

Palmer, M.L., 1990, *A ciência do ensino da natação*, (São Paulo, Editora Manole).

Xavier Filho, E. and Manoel, E.J., 2002. Desenvolvimento do comportamento motor aquático: implicações para a pedagogia da Natação, *Revista Brasileira de Ciência e Movimento*, **10** pp. 85–94.

IMPORTANCE OF THE SOCIAL ENVIRONMENT IN THE DEVELOPMENT OF FIELD HOCKEY EXPERTISE

K. M. Nieuwenhuis[1], M. T. Elferink-Gemser[1,2], S.C. M. Te Wierike[1], W. Idema[2], and C. Visscher[1]

[1] University Medical Center Groningen, University of Groningen, The Netherlands; [2] Institute for Studies in Sports and Exercise, HAN University of Applied Sciences, The Netherlands

39.1 INTRODUCTION

Talented athletes perform better in their sports than peers and have the potential to compete at the highest level (Howe *et al.*, 1998; Helsen *et al.*, 2000). To reach optimal performance levels, talented athletes should possess well-developed anthropometric, physiological, technical, tactical and psychological performance characteristics (Elferink-Gemser, 2005). It is important that talent identification and development procedures acknowledge the interaction between these performance characteristics and the social environment of athletes (Abbott and Collins, 2004). Several studies have emphasized the important roles of parents (Bloom *et al.*, 1985; Côté, 1999; Csikszentmihalyi *et al.*, 1993; Lauer *et al.*, 2010), trainers (Wolfenden and Holt, 2005), peers (Côté *et al.*, 2003; Côté and Fraser-Thomas, 2007) and siblings (Côte, 1999) in different stages of talent development in sports. Furthermore, Wolfenden and Holt (2005) stated that the involvement in elite performance levels in tennis is a team effort in which the player, parents, and the coach fulfil specific roles. A highly experienced coach who participated in Wolfenden and Holt's study (2005, p.124) said: "To get to the top in any sport it's all about teamwork (…). The most important person is the player and everyone around (…), be it coaches, parents, siblings, friends, fitness trainers, [they] have to work together to provide the optimal conditions to nurture this individual's talent (…)". These studies suggest that the social environment can facilitate talents to improve their performance. Thus, understanding the role of the social environment is crucial in talent development. However, to our knowledge, little research has been conducted that investigates players' own perception of important persons' influence on performance level from adolescence to adulthood, especially in field hockey. Therefore, the purpose of the current study is to examine which people talented field hockey players consider most important in their sports career during adolescence and adulthood. With this knowledge, an optimal interaction between athlete and environment can be created to improve the effectiveness of talent development programmes.

39.2 METHODS

The sample consisted of 21 athletes of the Dutch national female field hockey team (n = 21; Age = 25.24 ± 3.52 years), that won the silver medal in the Olympic final of 2004 in Athens, who filled out a questionnaire about the importance of social environment in their sports career during adolescence and adulthood. The hockey players were asked to indicate the importance of different persons by dividing a hundred percent over the categories partner, parents, trainers, siblings, friends, teachers and others. The question was answered by the same players for four different age categories: <15, <17, <19 and ≥19. At the moment of participation players were ≥19 and, therefore, looked back at their sports career to answer the questions. The category 'partner' was only available for the categories <19 and ≥19. Repeated measures ANOVA was performed with as dependent variables, partners, parents, trainers, siblings, friends, teachers, and others. The within subjects factor was age category (<15, <17, <19 and ≥19). For parents, siblings, and friends the assumption of sphericity was violated, so for these tests Greenhouse-Geisser values are reported. Level of significance was set at 0.05.

39.3 RESULTS

Table 39.1 presents the mean percentages allocated and standard deviations of all persons in the social environment of the athlete as well as corresponding effect sizes (Cohen's d) across age categories <15, <17, <19 and ≥19. Superscripts indicate which people are rated as most (1) to less (4) important for the four most important people in the four age categories.

Table 39.1 Mean percentages (± standard deviation) and effect sizes for all persons in the social environment of the athlete for age categories <15, <17, <19 and ≥19.

	<15		<17		<19		≥19
	(n=21)	d	(n=21)	d	(n=20)	d	(n=21)
Parents	50.0±19.6[1]	0.12[+]	47.6±18.8[1]	0.29[+]	42.5±17.1[1]	1.16[^]	25.7±11.3[2]
Trainer	21.2±12.4[2]	-0.37[°]	26.9±18.3[2]	-0.01[+]	27.0±18.2[2]	-0.16[+]	29.8±15.3[1]
Partner	-	-	-	-	4.23±9.9	-1.11[^]	21.2±19.1[3]
Friends	14.8±17.1[3]	0.04[+]	14.1±15.5[3]	-0.05[+]	14.8±13.6[3]	0.07[+]	13.8±14.7[4]
Siblings	12.1±13.8[4]	0.17[+]	10.0±11.5[4]	-0.04[+]	10.5±11.8[4]	0.20[+]	8.3±9.9
Teachers	0.2±1.1	-0.41[°]	1.2±3.1	0.06[+]	1.0±3.5	0.01[+]	1.0±3.4
Others	1.2±4.5	0.29[+]	0.2±1.1	0.31[+]	0.00±0.0	-0.36[+]	1.7±6.6

Note. d = 0.20 (small[+]), d = around 0.50 (moderate[°]), d = around 0.80 (large[^]); 1–4: indicating the importance of each category with 1 most important until 4 least important.

Parents are classified as the most important persons in the environment of players <15, <17 and <19, subsequently followed by the trainer, friends and siblings. A significant difference in rated importance for parents occurs over time (F=18.749; $p<0.001$), since a decline in importance was observed for ≥19 ($p<0.001$ between <15 and ≥19, $p=0.001$ between <17 and ≥19, and $p=0.005$ between <19 and ≥19). At the age of ≥19, partners play a more important role, rather than the parents (F=13.604; $p=0.002$). Players rated trainers and teachers as more important when they make the transition from <15 to <17, but no differences for trainers and teachers occur later on ($p>0.05$). Besides, the rated importance of friends, siblings, and others is fairly stable throughout adolescence ($p>0.05$).

Large effect sizes occur between parents and trainers for age categories <15, <17 and <19 ($d=1.76$ for <15, $d=1.12$ for <17 and $d=0.88$ for <19). Between trainers and friends large effect sizes were found for age categories <17 ($d=0.76$), and <19 ($d=0.76$) and a moderate effect for <15 ($d=0.43$). However, all effect sizes between friends and siblings are rather small ($d=0.17$ for <15, $d=0.30$ for <17 and $d=0.33$ for <19). For ≥19 the hierarchy changes to trainer as most important, followed by parents, partner, and friends. Nevertheless, influence of the top three is divided quite equally ($d=0.30$ between trainers and parents, $d=0.20$ between parents and partners, and $d=0.43$ between partners and friends).

39.4 DISCUSSION

The current study investigated which persons in the social environment of talented field hockey players are perceived as most important for their sports career. For age categories <15, <17 and <19 parents were perceived most important. This finding is confirmed in the studies of Côté (1999), and Lauer *et al.* (2010), who found that parents are involved in the sampling and specializing years (≤16) and become less important in the investment years (16+). Furthermore, Bloom (1985) showed that parents are often the key supporters, investing tangible and intangible resources to nurture their child's talent. A second result is the shift of perceived importance from parents to partner when athletes reach age category ≥19. Parents remain most important, but partners are now more important than friends and siblings. The shift of importance from parents to partner is reasonable, as according to Markiewicz *et al.* (2006) adolescents become more autonomous from parents. Besides, during adolescent development partners begin to emerge as attachment figures that are seen as a safe haven and base of support (Furman and Wehner, 1994). A third finding is that trainers were perceived equally important throughout adolescence. Although responsibility for training and competition was found to shift from trainer to athlete during later years of development (Bloom, 1985), trainers obviously are the guides of athletes' athletic development in their sports career (Côté, 1999). Fourth, for all age categories <19, friends and siblings were approximately equally important. Côté (1999) found that the encouragement of friends and siblings can be crucial for athletes in deciding to choose their sports over other activities. Results confirm the findings in the study of Wolfenden and Holt (2005), who stated that the involvement in elite performance levels is a team effort in which the player, parents, and the coach fulfil specific roles. The current study adds the important role of the partner when athletes are ≥19. To conclude, the importance of the social environment in the sports career of talented hockey players is an accumulation of different persons throughout adolescence and adulthood. This knowledge should be used to improve the effectiveness of talent development programmes; however, more research is needed to clarify the roles of different persons in the social environment of talented athletes.

39.5 REFERENCES

Abbott, A. and Collins., D., 2004, Eliminating the dichotomy between theory and practice in talent identification and development: considering the role of psychology. *Journal of Sports Sciences*, **22**, pp. 395–408.

Bloom, B.S., 1985, *Developing Talent in Young People*, (New York: Ballantine).

Côté, J., 1999, The influence of the family in the development of talent in sport. *The Sport Psychologist*, **13**, pp. 395–417.

Côté, J. and Fraser-Thomas, J., 2007, Youth involvement in sport. In *Introduction to Sport Psychology: A Canadian Perspective*, edited by Crocker, P.R.E., (Toronto: Pearson Prentice Hall), pp. 266–294.

Côté, J., Baker, J. and Abernethy, B., 2003, From play to practice: A developmental framework for the acquisition of expertise in team sport. In *Recent Advances in Research on Sport Expertise*, edited by Starkes, J. and Ericsson, K.A., (Champaign, IL: Human Kinetics), pp. 89–114.

Csikszentmihalyi, M., Rathunde, K. and Whalen, S., 1993, *Talented Teenagers: The Roots of Success and Failure*, (New York: Cambridge).

Elferink-Gemser, M.T., 2005, *Today's talented youth field hockey players, the stars of tomorrow? A study on talent development in field hockey*. Thesis Center for Human Movement Sciences, (Groningen: University of Groningen).

Furman, W. and Wehner, E.A., 1994, Romantic views: Toward a theory of adolescent romantic relationships. In *Advances in Adolescent Development: Relationships During Adolescence*, edited by Montemayor, R., Adams, G.R., and Gullota, G.P., (Sage, Thousand Oaks, CA), pp. 168–175.

Helsen, W.F., Hodges, N.J., Van Winckel, J. and Starkes, J.L., 2000, The roles of talent, physical precocity and practice in the development of soccer expertise. *Journal of Sports Sciences*, **18**, pp. 727–736.

Howe, M.J.A., Davidson, J.W. and Sloboda, J.A., 1998, Innate talents: Reality or myth. *Behavioral and Brain Sciences*, **21**, pp. 399–442.

Lauer, L., Gould, D., Roman, N. and Pierce, M., 2010, Parental behaviors that affect tennis player development. *Psychology of Sport and Exercise*, 11, pp. 487–496.

Markiewicz, D., Lawford, H., Doyle, A.B. and Haggart, N., 2006, Developmental differences in adolescents' and young adults' use of mothers, fathers, best friends, and romantic partners to fulfill attachment needs. *Journal of Youth and Adolescence*, **35**, pp. 127–140.

Wolfenden, L. E. and Holt, N. L., 2005, Tennis development in elite junior tennis: perceptions of players, parents and coaches. *Journal of Applied Sport Psychology*, **17**, pp. 108–126.

COACHES' JUDGMENT ABOUT CURRENT AND FUTURE PERFORMANCE LEVEL OF BASKETBALL PLAYERS

S.C.M. te Wierike[1], E.J. Yvonne-Tromp[1], J. Valente-dos-Santos[2], M. T. Elferink-Gemser[1,3], and C. Visscher[1]

[1]University Medical Center Groningen, University of Groningen, The Netherlands; [2]Faculty of Sport Sciences and Physical Education, University of Coimbra, Portugal; [3]Institute for Studies in Sports and Exercise, HAN University of Applied Sciences, The Netherlands

40.1 INTRODUCTION

Talented athletes, i.e., those who perform better than their peers and have the potential to reach the top (Howe *et al.*, 1998; Helsen *et al.*, 2000), are often selected for a talent development programme. The ultimate goal of these programmes is to guide talented youth athletes towards elite athletes in adulthood. To reach this goal, the 'right' athletes should be identified to enter the development programme. It is highly important to look further than the current performance and give extra attention to the potential and possible future performance level of youth athletes (Elferink-Gemser *et al.*, 2011). Unfortunately, it is very difficult to predict future level of performances, especially when the timespan to predict increases (Baker *et al.*, 2012; Vaeyens *et al.*, 2008). It is therefore often that athletes who may have the potential to reach the top are not identified as such (i.e., false-negatives) by coaches and scouts and the other way around in that athletes are identified as talented whereas they do not have the potential to reach the top (i.e., false-positives). The first scenario will decrease the chance for players of reaching elite level because they do not receive the extra facilities to develop themselves. Whether players are selected for a talent development programme mainly depends on the judgment of coaches. This indicates that coaches ought to be able to judge whether or not someone is a talented athlete. However, the question is whether this really is the case. Are coaches able to make a good judgment about the current and future performance level of their athletes and which characteristics are important for their judgment? To investigate this, the aim of this study is to examine the relation between coaches' overall judgment about the youth level of performances and the actual achieved performance level of players when they have become adults (i.e., ≥ 18 years). In addition, the relation between the predicted performance level and the actual achieved performance level of players will be investigated. It is also aimed to investigate which characteristics underlie the overall judgment of coaches about the performance level of young, talented basketball players.

40.2 METHODS

Four experienced coaches judged the talented youth basketball players (Mean age 15.90 ± 1.12 years; range 14–17 years) of their own team in season 2008–2009 or 2009–2010. Five multidimensional characteristics of the players were judged regardless of their playing position: technical, tactical, psychological, and two physiological characteristics (sprint performances and endurance). In addition, an overall judgment about the level of performance of the players was made. Coaches judged each of the characteristics on a 6-point Likert scale from 1 indicating 'very poor' to 6 indicating 'very good'. Coaches also predicted the level of performance of players in adulthood (i.e., ≥ 18 years). The response options of this question consisted of 'drop out', 'amateur level', 'third league', 'second league', 'first league', 'international level', and 'NBA'. In season 2012–2013, the actual achieved performance level of these same players, who became adult basketball players (i.e., ≥ 18 years), was estimated.

A Spearman correlation coefficient was calculated between the overall judgment of coaches concerning the youth level of performance of players (2008–2009/2009–2010) and the actual achieved level of performance in adulthood (2012–2013). A Spearman correlation coefficient was also calculated to estimate the relation between the predicted level of performance (2008–2009/2009–2010) and the actual achieved level of performance when players became adult basketball players (2012–2013). Magnitude of correlations was interpreted as follows: trivial ($r < 0.1$), small ($0.1 < r < 0.3$), moderate ($0.3 < r < 0.5$), large ($0.5 < r < 0.7$), very large ($0.7 < r < 0.9$), and nearly perfect ($r > 0.9$) (Hopkins et al., 2009). A forward stepwise multiple linear regression analysis was performed to determine the contribution of the five multidimensional characteristics to the overall judgment of coaches. Level of significance was set at .05.

40.3 RESULTS

Spearman correlation revealed that the relation between the overall judgment of coaches on youth level of performance (2008–2009/2009–2010) and the actual achieved performance level of players (season 2012–2013) was very low ($\rho = -.043$). In line with this, the correlation between the predicted (2008–2009/2009–2010) and actual achieved performance level of players (2012–2013) was also very low ($\rho = .015$). Regression analysis ($F = 19.32$; $p < .001$) showed that sprint performances (physiological) ($p = .005$) and tactical characteristics ($p < .001$) made a significant contribution to the overall judgment of coaches regarding the youth level of performances. Overall, 65.9 % of the variance in the overall judgment of the coach could be explained by the five multidimensional characteristics.

40.4 DISCUSSION

The main aim of this study was to investigate the relation between the current and future performance level of elite youth basketball players. In addition, it was aimed to examine which characteristics underlie this judgment of coaches.

Results showed a low correlation between the overall judgment of coaches concerning the youth performance level of players and their actual performance level, and between the predicted and actual achieved performance level. This indicates that coaches have difficulties with predicting the future performance level of youth basketball players. It might therefore be necessary for talent identification and development purposes to use more objective/other criteria for the selection of the 'right' talents in addition to the subjective criteria of coaches. A possible explanation for the low correlation between the predicted and actual achieved performance level might be related to the answer options we used in this study. Probably, other factors than these five multidimensional characteristics are important to possess as a player. Another explanation can be found in the fact that the performance of players is judged at one moment, while Vaeyens *et al.,* (2008) suggest that for identifying players that will eventually reach elite level of performance, coaches should look at the progress players make.

Results further revealed that sprint and tactical performances of players have a significant influence on the overall judgment of coaches regarding the current performance level of players. The influence of sprint performances is not remarkable since sprinting is one of the most common activities of basketball players during a game (Abdelkrim *et al.,* 2007). In addition, Torres-Unda *et al.* (2012) showed that elite basketball players are faster on sprint tests compared to non-elite players, indicating that sprinting is important in reaching elite level of performances.

Regarding the tactical characteristics of basketball players, the results of this study are in line with the results of Leite *et al.* (2011) which showed that experienced basketball coaches mainly focused on the tactical development of their players. In addition, research showed that tactical skills are important for reaching elite level in team sports (Kannekens *et al.,* 2009; Elferink-Gemser *et al.,* 2010).

In conclusion, this study revealed that coaches have some difficulties with predicting the future performance level of players. So, in talent development programmes, it is advised to apply additional tests to select the 'right' talents in order to eventually reach elite level of performances.

40.5 REFERENCES

Abdelkarim, N.B., El Fazaa, S., and El Ati, J., 2007, Time–motion analysis and physiological data of elite under-19-year-old basketball players during competition. *British Journal of Sports Medicine,* **41**, pp. 69–75.

Baker, J., Schorer, J. and Cobley, S., 2012, Lessons learned – the future of research in talent identification and development. In *Talent Identification and Development in Sport – International Perspectives,* edited by Baker, J., Cobley, S. and Schorer, J., (London: Routledge), pp. 167–173.

Helsen, W.F., Hodges, N.J., Van Winckel, J. and Starkers, J.L., 2000, The roles of talent, physical precocity and practice in the development of soccer expertise. *Journal of Sports Sciences*, **18**, pp. 727–736.

Hopkins, W.G., Marshall, S.W., Batterham, A.M. and Hanin, J., 2009, Progressive statistics for studies in sports medicine and exercise science. *Medicine and Science in Sports and Exercise*, **41**, pp. 3–13.

Howe, M.J.A., Davidson, J.W. and Sloboda, J.A., 1998, Innate talents: reality or myth. *Behavioral and Brain Sciences,* **21**, pp. 399–442.

Elferink-Gemser, M.T., Jordet, G., Coelho-E-Silva, M.J. and Visscher, C., 2011, The marvels of elite sports: how to get there? *British Journal of Sports Medicine*, **45**, pp. 683–684.

Elferink-Gemser, M.T., Kannekens, R., Lyons, J., Tromp, Y. and Visscher, C., 2010, Knowing what to do and doing it: Differences in self-assessed tactical skills of regional, sub-elite, and elite youth field. *Journal of Sports Sciences*, **28**, pp. 521–528.

Kannekens, R., Elferink-Gemser, M.T. and Visscher, C., 2009, Tactical skills of world-class youth soccer teams. *Journal of Sports Sciences*, **27**, 807–812.

Leite, N., Coelho, E. and Sampaio, J., 2011, Assessing the importance given by basketball coaches to training contents. *Journal of Human Kinetics*, **30**, pp. 123–133.

Torres-Unda, J., Zarrazquin, I., Gil, J., Ruiz, F., Irazusta, A., Kortajarena, M., Seco, J. and Irazusta, J., 2013, Anthropometric, physiological and maturational characteristics in selected elite and non-elite male adolescent basketball players. *Journal of Sports Sciences,* **31**, pp. 196–203.

Vaeyens, R., Lenoir, M., Williams, A.M. and Philippaerts, R.M., 2008, Talent identification and development programmes in sport. *Sports Medicine*, **38**, pp. 703–714.

BIOLOGICAL MATURATION AT TIME OF SELECTION AND SWIMMING CAREER PATHS IN FLEMISH SWIMMERS

T. Martine[1], G. Ariane[2], R. Stien[1], and L. Matthieu[3]

[1]Departement of Kinesiology, Physical Activity, Sports & Health Research Group, Faculty of Kinesiology and Rehabilitation Sciences, Belgium; [2]Faculty of Physical Education and Physical Therapy, Belgium; [3]Dept. Movement and Sports Sciences, Faculty of Medicine and Sports Sciences, Ghent University, Belgium

41.1 INTRODUCTION

Swimming is a very technical sport with high training loads. Talented swimmers are selected at a fairly young age. This selection is mostly based on performances in chronological age groups. This strategy can be problematic as it does not take into account the effects of biological maturation on performance. However there is little evidence available about the relationship between the level of sport career success and the maturity status of a swimmer at the time of selection, partly due to problems with the assessment of the maturity status. Skeletal maturity may be the best method to assess maturity, however, it is invasive, costly and requests expert ratings which make this method hard to implement in talent identification programmes. Therefore, researchers developed other, non-invasive methods to determine maturity in athletes (Malina *et al.,* 2012). This study determined interrelations among invasive and non-invasive indicators of biological maturation and related maturity status at time of selection of a Belgian swimming sample with the success of their swimming career.

41.2 METHODS

The sample consists of 49 swimmers aged 10.3–14.4 years, who were selected to enter the elite swimming school from the Flemish Swimming Federation, Belgium. All maturity measurements were conducted between 2006 and 2009, with a follow up of the swimming career up to 2012. Skeletal maturity was determined using the TWIII-method (Tanner *et al.,* 2001). Age at peak height velocity (APHV, yr) was estimated to determine maturity offset (Mirwald *et al.,* 2002), while percentage of predicted adult height quantifies how far the swimmer is progressed in his or her growth process (Khamis and Roche, 1994). All three measures were used to classify each individual as an early, on time or late maturer based on earlier methodology (Malina *et al.*, 2012). Interrelationships among maturity categorisation based on invasive (SA-CA) and non-invasive (percentage of predicted height (KR) and maturity offset) maturity indicators were evaluated (Cohen unweighted Kappa coefficients). Performance at time of selection (PS), best performance ever (BPE) and best performance during the last year of the swimming career (LYP) were objectively assessed by Rudolph-scores, an age and gender-specific swim ranking system (maximum score=20) (European Swim Federation, 2013). Three career paths were defined: positive development path (PDP: PS < BPE=LYP), a negative development path (NDP: PS > BPE > LYP) and a non-successful path (NSP: PS < BPE > LYP) (see Figure 41.1). One-way ANOVA was used to determine anthropometric and performance differences between early, average and late maturity groups, between PDP, NDP and NSP groups and between swimmers within or outside the Flemish elite swimming school programme.

Table 41.1 Frequencies and cross-tabulations of maturity status classifications between pairs of maturity indicators in swimmers aged between 10.3 and 14.4 years old.

Maturity indicators and categories	Maturity indicators and categories						
	Early	Average	Late	**Total**	$\%^a$	r_s	κ
Maturity offset		Skeletal maturity					
Early	2	2	0	4			
Average	3	32	9	44			
Late	0	0	1	1			
Total	5	34	10	49	71 [59;84]	0.39**	0.22
%Predicted height KR		Skeletal maturity					
Early	4	8	0	12			
Average	0	14	3	17			
Late	0	5	2	7			
Total	4	27	5	36	56 [41;80]	0.49**	0.31
Maturity offset		%Predicted height KR					
Early	3	1	0	4			
Average	9	16	6	31			
Late	0	0	1	1			
Total	12	17	7	36	56 [41;80]	0.38*	0.13

*P<0.05;**P<0.01; a percentage agreement [95% confidence interval].

41.3 RESULTS

Table 41.1 shows low agreement between invasive and non-invasive assessments of maturation status (κ=013-0.31), although significant correlations are found (r$_s$=0.39-0.49). Associations between maturity and performance indicators were higher in males compared to females, with advanced maturity related to better performance: e.g. CA-SA and best performance relationship (r_{males}=-0.66; P=0.005, $r_{females}$=-0.47; P= 0.006)(data not shown). Early and average maturers showed higher anthropometric measures and better performance (P= 0.04-0.01) compared to late maturers (Table 41.2). However, maturity indicators at time of selection were not found to be different between swimmers of different career paths (see Figure. 41.1). Swimmers within the Flemish elite school programme were more advanced at time of selection (CA-SA=-0.92 ± 1.3 yr, compared to 0.25±0.9 yr for other swimmers) and had higher performance scores.

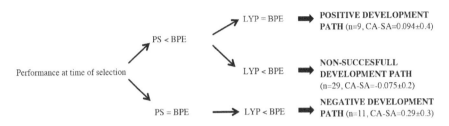

Figure 41.1 Representation of career paths (PS= performance at selection, BPE= best performance ever, LYP= last year performance; CA-SA= difference between chronological age and skeletal age).

41.4 DISCUSSION

Non-invasive maturity assessments showed limited agreement with skeletal maturity. Our findings with regards to predicted age at peak height velocity (maturity offset) are consistent with previous research (Malina *et al.*, 2006). These results suggest that the prediction equation developed on a non-athletic sample is not necessarily applicable to a sample of swimmers. When using this method, one must remember that care is warranted when interpreting the results, because maturity classification based on predicted APHV tends to overestimate maturity of swimmers.

Early maturers' advances in growth and performance at time of selection were confirmed, with larger effects in males compared to females. Swimmers selected for the Flemish elite swimming school programme were advanced in maturity although advanced maturity status per se was not predictive for a positive career development path. Our career path-determination was based on age and gender-specific relative performance scores, however, swimmers with a high Rudolph-score as personal best could be classified as non-successful when there was only a slight decrease in this score during their last performance year. Also we based career paths on within-subject patterns of performance scores without comparisons to other swimmers, a non-successful development path could therefore still be at a higher performance level then a positive development path.

Table 41.2 Anthropometric and performance characteristics (mean ± sd) of swimmers with different maturity status.

Males (n=16)	Early	Average	Late	F	P
	3	9	4		
CA (yr)	11.8 ± 1.3	13.2 ± 0.7	12.0 ± 0.9	5	0.02
SA (yr)	14.2 ± 0.8	13.4 ± 0.7	10.7 ± 1.0	19.16	0.0001[b,c]
Standing height (cm)	169.1 ± 2.7	168.6 ± 8.9	153.9 ± 6.8	5.44	0.02[c]
Sitting height (cm)	88.2 ± 3.0	87.2 ± 3.9	79.5 ± 3.7	6.58	0.01[b,c]
Body Mass (kg)	55.1 ± 0.3	52.9 ± 8.2	39.4 ± 3.2	6.76	0.01[b,c]
PS	12.5 ± 1.3	11.5 ± 2.8	7.5 ± 3.4	3.76	0.05
BPE	17.4 ± 2.3	15.7 ± 3.7	9.4 ± 5.4	6.52	0.011[b,c]
LYT	16.1 ± 1.3	12.3 ± 3.6	6.5± 5.4	5.64	0.017[b]
Female (n=33)	Early	Average	Late	F	P
	2	25	6		
CA(yr)	12.8 ± 1.0	12.3 ± 0.7	11.9 ± 0.5	1.36	0.2723
SA(yr)	14.1 ± 1.0	12.3 ± 0.9	10.4 ± 0.8	17.76	<.0001[a,b,c]
Standing height (cm)	169.2 ± 6.0	158.8 ± 8.9	152.6 ± 10.4	2.61	0.0901
Sitting height (cm)	92.1 ± 2.8	82.7 ± 4.8	79.0 ± 5.6	5.47	0.0095[a,b]
Body Mass (kg)	55.1 ± 1.7	46.2 ± 8.2	38.8 ± 10.6	3.26	0.0523
PS	11.6 ± 0.1	10.6 ± 3.8	6.7 ± 4.1	2.78	0.0780
BPE	14.1 ± 3.6	13.7 ± 2.5	10.6 ± 2.4	3.63	0.0388[c]
LYT	12.8 ± 5.1	11.0 ± 3.5	9.4 ± 2.9	0.87	0.4290

[a] Significant difference between early and average mature; [b] between early and late; [c] between average and late (based on CA-SA)

41.5 REFERENCES

European Swim Federation, 2013, *Swimrankings*. Retrieved 5 of March, 2013, from http://www.swimrankings.net/.

Khamis, H.J. and Roche, A.F., 1994, Predicting adult stature without using skeletal age: the khamis-roche method. *Pediatrics*, **94**, pp. 504–507.

Malina, R.M., Claessens, A.L., Van Aken, K., Thomis, M., Lefevre, J., Philippaerts, R. and Beunen, G.P., 2006, Maturity offset in gymnasts: application of a prediction equation. *Medicine and Science in Sports and Exercise*, **38**, pp. 1342–1347.

Malina, R.M., Coelho E Silva, M.J., Figueiredo, A.J., Carling, C. and Beunen, G.P., 2012, Interrelationships among invasive and non-invasive indicators of biological maturation in adolescent male soccer players. *Journal of Sports Sciences*, **30**, pp. 1705–1717.

Mirwald, R.L., Baxter-Jones, A.D., Bailey, D.A. and Beunen, G.P., 2002, An assessment of maturity from anthropometric measurements. *Medicine and Science in Sports and Exercise*, **34**, pp. 689–694.

Tanner, J., Healy, M., Goldstein, H. and Cameron, N., 2001, *Assessment of Skeletal Maturity and Prediction of Adult Height (TW3)*, (London: WB Saunders).

PEAK VO$_2$ IN PREPUBERTAL SWIMMERS

M.A. Rodrigues Ferreira[1, 2], J. Mendes[1, 2], R. Fernandes[2], C. Fernando[1], and A.M. Vences Brito[2]
[1]University of Madeira, Portugal; [2]Sport Sciences School of Rio Maior, Polytechnic Institute of Santarém, Portugal

42.1 INTRODUCTION

Children's participation in competitive sports frequently begins at an earlier age, going through training and competition process, so it's important to understand the physiological responses to training in prepubertal athletes (Armstrong and McManus, 2011; McManus and Armstrong, 2011). Swimming is characterized by high training volumes and a higher peak VO$_2$ in prepubertal boys and girls swimmers compared with children not involved in any regular sport practice is expected. The future of peak aerobic power research seems to focus on the VO$_2$ kinetics during sport specific tests in young athletes.

42.2 METHODS

Twenty-four prepubertal children participated in the study (Stage 1; Tanner, 1962). The experimental group was composed of 12 young swimmers, 6 boys (SB) and 6 girls (SG), with an average training experience of 2.5 ± 0.55 and 2.3 ± 0.52 years, respectively. The control group had 12 young children, 6 boys (CB) and 6 girls (CG), not involved in any regular sport practice. The physical characteristics of the participants are shown in Table 42.1. The study was approved by the scientific committee of the University of Madeira and the Sport Sciences School of Rio Maior, Polytechnic Institute of Santarém. Written informed consent was obtained from all the parents or guardians of the participants. All participants were volunteers and gave their assent to participate in the study. The data collection was performed at the Laboratory for Research in Sport (Sport Sciences School of Rio Maior, Polytechnic Institute of Santarém), where temperature ranged between 18 and 23°C and humidity between 40 and 60%. Instructions were given to participants about the objectives, protocol and experimental procedures, including safety rules; there were also a period for habituation to the instruments and encouragement during the test, mainly during the last few minutes (Malina et al., 2004; Gore et al., 2013).

Anthropometric measurements were performed according to the International Working Group on Kinanthropometry, described by Fragoso and Vieira (2011). The maturity stage given by public hair development was evaluated (Tanner, 1962). Peak VO_2 was measured with direct gas analysis, breath-by-breath (Cosmed K4b^2, Rome, Italy), during a continuous progressive protocol (Modified Balke for Children's) on a treadmill (Technogym Runrace Treadmill HC1200), until exhaustion. Data were recorded using a telemetric system and the heart rate was measured with Polar S 610ws. The calibration procedures of the gas analyzer Cosmed K4B^2 were according to the guidelines from the manufacturer: room air; reference gas (16% O_2 and 5% CO_2); delay (gas transition time); and turbine (with a 3000ml syringe). The criteria used to guarantee the attainment of peak VO_2 were: a respiratory exchange ratio value greater than 1.10; achieving the maximal heart rate estimated; plateau in VO_2 (increase of not more than 2 ml $\cdot$ kg^{-1} $\cdot$ min^{-1}) despite an increase in work rate; and the volitional fatigue of the participant, that is, if the participant cannot follow the required speed despite continuous encouragement of the investigator (Malina et al., 2004; Gore et al., 2013). Data were filtered and values averaged every 5 seconds (Duffield et a., 2994)

Descriptive data are presented as means and standard deviation. Normality (Shapiro-Wilks test) and homogeneity (Levene's test) were satisfied for a significance level of .05. The one-way analysis of variance (ANOVA) and LSD Post-Hoc was used (SPSS, version 17.0), with a significance level of p <0.05.

Table 42.1 Physical characteristics of the participants.

	SB	SG	CB	CG
Age (yr.)	10.8 ± 0.41	10.2 ± 0.41	11.0 ± 0.63	10.3 ± 0.52
Height (cm)	147.27 ± 8.45	147.08 ± 7.07	145.13 ± 7.26	143.9 ± 8.65
Weight (kg)	42.23 ± 9.72	40.85 ± 7.66	50.6 ± 12.87	41.05 ± 10.31

42.3 RESULTS

A significantly higher relative peak VO_2 (p = .000; Table 42.2) and peak respiratory exchange ratio (p = .041; Table 42.2) were observed in male and female swimmers compared to boys and girls not involved in any regular sport practice. Peak expired ventilation was significantly higher in boys (p = .013) and girls (p = .009) swimmers compared to girls not involved in any regular sport practice.

254

Table 42.2 Variables of the maximal oxygen consumption test.

	SB	SG	CB	CG	F	Sig.
Peak VO$_2$	68.6±9.43	63.3±5.55	42.8±5.38	43.7±7.31	22.663	.000
Peak VE	88.1±23.26	84.6±12.84	68.8±16.61	60.4±13.31	3.864	.025
Peak HR	192.0±9.44	196.6±6.69	196.3±11.59	193.5±8.89	0.321	.810
Peak RER	1.36±0.18	1.36±0.14	1.21±0.07	1.18±0.12	3.324	.041

Peak VO2: peak oxygen consumption (mL.kg^{-1}.min^{-1}); Peak VE: peak expired ventilation (L.min^{-1}); Peak HR: peak heart rate (beats.min^{-1}); Peak RER: peak respiratory exchange ratio.

42.4 DISCUSSION

Prepubertal swimmers present better maximal aerobic performance compared with the control group. The mean values for the different variables analysed were in agreement with the literature of trained (Falgairette *et al.*, 1993; Al-Hazzaa *et al.*, 1998) and untrained children (Falk and Bar-Or, 1993; Armstrong *et al.*, 1995). Despite the small sample size, the results of the present study might be due to the differences in sport practice between the groups. A higher peak VO$_2$ is important for elite performance in many sports (Armstrong *et al.*, 2011, Armstrong and Barker, 2011), and the results of the present study were in agreement with enhanced aerobic performance in prepubertal swimmers (Sperlich *et al.*, 2010). Furthermore, the swimming training fits the principles of endurance training by inducing an improvement in aerobic performance (Baquet *et al.*, 2010; Armstrong *et al.*, 2011; Armstrong and Barker, 2011). Further studies are needed to access the peak aerobic power from sport specific tests in prepubertal swimmers, especially the VO$_2$ kinetics.

42.5 REFERENCES

Al-Hazzaa, H.M., Al-Tefaee, S.A., Sulaiman, M.A., Dafterdar, M.Y., Al-Herbish, A.S. and Chekwuemeka, A.C., 1998, Cardiorespiratory responses of trained boys to treadmill and arm ergometry: effect of training specifity. *Pediatric Exercise Science*, **10**, 264–276.

Armstrong, N. and Barker, A.R., 2011, Endurance training and elite young athletes. *Medicine and Sport Science*, **56**, pp. 59–83.

Armstrong, N. and McManus, A.M., 2011, Physiology of elite young male athletes. *Medicine and Sport Science*, **56**, pp. 1–22.

Armstrong, N., Tomkinson, G. and Ekelund, U., 2011, Aerobic fitness and its relationship to sport, exercise training and habitual physical activity during youth. *British Journal of Sports Medicine*, **45**, 849-858.

Armstrong, N., Kirby, B.J., McManus, A.M. and Welsman, J.R., 1995, Aerobic fitness of prepubescent children. *Annals of Human Biology*, **22**, 427–441.

Baquet, G., Gamelin, F.X., Mucci, P., Thévenet, D., Van Praagh, E. and Berthoin, S., 2010, Continuous vs. interval aerobic training in 8- to 11-year-old children. *Journal of Strength and Conditioning Research*, **24**, pp. 1381–1388.

Duffield, R., Dawson, B., Pinnington, H.C. and Wong, P., 2004, Accuracy and reliability of a Cosmed K4b2 portable gas analysis system. *Journal of Science in Medicine and Sport*, **7**, pp. 11–22.

Falgairette, D., Duche, P., Bedu, M., Fellman, N. and Coubert., J., 1993, Bioenergetic characteristics in prepubertal swimmers. *International Journal of Sports Medicine*, **14**, 444–448.

Falk, B. and Bar-Or, O., 1993, Longitudinal changes in peak aerobic and anaerobic mechanical power of circumpubertal boys. *Pediatric Exercise Science*, **5**, 318–331.

Fragoso, I. and Vieira, F., 2011, *Cinantropometria: curso prático*, (Cruz Quebrada: FMH).

Gore, C.J., Tanner, R.K., Fuller, K.L. and Stanef, T., 2013, Determination of maximal oxygen consumption (VO$_2$max). In *Physiological Tests for Elite Athletes*, 2nd ed., edited by Tanner, R.K. and Gore, C.J. (Champaign: Human Kinetics), pp. 103–122.

Malina, R., Bouchard, C. and Bar-Or, O., 2004, *Growth, Maturation and Physical Activity*, 2nd ed., (Champaign: Human Kinetics).

McManus, A.M. and Armstrong, N., 2011, Physiology of elite young female athletes. *Medicine and Sport Science*, **56**, pp. 23–46.

Sperlich, B., Zinner, C., Heilemann, I., Kjendlie, P.L., Holmberg, H.C. and Mester, J., 2010, High-intensity interval training improves VO2peak, maximal lactate accumulation, time trial and competition performance in 9–11-year-old swimmers. *European Journal of Applied Physiology*, **110**, pp. 1029–1036.

Tanner, J.M., 1962, *Growth at Adolescence*, 2nd ed., (Oxford: Blackwell).

ABSOLUTE AND SCALED PEAK POWER ASSESSMENTS IN YOUNG MALE SOCCER PLAYERS: VARIATION BY PLAYING POSITION

V. Severino[1], M.J. Coelho-e-Silva[1], J.P. Duarte[1], J.R. Pereira[1], F. Simões[1]†, R. Rebelo-Gonçalves[1], J. Valente-dos-Santos[1], C. Castagna[2], and A.J. Figueiredo[1]

[1]University of Coimbra, Portugal; [2]Italian Football Federation (FIGC), Technical Department, Italy

43.1 INTRODUCTION

Due to the length of the game, aerobic metabolism is the main energy source in soccer (Stølen *et al.*, 2005). Although episodes of anaerobic effort occur on a smaller scale during the game, they play a decisive role in performance and can make the difference between winning and losing a game (Reilly, 2007). Total distance covered in youth soccer matches ranged from 5715–7672 m, and high-intensity distance was 1713 m in U12 and 2481 m in U16 (Harley *et al.*, 2010). In addition, elite athletes performed more high-intensity running episodes during a match (Mohr *et al.*, 2003) compared to their non-elite peers. Variation in physical and functional characteristics of young soccer players by position is not well documented and the literature does not systematically control for variation in body size when profiling players by field position. This study aims to examine variation of Peak Power (WAnT) by position before and after normalizing for body size.

43.2 METHODS

The sample consisted of 41 Portuguese male soccer players aged 12.3–14.9 years from the academy of a club that participates in the national professional league and also in UEFA Europa League at the time of the study. Training experience (range: 2–6 years) was obtained by interview and subsequently confirmed in the archives of the *Portuguese Soccer Federation*. Stature (H) was measured to the nearest 0.1 cm with a Harpenden stadiometer (model 98.603, Holtain Ltd, Crosswell, UK). Body mass (BM) was measured to the nearest 0.1 kg with a SECA balance (model

770, Hanover, MD, USA). The same trained observer collected all measurements needed to estimate thigh volume (TV) by anthropometry (Jones and Pearson, 1969). Fat mass (FM) and fat-free mass (FFM) were derived from air displacement plethysmography (Bod Pod, Life Measurement, Inc., Concord, CA). Predicted mature stature (PMS) was obtained (Khamis & Roche, 1994, 1995) and current stature expressed as a %PMS to provide an estimate of biological maturity status (ranged 84.7% to 96.9%). The Wingate anaerobic test (WAnT) was performed on a cycle ergometer (Monark 824 E, Monark, Sweden) equipped with a 1.0-kg-resistance basket and interfaced with a computer. Verbal encouragement was given throughout all tests. Peak power output (WAnT-P) was defined as the highest average power output obtained during any 1-second interval during the 30-second WAnT. Descriptive statistics were determined and correlations between WAnT-P and size descriptors (k) calculated. Allometric coefficients were obtained using linear regression analyses from log-transformed variables (Log-WAnT-P, Log-H, Log-BM, Log-TV) in order to permit size independent performance. Variation by playing position was tested using ANOVA for body size and ANCOVA (chronological age as covariate) on absolute values of WAnT-P, traditional ratio ($W \cdot kg^{-1}$) and also using power function ratios ($W \cdot K^{-b}$).

43.3 RESULTS

Table 43.1 summarizes mean and standard deviation for stature, body mass, estimated FFM, estimated thigh volume and WAnT-P. Data suggest a substantial relationship between performance (WAnT-P) and size descriptors (right portion of Table 43.1) and also with CA (r=+0.581, 95%CI: 0.333 to 0.754), TE (r=+0.221, 95%CI: -0.093 to 0.495). Allometric exponents for three size descriptors (BM, FFM, TV) are presented in Table 43.2 that also includes the coefficients of correlation between scaled performance and the respective size descriptor.

Table 43.1 Descriptive statistics for the young soccer players aged 13–14 years (*n*=41), test of normality on body size descriptors and correlation between WAnT peak power and size descriptors.

	Mean±St Dev	K-S value (p)	$r_{WAnT-P, K}$ (95% CI)
Stature (cm)	164.4±9.3	0.078 (0.200)	
Body Mass (kg)	53.9±10.3	0.090 (0.200)	0.898 (0.816 to 0.945)
Fat Free Mass (kg)	47.7±9.8	0.076 (0.200)	0.900 (0.819 to 0.946)
Thigh Volume (L)	4.00±1.00	0.102 (0.200)	0.850 (0.734 to 0.918)
WAnT-peak (W)	671.9±178.2	0.080 (0.200)	-

K-S (Kolmogorov-Smirnov test value); WAnT-peak (peak output obtained from the Wingate test); k (size descriptors).

Table 43.2 Allometric exponents for different descriptors and correlations between size descriptors (X_i) and scaled performance (Y/X_i^b) after determination of power function ratios among young soccer players aged 13–14 years (n=41).

Descriptors (X_i)	Allometric exponent [Log Y = Log a+b·Log X+Log ε]			Correlation between X_i and (Y/X^k)	
	b	95% CI	R^2	r	95% CI
Body Mass	1.210	1.021 to 1.399	0.81	0.068	-0.245 to 0.368
Fat Free Mass	1.170	1.000 to 1.341	0.83	-0.213	-0.101 to 0.489
Thigh Volume	0.911	0.706 to 1.115	0.67	0.007	-0.301 to 0.314

WAnT-peak (peak output obtained from the 30-s Wingate test); 95%CI (confidence interval at 95%); * (p<.05), ** (p<.01)

Table 43.3 presents estimated means and standard errors in WAnT-P outputs with chronological age as covariate and also the results of comparisons between defenders, midfielders and attackers. A significant effect of playing position as an independent variable was noted on performance when WAnT-P is expressed in its absolute format. When peak output of the WAnT is expressed in watts per unit of the selected size descriptor, differences between groups were only significant for thigh volume as descriptor. The previous note was valid both using the traditional ratio $(W \cdot L_{TV})$ and the obtained power function $(W \cdot L_{TV}^{-0.911})$.

43.4 DISCUSSION

Specialization by playing position is a relevant topic in the discussion of long-term athletic development. Physical and functional characteristics of young soccer players by playing position are less extensive in the literature compared to available information in adult soccer. The present study showed that the defenders were the tallest and heaviest among the sample, which supports the idea that players with a particular morphology are often oriented towards certain playing positions. A previous study (Al-Hazzaa *et al.*, 2001) assessed anaerobic performance (WAnT) on 23 elite soccer players, and comparisons by playing position were made. Considering peak power, centre-backs attained significantly the highest value but, on the other hand, when anaerobic power was expressed relative to body mass there were no significant differences among players of different positions. In our study the same trend was noted. However, when performance was considered in relation to thigh volume, both using the traditional ratio (watt . L_{TV}) and the obtained power function $(W \cdot L_{TV}^{-0.911})$, differences between groups were significant but with an opposite gradient (midfielders>attackers>defenders). This study proposes the adoption of adequate analytical techniques to compare functional capacities by playing position, especially in variables that are correlated with body size and during years of maximal growth. Research is needed to examine the interrelationship of playing position with growth, maturation, and training effects on functional capacities.

Table 43.3 Estimated means and standard errors by playing position and results of analysis of covariance (ANCOVA) to test the variation associated to position among soccer players aged 13–14 years after controlling for chronological age (n=41).

Y_i, units	Playing position			F (p)	ES-r
	Defenders (n=15)	Midfielders (n=14)	Attackers (n=12)		
WAnT-P (W)	713.8	689.7	611.6	8.254	
	(37.0)	(41.4)	(38.3)	(0.000)	0.63
WAnT-P (W·kg$_{BM}^{-1}$)	11.6	12.2	12.3	0.859	
	(0.4)	(0.4)	(0.4)	(0.471)	0.26
WAnT-P (W·kg$_{BM}^{-1.210}$)	5.2	5.6	5.4	1.457	
	(0.2)	(0.2)	(0.2)	(0.242)	0.33
WAnT-P (W·kg$_{FFM}^{-1}$)	13.9	14.4	13.7	1.826	
	(0.4)	(0.5)	(0.4)	(0.159)	0.36
WAnT-P (W·kg$_{FFM}^{-1.170}$)	5.0	5.1	5.1	0.546	
	(0.8)	(0.9)	(0.8)	(0.654)	0.21
WAnT-P (W·L$_{TV}^{-1}$)	161.4	183.3	165.5	3.478	
	(6.1)	(6.8)	(6.3)	(0.025)	0.47
WAnT-P (W·L$_{TV}^{-0.911}$)	183.9	205.8	185.5	4.234	
	(6.6)	(7.4)	(6.8)	(0.011)	0.51

WAnT-peak (peak output obtained from the 30-s Wingate test); BM (body mass); FFM (fat-free mass); TV (thigh volume); ES-r (magnitude of the effect size).

43.5 ACKNOWLEDGMENTS AND CONTRIBUTIONS

VS is granted by *Fundação para a Ciência e a Tecnologia*: SFRH/BD/69447/2010] and is being supervised by AF, MJCS, CC. Data collected by JPD, JRP, FS, RRG, VS, JVS and MJCS. Analyses were performed by VS and MJCS. All authors critically reviewed the chapter and approved the final version.

43.6 REFERENCES

Al-Hazzaa, H.M., Almuzaini, K.S., Al-Refaee, S.A., Sulaiman, M.A., Dafterdar, M.Y., Al-Ghamedi, A. and Al-Khuraiji, K.N., 2001, Aerobic and anaerobic power characteristics of Saudi elite soccer players. *Journal of Sports Medicine and Physical Fitness*, **41**, pp. 54–61.
Harley, J.A., Barnes, C.A., Portas, M., Lovell, R., Barrett, S., Paul, D. and Weston, M., 2010, Motion analysis of match-play in elite U12 to U16 age-group soccer players. *Journal of Sports Sciences*, **28**, pp. 1391–1397.

Jones, P.R. and Pearson, J., 1969, Anthropometric determination of leg fat and muscle plus bone volumes in young male and female adults. *The Journal of Physiology*, **204**, pp. 63–66.

Khamis, H.J. and Roche, A.F., 1994, Predicting adult stature without using skeletal age: The Khamis-Roche method. *Pediatrics,* **94**, pp. 504–507.

Khamis, H.J. and Roche, A.F., 1995, Predicting adult stature without using skeletal age: The Khamis-Roche method. *Pediatrics – erratum*, **95**, pp. 457.

Mohr, M., Krustrup, P. and Bangsbo, J., 2003, Match performance of high-standard soccer players with special reference to development of fatigue. *Journal of Sports Sciences*, **21**, pp. 519–528.

Reilly, T., 2007, *The Science of Training – Soccer. A Scientific Approach of Developing Strength, Speed and Endurance*, (London: Routlegde).

Stølen T., Chamari, K., Castagna, C. and Wisløff, U., 2005, Physiology of soccer: an update. *Sports Medicine*, **35**, pp. 501–536.

TRAINING BEHAVIOUR IN RELATION TO PERFORMANCE DEVELOPMENT IN TALENTED SPEED SKATERS: A DESCRIPTIVE STUDY

M.T. Elferink-Gemser[1,2], I.M. de Roos[1], M. Torenbeek[2], W. Idema[2], L. Jonker[1], and C. Visscher[1]

[1] University Medical Center Groningen, University of Groningen, The Netherlands; [2] Institute for Studies in Sports and Exercise, HAN University of Applied Sciences, The Netherlands

44.1 INTRODUCTION

Athletes in talent development programmes must improve their performance enormously to reach the top. Multidimensional personal characteristics such as anthropometric, physiological, technical, tactical, and psychological skills underlie their development; always in and with the environment. Although the value of training is acknowledged and the theory of deliberate practice (i.e., 10.000 hours or 10 years to reach elite level) well known (Ericsson, 1996) relatively little is known about which training behaviour is beneficial for performance development. This is also true for speed skating, a popular sport in the Netherlands. Recent studies on self-regulated learning in talented athletes have revealed that self-regulated learning skills play a distinguishing role at the highest levels of performance (Jonker *et al.*, 2010; Toering *et al.*, 2009). Moreover, studies examining self-regulated learning in sport training showed that experts have a higher degree of self-regulated learning skills than non-experts or novices (Cleary and Zimmerman, 2001; Kitsantas and Zimmerman, 2002). Especially, reflection is a very important self-regulatory skill in talented athletes (Jonker *et al.*, 2012). Additionally, goal orientation is related to the level of performance. The research of Van Yperen and Duda (1999) among talented soccer players showed that an increase in skilled performance over the season corresponded to a stronger task orientation. However, the knowledge of theoretical processes underpinning behaviour will only be meaningful if it can be related to real-world, overt behavior (Toering *et al.*, 2011). Specifically, for practical application and implementation of psychological constructs in talent development, it is important to know how these theoretical constructs are expressed in the actual behaviour of an athlete. Moreover, there is very little research with respect to behaviour in the sport context (Toering *et al.*, 2011; Young and Starkes, 2006a; Young and Starkes, 2006b).

44.2 METHODS

Eight international level talented speed skaters (mean = 17.00 ± 0.76) from the Dutch National Junior Team filled out questionnaires for training volume, reflection and goal orientation. Reflection was measured using the 5-item reflection subscale of the Self-Regulated Learning—Self-Report Scale (SRL-SRS; Toering *et al.*, 2012). This subscale was originally based on the Reflective Learning Continuum (Peltier *et al.*, 2006). Goal orientation was measured using the Dutch Task and Ego Orientation in Sport Questionnaire (TEOSQ; Van Yperen and Duda, 1999). This instrument, originally developed by Duda and Nicholls (1992), measures task orientation (7 items) and ego orientation (6 items). Participants had to score all items on a 5-point Likert-scale, ranging from 'strongly disagree' to 'strongly agree'.

To examine performance development, the best times of two subsequent seasons were extracted from the database of the Dutch National Speed Skating Association (SARA database; www.knsb.nl). For each speed skater we extracted the season best times on all regular distances (i.e., for males 500, 1000, 1500, 3000 and 5000 metres; for females 500, 1000, 1500 and 3000 metres). All speed skating times in seconds were corrected for the ice rink on which the competition was held, using the estimated rink parameters calculated by Kamst (2010), so that all speed skating times were comparable. Subsequently, we converted all corrected speed skating times to 500 metre times. For all speed skaters the difference between season best times in the subsequent seasons were calculated. Thereafter, we were able to identify the distance on which the most progression or the least decline was made for each speed skater. Finally, the progression or decline on this distance was calculated both in absolute terms (progression or decline in seconds, converted to 500 metre time) and in relative terms (progression or decline in percentages).

To identify characteristics of behaviour, semi-structured interviews with 4 male expert speed skating coaches were conducted (N = 4, mean = 37.33 years, SD = 10.69). They had 5 to 22 years of experience as speed skating coaches (M = 11.00 years, SD = 9.54). Three of the four coaches had experience in coaching at international level. The expert coaches were interviewed and asked to describe behaviours of talented speed skaters aged 16 to 19 years, that according to them led to performance development. The interviews concerned behaviours both before, during and after practice and competition, as well as behaviours in daily life, for example combining high level sports with educational activities, and coping with injuries. The coach interviews were transcribed verbatim. Behavioural items reflecting the same content were grouped together. Subsequently, only behaviours that were mentioned by at least two coaches were included in the list of behavioral items. The identified behavioral items were then scored by the main coach (male, former international speed skater, experienced coach) of the Dutch National Junior Team for each speed skater at the end of the competitive season on a 10-point Likert-scale. This score formed the measure of behaviour. To provide a description of behaviour in speed skating in relation to performance development, we described the cases of two speed skaters. The first case description concerned the speed skater who made the most progression in performance during two subsequent seasons, while the second case concerned the speed skater who made the least progression in performance.

44.3 RESULTS

The speed skater with most progression (case 1) trained less hours per week and scored lower on ego orientation but had higher scores on reflection and task orientation than the group means and the speed skater with least progression (case 2; see Table 44.1). Based on the outcomes of the semi-structured interviews, 22 behavioural items were defined which were judged for case 1 and 2 (see Table 44.2). In contrast to case 2, case 1 scored very high (i.e., score 9 or 10) on the behavioural items 'taking responsibility for own behaviour and performance', 'being able to combine high level sport with educational activities' and 'being on time for practice'. Furthermore, the cases differed largely (>3 points) on the items 'being self-directed', 'being able to work autonomously', 'taking initiative', 'using previous experiences to learn from' and 'being prepared for practice and competition', with case 1 outscoring case 2. In contrast, case 2 outscored case 1 on multiple items as well, e.g., taking sufficient rest during training trips.

Table 44.1 Descriptive statistics for the entire sample of international level talented speed skaters (n = 8) as well as for the speed skater who made most progression (case 1) and the one who made least progression (case 2).

	Mean	SD	Case 1	Case 2
Training volume (hours/week)	19.44	2.83	16.50	22.00
Absolute performance development (s)	0.83	0.52	1.80	0.20
Relative performance development (%)	2.05	1.20	4.09	0.52
Reflection (1–5)	4.34	0.40	4.80	4.20
Task orientation (1–5)	4.25	0.62	4.71	4.00
Ego orientation (1–5)	4.19	0.52	3.50	4.33

44.4 DISCUSSION

This study sought to describe the behaviour of international talented speed skaters and relate this to performance development. Because of the relatively small sample size which is inevitable at the highest level of performance, the results have to be interpreted with caution. Nevertheless, interesting results appeared. For example, it is notable that the speed skater with the most progression scored the highest possible score on the behavioural item 'taking responsibility for own behaviour and performance'. Self-regulated learning is reflected in taking responsibility for learning (Toering *et al.*, 2011). Moreover, the speed skater who improved most scored high on 'using previous experiences to learn from', which can be considered as an indicator of reflection. Another remarkable difference with the speed skater who made the least progression, was that this speed skater was less self-directed, not able to work autonomously and did not take initiative, compared to the speed skater who showed the largest performance development. Athletes who fail to self-regulate are less disciplined and motivated, and show less initiative (Young and Starkes, 2006a). Furthermore, the speed skater with the least progression did not score high on the self-regulated learning skill reflection, compared to the speed skater with most progression and the group average. Recently, Jonker *et al.* (2012) showed the importance of reflection for expertise. However, the speed skater with least progression outscored the skater with most progression on multiple relevant items as well, such as taking rest. On a high performance level there were differences in behaviour between speed skaters all performing at the international level. In combination with a high task orientation; i.e., experiencing success when improving yourself, more use of self-regulated learning skills, seems to lead to more performance development, in spite of a lower amount of deliberate practice. To conclude, task orientation and reflection seem positively related to performance development in contrast to quantity of training and ego-orientation (experiencing success when performing better than others). It is possible to identify behaviour which is related to performance development. This knowledge can be used to improve talent development, however, more research is needed.

Table **44.2** List of 22 behavioural items regarded important for performance development in international level talented speed skaters according to expert speed skating coaches.

The speed skater...		#1	#2
1	is able to combine high level sport with school	9	2
2	takes responsibility for own behavior and performance	10	6
3	is on time for practice	9	5
4	takes sufficient rest during training trips	4	8
5	uses previous experiences to learn from	8	5
6	takes care for nutrition	5	8
7	is self-directed, able to work autonomously	7	4
8	is prepared for practice and competition	6	3
9	applies instructions and advices directly	8	6
10	asks substantive questions to the coach	5	7
11	is conscious of own behaviour	7	5
12	does everything needed to recover from injuries	4	6
13	knows training intensities needed for practice	5	7
14	asks for feedback to the coach on own initiative	7	8
15	creates optimal conditions for performance	6	7
16	takes care of rest times during practice	7	6
17	sets clear goals, monitors progress and evaluates	6	5
18	evaluates with the coach after practice and races	7	7
19	behaves optimally to benefit from practice and races	7	7
20	has a goal and plan for both practice and competition	6	6
21	keeps a logbook, even when it's not mandatory	5	5
22	executes a warm up and cool down on own initiative	5	5

44.5 REFERENCES

Cleary, T.J. and Zimmerman, B.J., 2001, Self-regulation differences during athletic practice by experts, non-experts, and novices. *Journal of Applied Sport Psychology,* **13**, pp. 185–206.

Ericsson, K. A., Krampe, R. Th. and Tesch-Römer, C., 1993, The role of deliberate practice in the acquisition of expert performance. *Psychological Review,* **100**, pp. 363–406.

Jonker, L., Elferink-Gemser, M.T. and Visscher, C., 2010, Differences in self-regulatory skills among talented athletes: the significance of competitive sport level and type of sport. *Journal of Sports Sciences,* **28**, pp. 901–908.

Jonker, L., Elferink-Gemser, M.T., de Roos, I.M. and Visscher, C., 2012, The role of reflection in sport expertise. *The Sports Psychologist,* **26**, pp. 224–242.

Kamst, R., 2010, Talent development tracking for speed skating. Unpublished Master Thesis, University of Groningen, Groningen.

Kitsantas, A. and Zimmerman, B.J., 2002, Comparing self-regulatory processes among novice, non-expert, and expert volleyball players: a microanalytic study. *Journal of Applied Sport Psychology,* **14**, pp. 91–105.

Peltier, J.W., Hay, A. and Drago, W., 2006, Reflecting on self-reflection: scale extension and a comparison of undergraduate business students in the United States and the United Kingdom. *Journal of Marketing Education,* **28**, pp. 5–16.

SARA-database KNSB, 2011, Retrieved from: www.knsb.nl

Toering, T.T., Elferink-Gemser, M.T., Jordet, G., Jorna, C., Pepping, G.J. and Visscher, C., 2011, Self-regulation of practice behavior among elite youth soccer players: an exploratory observation study. *Journal of Applied Sport Psychology,* **23**, pp. 110–128.

Toering, T.T., Elferink-Gemser, M.T., Jordet, G. and Visscher, C., 2009, Self-regulation and performance level of elite and non-elite youth soccer players. *Journal of Sports Sciences,* **27**, pp. 1509–1517.

Toering, T.T., Elferink-Gemser, M.T., Jordet, G., Pepping, G.J. and Visscher, C, 2012, Self-regulation of learning and performance level of elite youth soccer players. *International Journal of Sport Psychology,* **43**, pp. 312–325.

Van Yperen, N.W. and Duda, J.L, 1999, Goal orientations, beliefs about success, and performance improvement among young elite Dutch soccer players. *Scandinavian Journal of Medicine and Science in Sports,* **9**, pp. 358–364.

Young, B.W. and Starkes, J.L, 2006a, Coaches' perceptions of non-regulated training behaviors in competitive swimmers. *International Journal of Sports Science and Coaching,* **1**, pp. 53–68.

Young, B.W. and Starkes, J.L., 2006b, Measuring outcomes of swimmers' non-regulation during practice: relationships between self-report, coaches' judgments, and video observation. *International Journal of Sports Science and Coaching,* **1**, pp. 131–148.

THE ANTHROPOMETRIC CHARACTERISTICS OF YOUNG PADDLERS AND THEIR RELATIONSHIP WITH PADDLE SET-UP AND PERFORMANCE

R.A. Fernandes, B.B. Gomes, R. Rebelo–Gonçalves, J.P. Duarte, J.R. Pereira, and A. Cupido-dos-Santos

University of Coimbra, Portugal

45.1 INTRODUCTION

As sports become more specialized identification and selection of young talent tends to occur in increasingly younger ages (Helsen *et al.*, 2000). In canoeing, although there are studies which describe attributes, whether anthropometric or physiological of elite (Michael *et al.*, 2008) and young kayakers (Alacid *et al.*, 2011) few normative data exist on the optimization of the equipment set-up. According to human morphology in sprint kayaking and the existing studies focusing on adult athletes (Ong *et al.*, 2005), it seems that an incorrect adjustment of the equipment will affect the comfort of the athlete, his ability to execute the technical movement, and consequently his performance (Burke and Pruitt, 2003). Thereby the aim of this study was to describe the anthropometric characteristics of athletes competing at the level of 15 and 16 years old and their relationship with the paddle set-up and performance.

45.2 METHODOLOGY

This study involved 23 young male kayakers (15.39 ± 0.46 years). All athletes participated in the national control of 1000 metres and was assessed for body mass, stature, sitting height, lengths (arm span, arm, forearm and hand), circumferences (brachial, brachial in maximum contraction and chest), diameters (biacromial) and skinfolds (triceps and subscapular), we adopted the procedures described by Lohman *et al.* (1988). We also assessed the upper limb volume in the dominant limb (Rogowski *et al.*, 2008) and the body composition (Slaughter *et al.*, 1988). Technical error of measurement ranged from 0.1% to 2% and reliability ranged from 97.1% to 100% (Perini *et al.*, 2005). The equipment set-up measured was paddle length; blade length; blade width; hand grip distance; frontal blade area; angle between blades and diameter of the shaft. The physical fitness of the athletes was assessed by performing a test of sit-ups, push-ups, pull-ups (The Cooper Institute for Aerobics Research, 1999) and handgrip strength (Council of Europe, 1988). Prior to the assessment of physical fitness, a standardized 5 min warm-up was performed. Biological maturation was assessed by maturity offset (Mirwald *et al.*, 2002) and percentage of predicted mature stature (Khamis and Roche, 1994, 1995). Statistical analysis included descriptive statistics and a Shapiro-Wilk (*SW*) test for total sample a linear regression analysis for test relationship between anthropometry, paddle set-up and performance and a Spearman correlation coefficient was calculated to ascertain the strength of the correlations and facilitate the selection of independent variables as input data for regression analysis. A significance level of $p < 0.05$ was selected. The Statistical Programme for Social Sciences, version 20.0 for Windows was used.

45.3 RESULTS

An association was found between better performances at 1000m and body mass (*rho* $\leq$ 0.05), brachial circumference (*rho* $\leq$ 0.01), brachial circumference in maximum contraction (*rho* $\leq$ 0.01), chest circumference (*rho* $\leq$ 0.01), upper limb volume (*rho* $\leq$ 0.05), arm volume (*rho* $\leq$ 0.01) and pull-ups (*rho* $\leq$ 0.01). The predictive model for paddle length, derived from total sample assessment (equation 3.1), shows that 48% of this parameter is explained by the variation of the sitting height, maturity offset or handgrip strength ($R^2 = 0.480$; Std. Error Estimate= 2.189; $F = 5.840$; $p = 0.005$). Statistical differences between the three best times *vs.* three worst times was established for training experience ($p \leq 0.05$); body mass ($p \leq 0.05$); brachial circumference ($p \leq 0.05$); brachial circumference in maximum contraction ($p \leq 0.05$); chest circumference ($p \leq 0.05$); arm length ($p \leq 0.05$); angle between blades ($p \leq 0.05$); pull-ups ($p \leq 0.05$) and time at 1000 meters ($p \leq 0.05$). Table 45.1 shows descriptive statistics and *SW* test results.

45.4 CONCLUSIONS

This study aimed to identify the anthropometric characteristics of young paddlers who better associate with the equipment set-up for a physical fitness test battery and the performance achieved in real race conditions. The results obtained respecting anthropometric characteristics are similar to those obtained by Alacid *et al.* (2011) and with respect to predictive models of equipment set-up, our results are in accordance with Ong *et al.* (2005) and Diafas *et al.* (2012) since the regression analysis in our study also showed a significant relationship between anthropometric variables and equipment set-up. The results obtained: (1) offer the anthropometric profile of the young male paddler, and uncover that athletes with slightly larger upper body dimensions and better results in pull-up test have better performance in flatwater racing, (2) could be used more objectively in initial equipment set-up selection, (3) allow coaches and athletes to explore the feasibility of customizing the dimensions of the paddle, and (4) can be used as a guide in the process of talent identification.

Table 45.1 Descriptive statistic and the Shapiro-Wilk (SW) test for total sample (n=23).

Variables	Units	Mean	SD	SW value	p
Training	years	3.4	2.2	0.948	0.262
Estimated mature stature	%	96.0	2.3	0.952	0.326
Maturity offset	years	1.7	0.5	0.972	0.745
Stature	cm	172.8	6.4	0.945	0.232
Sitting height	cm	91.6	2.8	0.985	0.968
Body mass	kg	63.6	7.1	0.977	0.847
Fat mass	%	15.1	3.4	0.970	0.685
Arm span	cm	177.7	7.5	0.938	0.165
Arm	cm	34.1	1.9	0.962	0.498
Forearm	cm	28.5	1.2	0.980	0.900
Hand	cm	18.6	0.7	0.887	0.014
Brachial	cm	27.2	1.8	0.987	0.986
Brachial maximum contraction	cm	30.6	2.1	0.961	0.474
Chest	cm	92.3	5.0	0.975	0.812
Biacromial	cm	38.6	1.9	0.956	0.379
Upper limb volume	L	3327.8	436.4	0.960	0.473
Arm volume	L	2184.8	315.5	0.957	0.401
Forearm volume	L	1143.0	133.5	0.955	0.368
Paddle length	cm	212.2	2.8	0.930	0.112
Blade length	cm	48.3	1.2	0.756	0.000
Blade width	cm	15.8	0.5	0.918	0.061
Handgrip distance	cm	70.1	4.2	0.961	0.492
Frontal blade area	cm^2	650.8	34.1	0.949	0.285
Angle between blades	gr^o	60.7	8.9	0.955	0.375
Shaft diameter	mm	28.8	1.5	0.817	0.001
Push-ups	#	34.1	11.7	0.903	0.030
Pull-ups	#	9.8	6.1	0.933	0.124
Sit-ups	#	67.6	16.9	0.494	0.000
Handgrip strength	kg/f	44.1	6.7	0.949	0.277
1000 metres	min:s	5:34	0.6	0.910	0.042

45.5 REFERENCES

Ackland, T.R., Ong, K.B., Kerr, D.A. and Ridge, B., 2003, Morphological characteristics of Olympic sprint canoe and kayak paddlers. *Journal of Science and Medicine in Sport*, **6**, pp. 285–94.

Alacid, F., Muyor, J.M. and López-Miñarro, P.A., 2011, Perfil antropométrico del canoísta joven de aguas tranquilas. *International Journal of Morphology*, **29**, pp. 835–841.

Burke. E.R. and Pruitt, A.L., 2003, Body positioning for cycling. In *High-tech Cycling*, 2nd ed., edited by Burke, E. (Champaign: Human Kinetics), pp. 69–92.

Council of Europe, 1988, *Eurofit: Handbook for the Eurofit tests of Physical Fitness*, (Rome: Council of Europe).

Diafas, V., Kaloupsis, S., Dimakopoulou, E., Zelioti, D., Diamanti, V. and Alexiou, S., 2012. Selection of paddle length in flatwater kayak: Art or science?, *Biology of Exercise*, **8**, pp. 17–26.

Helsen, W.F., Hodges, N.J., Van Winckel, J. and Starkes, J.L., 2000, The role of talent, physical precocity and practice in the development of soccer expertise. *Journal of Sports Sciences*, **18**, pp. 727–736.

Khamis, H.J. and Roche, A.F., 1994; 1995 – erratum, Predicting adult stature without using skeletal age. *Pediatrics*, **94**, pp. 504–507.

Michael, J.S., Rooney, K.B. and Smith, R., 2008, The metabolic demands of kayaking : A review. *Journal of Sports Sciences and Medicine*, **2**, pp. 1–7.

Mirwald. R.L., Baxter-Jones, A.D., Bailey, D.A. and Beunen. G.P., 2002, An assessment of maturity from anthropometric measurements. *Medicine and Science in Sports and Exercise*, **34**, pp. 689–694.

Ong, K.B., Ackland, T.R., Hume, P.A, Ridge, B., Broad, E. and Kerr, D.A., 2005, Equipment set-up among Olympic sprint and slalom kayak paddlers. *Sports Biomechanics*, **4**, pp. 47–58.

Perini, T.A., Oliveira, G.L., Ornellas, J.S. and Oliveira, F.P., 2005, Technical error of measurement in anthropometry. *Revista Brasileira de Medicina do Esporte*, **11**, pp. 86–90.

Rogowski, I., Ducher, G., Brosseau, O. and Hautier, C., 2008, Asymmetry in volume between dominant and nondominant upper limbs in young tennis players. *Pediatric Exercise Science*, **20**, pp. 263–72.

Slaughter M.H., Lohman, T.G., Boileau, R.A., Horswill, C.A., Stillman, R.J., Van Loan, M.D. and Bemben, D.A., 1988, Skinfold equations for estimation of body fatness in children and youth. *Human Biology,* **60**, pp. 709–723.

The Cooper Institute for Aerobics Research, 1999, *Fitnessgram : Test Administration Manual,* 2nd ed., edited by Meredith, M.D. and Welk, G.J. (Champaign: Human Kinetics), pp. 21–27.

CORRELATION BETWEEN CRITICAL VELOCITY AND MAXIMAL LACTATE STEADY STATE IN ADOLESCENT ELITE SWIMMERS

M.V. Machado[1,2], O.A. Junior[3], A. Marques[3], E. Colantonio[4], L.R. Altimari[2,5], E.S. Cyrino[2,5], and M.T. de Melo[4]

[1]Laboratory of Cardiovascular Investigation, Oswaldo Cruz Foundation, Brazil; [2]Group for Study and Research in Metabolism, Nutrition and Exercise, Brazil; [3]Campinas State University, Brazil; [4]São Paulo Federal University; [5]Londrina State University, Brazil

46.1 INTRODUCTION

The Critical Power (CP) is a theoretical concept that assumes the existence of a maximum power of exercise that can be maintained indefinitely (Monod and Scherrer, 1965). The method was originally proposed for evaluating muscle groups synergists (Monod and Scherrer, 1965), and later extended to the assessment of large muscle groups (Moritani et al., 1981). In the early 90s, the CP was used in swimming and the term critical velocity (CV) was proposed to represent the swimming speed which theoretically could be maintained for a long period of time without depletion (Wakayoshi et al., 1992a). Over the years the CV has received different experimental approaches to confirm its validity (Wakayoshi et al., 1992b; Denadai and Greco, 2005; Machado et al., 2011), in swimmers of different ages (between 8 and 18 years) (Hill et al., 1995). However, the behaviour of CV as a predictor of aerobic performance in adolescent athletes of high competitive level has not yet been evaluated. Thus, the present study aimed to verify whether the CV corresponds to maximal lactate steady state (MLSS) in adolescent athletes characterized as elite swimmers in the child and youth categories.

46.2 METHODS

The study was approved by the Research Ethics Committee of the Faculty of Medical Sciences, State University of Campinas (#774/2007), according to Resolution #196/96 of the National Health Council on research involving human beings. Twelve swimmers (6 boys and 6 girls) participated in the study (13.92 ± 0.90 years, 5.75 ± 1.92 years of training experience; 54.86 ± 6.55 kg, 13.57 ± 4.99 % fat). All swimmers were ranked in the top four in the Rio de Janeiro State Championships in child and youth categories between the years 2006 and 2007. Of these, two won the 100-m backstroke, 100 and 200-m freestyle. Two swimmers won first place in the Brazilian Championship Youth in 2008 on 200-m medley and 200-m freestyle, and another won the 3er place in the 200-m freestyle.

CV was determined through four front crawl sprints of 50, 100, 200, and 400 m respectively with 24 h between sprints. All repetitions were performed in random order during the training sessions. CV was determined by the slope (b) of the linear regression line between the distances and the times obtained during each repetition (Wakayoshi et al., 1992a; Wakayoshi et al., 1992b), and anaerobic work capacity (AWC) was determined by extending the line of linear regression (di Prampero, Dekerle et al. 2008). Determination of MLSS was performed according to the methodology proposed by Wakayoshi et al. (1993). The participants performed three series of four sprints of 400 m (3 x 4 x 400- m) in random order with constant speed corresponding to 98%, 100%, and 102% of CV, with breaks of 45–60s among sprints to collect blood and 48 h among the series. Arterialized capillary blood (25 μl) was collected and transferred through a Kacil® fixed volume pipette to a micro Eppendorf® tube containing 50 μl of 1% sodium fluoride. Blood lactate concentration was determined in an electrochemical analyser (YSL 2300, STAT Yellow Spring Co., USA). Intensity at MLSS was defined as the highest workload that could be maintained for a long period of time without a continuous rise in blood lactate accumulation (Beneke, 2003).

Data are presented as mean ± standard deviations. Student's t-test was used for comparisons among the CV and MLSS. CV and MLSS were assessed using Pearson's correlation coefficient. Two-way ANOVA was used to compare the blood lactate concentration in the 400-m shots in three intensities (98, 100 and 102%) and Tukey's post-hoc test where appropriate. Statistical significance was set at p <0.05.

46.3 RESULTS

Figure 46.1 shows the values of CV and MLSS in metres per second (m/s). The CV was significantly higher than the MLSS (1.32± 0.06 vs 1.29 ± 0.05 m/s, p <0.05), overestimating their speed by 2.27%. However, a high correlation was found between the methods.

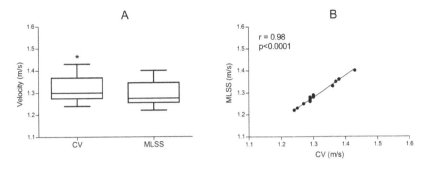

Figure 46.1 Comparisons among the CV and MLSS (A), and correlation coefficient between CV and the velocity at MLSS (B).

The Figure 46.2 shows the blood lactate values obtained in the range of 3 x 4 x 400-m intensities of 98, 100 and 102% of CV. The exercise intensity that characterizes the MLSS intensity was observed in 98% (3.60 ± 1.05, 3.76 ± 1.26, 3.71 ± 1.46, 3.83 ± 1.56 mM). The intensities of 100% and 102% of CV were not observed in a dynamic equilibrium concentration of lactate.

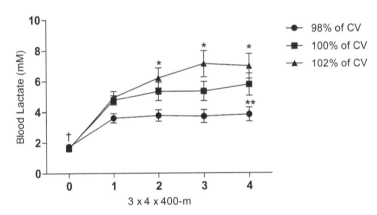

Figure 46.2 Relationship between blood lactate concentration and the three series of 400-m sprints (98%, 100%, and 102% of CV) for the determination of MLSS. † $p < 0.05$ vs all sprints. ** $p < 0.05$ vs 98% and 100%. * $p < 0.05$ vs 98% e 102%.

46.4 CONCLUSION

In conclusion, our results indicate that the CV overestimates the MLSS in adolescent elite swimmers. However, the high correlation between the methods suggests that CV is reliable when used to prescribe and monitor the training of adolescent athletes.

46.5 REFERENCE

Beneke, R., 2003, Methodological aspects of maximal lactate steady state-implications for performance testing. *European Journal of Applied Physiology*, **89**, pp. 95–99.

Denadai, B. and Greco, C., 2005, Critical speed endurance capacity in young swimmers: effects of gender and age. *Pediatric Exercise Science*, **17**, pp. 353–363.

di Prampero, P.E., Dekerle, J., Capelli, C. and Zamparo, P., 2008, The critical velocity in swimming. *European Journal of Applied Physiology.* **102**, pp. 165–171.

Hill, D.R., Steward, R.P. and Jane, C.J., 1995, Application of the critical power concept to young swimmers. *Pediatric Exercise Science*, **7**, pp. 281–293.

Machado, M.V., Júnior, O.A., Marques, A.C., Colantonio, E., Cyrino, E.S. and De Mello, M.T., 2011, Effect of 12 weeks of training on critical velocity and maximal lactate steady state in swimmers. *European Journal of Sport Science*, **11**, pp. 165–170.

Monod, H. and Scherrer, J., 1965, The work capacity of a synergic muscular group. *Ergonomics*, **8**, pp. 329–338.

Moritani, T., Nagata, A., deVries, H.A. and Muro, M., 1981, Critical power as a measure of physical work capacity and anaerobic threshold. *Ergonomics*, **24**, pp. 339–350.

Wakayoshi, K., Ikuta, K., Yoshida, T., Udo, M., Moritani, T., Mutoh, Y. and Miyashita, M., 1992a, Determination and validity of critical velocity as an index of swimming performance in the competitive swimmer. *European Journal of Applied Physiology and Occupational Physiology*, **64**, pp. 153–157.

Wakayoshi, K., Yoshida, T., Udo, M., Harada, T., Moritani, T., Mutoh, Y. and Miyashita, M., 1993, Does critical swimming velocity represent exercise intensity at maximal lactate steady state? *European Journal of Applied Physiology and Occupational Physiology*, **66**, pp. 90–95.

Wakayoshi, K., Yoshida, T., Udo, M., Kasai, T., Moritani, T., Mutoh, Y. and Miyashita, M., 1992b, A simple method for determining critical speed as swimming fatigue threshold in competitive swimming. *International Journal of Sports Medicine*, **13**, pp. 367–371.

AGREEMENT BETWEEN PEAK POWER OUTPUTS OBTAINED FROM THE APPLICATION OF COMMON BRAKING FORCE AND THE ESTIMATED OPTIMAL LOAD IN SOCCER GOALKEEPERS

R. Rebelo-Gonçalves[1], A.J. Figueiredo[1], J.P. Duarte[1], J.R. Pereira[1], R.A. Fernandes[1], F. Simões[1]†, V. Severino[1], J. Valente-dos-Santos[1], V. Vaz[1], A. Cupido-dos-Santos[1], M.J. Coelho-e-Silva[1], A. Tessitore[2], and N. Armstrong[3]

[1]University of Coimbra, Portugal; [2]University of Rome 'Foro Italico, Italy, [3]University of Exeter, UK

47.1 INTRODUCTION

Soccer specific tasks such as sprinting, changing of direction, jumping and running demand the ability to generate energy anaerobically. Maximal short-term fitness is often assessed by the Wingate anaerobic test (WAnT) which provides an estimation of the peak power output of the legs. An alternative to the WAnT protocol is provided by a series of short "all out" sprints against a range of braking forces on a friction-braked cycle ergometer (Force-velocity test, FVT). The latter protocol is a promising alternative for investigation, although the literature comparing the peak power outputs from the two protocols has not been exhaustively explored. Therefore, the purpose of this study was to examine agreement between peak power outputs derived from the two cycle-ergometer tests.

47.2 METHODS

The participants were 33 young male soccer goalkeepers aged 12.73–18.67 years who visited the laboratory three times. Data collected included years of training obtained by interview, chronological age (CA), stature, sitting height, body mass and anthropometric variables needed to calculate thigh volume (Jones and Pearson, 1969). Fat mass and fat-free mass were assessed by air-displacement plethysmography. The percentage of predicted mature stature (PMS) was used as an indicator of maturation (Khamis and Roche, 1995). A standardized warm up routine was applied before the completion of all protocols on a friction-loaded ergometer (Monark 824E Peak Bike, Monark AB, Vargerg, Sweden) interfaced with a microcomputer. Each participant completed the WAnT adopting a standardized load of 0.74 N·kg^{-1}. In the second visit a series of 3–5 maximal bouts against a range of braking forces (0.19 to 1.06 N·kg^{-1}; initial braking force [Fb] set at 0.74 N·kg^{-1} with subsequent Fb above and below this intensity) was performed. Based on estimated optimal load (OL), participants completed an additional 30-s all-out maximal exercise. Descriptive statistics were calculated and the assumption of normality was checked using the Kolmogorov–Smirnov test. Bivariate correlations were used to examine the association between peak power outputs, and between P_{WAnT}, P_{OL} and other variables.

Table 47.1 Descriptive statistics ($n = 33$) and bivariate correlations between P_{WAnT}, P_{OL}, and training years, chronological age (CA), predicted mature stature (PMS) and body size variables.

| | Descriptive | | Correlations | |
| | | | P_{WAnT} (watt) | P_{OL} (watt) |
	(min–max)	Mean±sd	r (p)	r (p)
Training years (y)	0.00–12.00	5.61±2.65	0.287 (0.105)	0.303 (0.087)
CA (y)	12.73–18.67	15.56±1.86	0.654 (0.000)	0.702 (0.000)
PMS (%)	87.4–100.2	95.7±3.5	0.663 (0.000)	0.688 (0.000)
Stature (cm)	159.0–184.7	173.5±6.7	0.580 (0.000)	0.691 (0.000)
Body mass (kg)	46.8–91.6	65.5±10.4	0.561 (0.001)	0.622 (0.000)
Sitting height (cm)	62.60–96.00	73.53±10.50	0.546 (0.001)	0.511 (0.002)
Leg length (cm)	75.80–91.80	83.39±3.73	0.414 (0.017)	0.557 (0.001)
Fat mass (%)	1.4–22.3	11.2±5.6	-0.393 (0.024)	-0.394 (0.023)
Fat-free mass (kg)	41.6–77.6	58.2±9.3	0.715 (0.000)	0.780 (0.000)
Mid thigh girth (cm)	37.60–52.80	45.03±3.62	0.550 (0.001)	0.618 (0.000)
Thigh volume (L)	3.40–6.90	5.05±0.92	0.577 (0.000)	0.622 (0.000)
OL (kg)	3.50–6.90	4.90±0.78		
P_{OL} (watt)	446.8–1298.8	792.5±215.7		
WAnT (kg)	2.40–8.90	5.31±1.40		
P_{WAnT} (watt)	533.0–1278.0	873.2±216.8		

A linear regression analysis was used to determine the relationship between both protocols. Upper and lower limits of agreement (ULOA and LLOA) were also determined by plotting the mean differences between methods (Bland and Altman, 1986). The paired samples t-test was used to compare the means of P_{OL} and P_{WAnT}. Finally, multiple linear regression (method stepwise) was used to estimate the relative contributions of training years, CA, PMS, stature, sitting height, leg length, body mass, fat mass, fat-free mass, mid thigh circumference and thigh volume to variation in peak power outputs. Correlation coefficients were considered trivial (r

< 0.1), small (0.1 < r < 0.3) moderate (0.3 < r < 0.5), large (0.5 < r < 0.7), very large (0.7 < r < 0.9), nearly perfect (r >0.9) and perfect (r = 1) (Hopkins, 2002).

47.3 RESULTS

Descriptive characteristics of the total sample are summarized in Table 47.1 which also presents the coefficients of correlations between peak power outputs obtained from the 30-s all-out maximal exercises and related variables. The association between peak power outputs ($r = 0.891$, $p = 0.000$) was very large. The mean difference between peak power outputs ($P_{OL}-P_{WAnT}$) was significant [mean difference=80.7, 95% CI: 45.0 to 116.5, $t_{(32)}$=4.598; $p<0.001$] with ULOA = 278.36; LLOA = -116.94 (Figure 47.2). Figure 47.1 illustrates the linear relationship between the power outputs derived from the common braking forces and the estimated OL ($r = 0.891$, 95% CI: 0.790 to 0.945). Multiple linear regression (stepwise mode) demonstrated a significant multiple correlation between the combination of leg length and WAnT peak power output, as independent variables, and P_{OL} as the predicted variable ($R = 0.904$, $R^2 = 0.816$, Adjusted $R^2 = 0.800$).

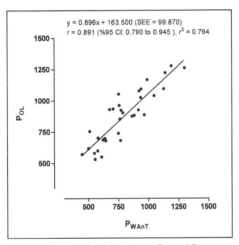

Figure 47.1 Relationship between P_{OL} and P_{WAnT}.

47.4 DISCUSSION

The issue of load optimization in cycle-ergometer testing has been mainly discussed through theoretical models (Dotan and Bar-Or, 1983; Santos *et al.*, 2003) and the present study examined the agreement between peak power outputs derived from two cycle-ergometer tests. The use of a fixed applied force of 0. 74 N·kg^{-1} may not be optimal for eliciting anaerobic peak outputs in cycle-ergometer tests, as this common braking force tends to underestimate peak power. Performance fluctuation in both protocols was determined by CA, maturation, body size, body composition and thigh volume. The independent variables in the regression model explained 80% of variance for P_{OL}, emphasizing the importance of body size and composition to variance in maximal power output in the 30-s cycle-ergometer test when using an estimated OL, which is consistent with previous results (Dotan and Bar-Or, 1983; Santos *et al.*, 2003). Future research should examine agreement for other measures derived from the two cycle-ergometer tests such as explosive power (ratio of peak power and time to when the peak power is reached, $W \cdot s^{-1}$).

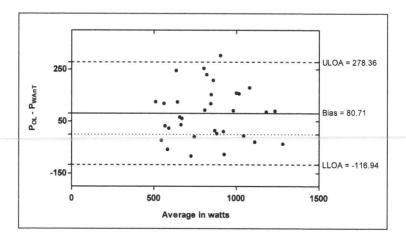

Figure 47.2 Differences in anaerobic peak outputs between protocols against the average performance. The bias line, upper and lower 95% limits of agreement (ULOA and LLOA) are also presented.

47.5 ACKNOWLEDGMENTS AND CONTRIBUTIONS

RRG is granted by *Fundação para a Ciência e a Tecnologia*: SFRH/BD/72111/2010] and is being supervised by AF, MJCS, AT. Data collected by RRG, JPD, JRP, RAF, FS, VS, JVS, VV. Analyses performed by RRG and MJCS. NA, ACS, AF critically reviewed the chapter. All authors approved the final version.

47.6 REFERENCES

Bland, J.M. and Altman, D.G., 1986, Statistical methods for assessing agreement between two methods of clinical measurement. *Lancet*, **1**, pp. 307–310.
Dotan, R. and Bar-Or, O., 1983, Load optimization for the Wingate Anaerobic Test. *European Journal of Applied Physiology and Occupational Physiology*, **51**, pp. 409–417.

Hopkins, W.G., 2002, *A scale of magnitudes for effect statistics. A new view of statistics*. [http://www.sportsci.org/resource/stats/index.html], accessed on December 25, 2011.

Jones, P.R. and Pearson, J., 1969, Anthropometric determination of leg fat and muscle plus bone volumes in young male and female adults. *Journal of Physiology*, **204**, pp. 63–66.

Khamis, H.J. and Roche, A.F., 1995, Predicting adult stature without using skeletal age: the Khamis and Roche method – erratum. *Pediatrics,* **95**, pp. 457.

Santos, A.C., Armstrong, N., De Ste Croix, M. B. A., Sharpe, P. and Welsman, J. R., 2003, Optimal peak power in relation to age, body size, gender, and thigh muscle volume. *Pediatric Exercise Science*, **15**, pp. 406–418.

AGREEMENT BETWEEN INVASIVE AND NON-INVASIVE INDICATORS OF BIOLOGICAL MATURATION IN ADOLESCENT SWIMMERS

L. Ribeiro[1, 2], M.J. Coelho-e-Silva[1], V. Vaz[1], A.J. Figueiredo[1], A. van der Sluis[3], M.T. Elferink-Gemser[3, 4], M.E. Peña-Reyes[5], and R.M. Malina[6, 7]

[1]University of Coimbra, Portugal; [2]University of Algarve, Portugal; [3]University of Groningen, The Netherlands; [4]HAN University of Applied Sciences, The Netherlands; [5]National School of History and Anthropology, Mexico; [6]University of Texas, USA; [7]Tarleton State University, USA

48.1 INTRODUCTION

Growth and maturation characteristics of young athletes are implicit in models of talent identification, selection and development. During pubertal years, male athletes in several sports include proportionally more players who are advanced in biological maturation and proportionally fewer players who are delayed (Malina, 2011). The ability to predict the timing of the adolescent growth spurt is also central to the Long Term Athlete Development model (Balyi et al., 2005), although empirical evidence supporting the model is lacking (Ford et al., 2011). This study evaluates the concordance between maturity classifications (early, on time, late) based on skeletal maturation and a non-invasive method, predicted age at peak height velocity (APHV).

48.2 METHODS

The sample included 76 Portuguese male swimmers. Radiographs of the left hand-wrist were taken and evaluated with the Fels method for assessing skeletal age (SA) (Roche et al., 1988). Two swimmers 13.6 and 15.6 years of age were skeletally mature and thus excluded. Predicted APHV was based on maturity offset, an estimate of time (years) before or after PHV (Mirwald et al., 2002). Offset and chronological age (CA) at observation were used to estimate APHV. Players were classified into three maturity groups on the basis of SA minus CA:

average or on time – SA within ±1.0 year of CA, late – SA behind CA by more than 1.0 year, and early – SA in advance of CA by more than 1.0 year. Contrasting maturity groups based on predicted APHV were defined relative to the mean and standard deviation for APHV of the three samples upon which the offset protocol was developed: on time – predicted APHV within ±1.0 SD of the sample mean (12.9 to 14.7 y), late - predicted APHV >14.7 y, and early – predicted APHV <12.9 y (Malina et al., 2012). Descriptive statistics and cross-tabulation of maturity classifications were calculated. Cohen Kappa and Spearman rank-order correlation coefficients were used to evaluate the concordance of classifications.

48.3 RESULTS

Descriptive characteristics of the 74 swimmers are summarized in Table 48.1. Cross-tabulation of maturity classifications with SA and predicted APHV is summarized in Table 48.2. Concordance between SA-CA classifications and the non-invasive criteria was 50% (95%CI: 38% – 62%). The Kappa coefficient (unweighted) was 0.04 (95%CI: 0 – 0.26) and the Spearman rank order correlation was 0.43 (p<0.01).

Table 48.1 Descriptive statistics for age, body size and maturity indicators for the 74 swimmers.

	Min	Max	Mean	Standard Deviation
Chronological age (y)	11.10	15.97	13.4	1.4
Skeletal Age – Fels (y)	10.33	17.88	14.0	1.7
Body weight (kg)	31.9	82.1	50.2	10.8
Height (cm)	139.1	184.6	161.2	10.0
Maturity offset (y)	-2.81	2.30	-0.74	1.26
Predicted APHV (y)	12.74	15.66	14.2	0.6

Table 48.2 Cross-tabulation of maturity status classifications based on skeletal age (SA) and predicted APHV.

		Maturity status based on predicted APHV			
		Late	Average	Early	TOTAL
Maturity status	Late	4	3	0	7
based on SA – Fels	Average	11	32	0	43
	Early	0	23	1	24
	TOTAL	15	58	1	74

284

48.4 DISCUSSION

The sample of adolescent swimmers was, on average, advanced in SA relative to CA by 0.52±1.14 years with a range of -2.84 to 3.11 years. The variation in SA exceeded the age range of the sample (Table 48.1). Predicted APHV, 14.2±0.6 years, was slightly later than modeled APHV for the three samples used to develop the maturity offset protocol, 13.8±0.9 years. The latter standard deviation approximates those for ages at PHV in longitudinal studies of European boys, ~1.0 year (Malina *et al.*, 2004), while that for predicted APHV in swimmers was reduced compared to that for the three longitudinal samples. The reduced standard deviation for predicted APHV was consistent with other studies applying maturity offset to samples of adolescent male athletes (Malina *et al.*, 2012).

The reduced variation in predicted APHV influenced classifications of swimmers into contrasting maturity groups using the mean and standard deviation for APHV of the samples used to develop the prediction protocol. The majority of swimmers (58 / 78%) were classified as on time (average) in maturation on the basis of predicted APHV in contrast to 43 (58%) classified as such by SA-CA. Only one swimmer was classified early maturing and 15 (20%) were classified late maturing on the basis of predicted APHV, which contrasts the somewhat advanced skeletal maturity status of the sample as a whole. This probably reflects the CA range of the sample and the trend for predicted APHV to increase with CA per se: 11 (n=14, 13.7±0.4 yrs), 12 (n=15, 14.1±0.5 yrs), 13 (n=16, 14.5±0.5 yrs), 14 (n=18, 14.4±0.6 yrs), and 15 (n=11, 14.3±0.8 yrs). The one early maturing swimmer based on predicted APHV was 11.43 years of age, while those classified as on time and late maturing by predicted APHV were 13.3±1.4 and 14.2±1.1 years of age, respectively, and differed significantly (F=3.801, p<0.05). Corresponding ages of late early (n=24), on time (n=43) and late (n=7) maturing swimmers based on SA-CA were 13.5±1.5, 13.4±1.3 and 13.8±1.2 years, respectively, which did not differ (F=0.332)

The SEE of the final prediction equation was 0.592 (Mirwald *et al.*, 2002), which translates to an estimated 95% CI of 1.18 years. Sampling variation and perhaps population variation in proportions of leg length and sitting height may also influence maturity offset and predicted APHV. Both variables are included in the prediction equation. Measurement error is an additional source of variation. Since leg length is derived by subtraction (height minus sitting height), two potential sources of measurement variation are involved.

As noted, two swimmers (13 and 15 years) were skeletally mature and excluded from the analysis. This is not unusual among a sample of adolescent male athletes (Malina, 2011). Skeletal maturity is attained at an SA of 18.0 years, and it is likely that growth in leg length has already ceased. Of interest, the predicted ages at PHV of the two boys were 13.56 and 13.82 years, respectively, which would classify both as on time. Although classifications are not expected to correspond exactly, the observation that predicted APHV classified the majority of Portuguese swimmers 11–15 years as on time in maturation has implications for application of the protocol to predict the maturity timing in developmental programmes for youth athletes. Similar results were noted among Portuguese soccer players 11–14 years of age (Malina *et al.*, 2012). The limitation of maturity offset to differentiate players at the extremes of the maturity continuum requires critical evaluation in samples of youth athletes.

48.5 ACKNOWLEDGMENTS AND CONTRIBUTIONS

LR was supervised by MJCS and AF. VV supported the data collection of the first author. Data collected by LR. MEPR completed two visits in the University of Coimbra and taught the FelS method to assess skeletal age. AJF assessed skeletal age from hand-wrist films. MEG, AVDL critically reviewed the chapter. RMM contributed in all phases of the project and chapter (design, training, analysis, review). All authors approved the final version.

48.6 REFERENCES

Balyi, I., Cardinal, C., Higgs, C., Norris, S. and Way, R., 2005, *Canadian Sport for Life: Long-term athlete development resource paper V2*, (Vancouver: Canadian Sport Centres).
[http://www.canadiansportforlife.ca/default.aspx?PageID=1076&LangID=en], accessed on December 25, 2011.
Ford, P., de Ste Croix, M., Lloyd, R., Meyers, R., Moosavi, M., Oliver, J., Till, K. and Williams, C., 2011, The long-term athlete development model: Physiological evidence and application. *Journal of Sports Sciences*, **29**, pp. 389–402.
Malina, R.M., 2011, Skeletal age and age verification in youth sport. *Sports Medicine*, **42**, pp. 925–947.
Malina, R.M., Bouchard, C. and Bar-Or, O., 2004, *Growth, Maturation, and Physical Activity*, 2nd ed., (Champaign, IL: Human Kinetics).
Malina, R.M., Coelho e Silva, M., Figueiredo, A., Carling, C. and Beunen, G., 2012, Interrelationships among invasive and non-invasive indicators of biological maturation in adolescent male soccer players. *Journal of Sports Sciences*, **30**, pp. 1705–1717.
Malina, R.M., Peña Reyes, M.E., Eisenmann, J.C., Horta, L., Rodrigues, J. and Miller, R., 2000, Height, mass and skeletal maturity of elite Portuguese soccer players 11–16 years. *Journal of Sports Sciences*, **18**, pp. 685–693.
Mirwald, R.L., Baxter-Jones, A.D., Bailey, D.A. and Beunen, G.P., 2002, An assessment of maturity from anthropometric measurements. *Medicine and Science in Sports and Exercise*, **34**, pp. 689–694.
Roche, A.F., Chumlea, C.W. and Thissen, D., 1988, *Assessing the Skeletal Maturity of the Hand-Wrist: Fels Method*, (Springfield, IL: C.C. Thomas).

REPRODUCIBILITY OF REPEATED DRIBBLING ABILITY

J.P. Duarte[1], V. Severino[1], J.R. Pereira[1], R.A. Fernandes[1], F. Simões[1] †, R. Rebelo-Gonçalves[1], J. Valente-dos-Santos[1], V. Vaz[1], A. Seabra[2], and M.J. Coelho-e-Silva[1]

[1]University of Coimbra, Portugal; [2]University of Porto, Portugal

49.1 INTRODUCTION

The intermittent nature of match performance in soccer requires the ability to repeatedly produce high-intensity actions (Bradley *et al.*, 2009). Additional evidence noted that 1.2% to 2.4% of the total covered distance is performed with ball possession. Sprinting and dribbling abilities are interrelated; however the skill of dribbling is more complex and, not surprisingly, previous research indicated that amateur and professional soccer players significantly differed in developmental changes in dribbling (Huijgen *et al.*, 2010). In parallel, the literature also noted the contribution of repeated sprint ability to distinguished players who dropped out from competitive soccer and those who continued and were promoted (Figueiredo *et al.*, 2009). The purpose of this study was to examine the reproducibility of a new test named repeated dribbling ability (RDA) in young soccer players. Additionally, the interrelationship between this new protocol and the traditional repeated sprint ability (RSA) protocol without the ball was explored.

49.2 METHODS

The sample included 25 soccer players aged 12.9–18.6 years. Chronological age (CA) was calculated at the date of the first visit to clubs. Body mass (BM) and stature (H) were measured to the nearest 0.1 kg and 0.1 cm using a balance (SECA 770, Hanover, MD, USA) and a stadiometer (Harpenden 98.603, Holtain Ltd, Croswell, UK), respectively. The triceps and geminal medial skinfolds were measured using a Lange Caliper (Beta Technology, Ann Arbor, MI, USA), and % fat mass estimated (Slaughter *et al.*, 1988). Fat mass (FM) and fat-free mass (FFM) were derived. Biological maturation was assessed as % of predicted mature stature (%PMS) based on the non-invasive method developed by Khamis and Roche (1994). The battery also included circumferences and lengths needed to estimate total thigh volume (TV) of the dominant leg (Jones and Pearson, 1969). Repeated

Sprint Ability (RSA: 7 x 34.2-m / 25″) and Repeated Dribbling Ability (RDA: 7 x 34.2-m / 25″) were assessed as described by Bangsbo (1994). The time for each sprint was recorded on a digital chronometer connected to photoelectric cells (Globus Ergo Timer Timing System, Codogné, Italy). The two protocols permitted the following information: total time, ideal time (best sprint x best trial) and decrement score (Bishop *et al.*, 2001). In addition, standing long jump and 60-s sit-ups were also assessed (Council of Europe, 1988). Information about sport experience was obtained by interviews and confirmed by the Portuguese Soccer Federation. Based on test and re-test design, the technical error of measurement (TEM) was calculated (Mueller and Martorell, 1988) for RDA, and intra-class correlation coefficients (ICC), % of coefficients of variation (CV), and their 95% confidence intervals (95% CI). Bland-Altman plots were used to examine the agreement between consecutive trials of scores derived from RDA test. Statistical significance was set to a p value < 0.05. Statistical analyses were performed using the software IBM SPSS v.20 for Mac OS (SPSS Inc., IBM Company, NY, USA).

49.3 RESULTS

Regarding the properties of RDA, values of ICC ranged from 0.543 to 0.808 for the trials, 0.878 for total time and 0.891 for ideal time. The coefficient for decrement score (RDA-DS) is very low. TEM fluctuates between 0.45 and 0.99 seconds for the singular trials and 2.78 s and 2.48 s for total time (RDA-TT) and ideal time (RDA-IT), respectively. Coefficients of reliability were below 0.80 for all single trials and > 0.80 for the composite variables, except for RDA-DS (decrement score). For RDA-TT and RDA-IT, %CV was 4.07% and 3.89%, respectively. Bivariate correlations between the variance in within subject in RDA scores and age, % of PMS, stature, BM, TV, FM (%) and FFM (kg) plus performance tests are presented in Table 49.2.

The magnitude of coefficients was low or very low. Regarding differences in RDA-TT (session 2 - session 1), the variable suggested an inverse correlation with training experience, CA, %PMS, TV and sit-ups and, in parallel, direct relationships with RSA-TT and RSA-IT. RDA-IT was directly related to standing long jump and RSA scores. Note that higher RSA scores correspond to poorer performances, which means that there is an inverse relationship, suggested between fitness in RSA and discrepancy between sessions. Figure 49.1 represents the plot of within-individual variation by the magnitude of the variable taking into account limits of agreement (1.96 std. deviation). In the left panel (A), it is possible to observe 2 critical cases, while in the right panel (B) two cases were also problematic. This corresponds to 8% of the total sample.

Table 49.1 Coefficients (ICC) obtained for repeated measurements, TEM, reliability coefficient and %CV in young soccer players (*n*=25).

Variables	ICC Coefficient	ICC 95% CI	TEM	Reliability Coefficient	%CV
RDA trial 1	0.643	0.332 to 0.828	0.70s	0.49	7.37
RDA trial 2	0.589	0.253 to 0.798	0.99s	0.44	10.16
RDA trial 3	0.656	0.352 to 0.835	0.72s	0.65	7.31
RDA trial 4	0.684	0.396 to 0.850	0.77s	0.54	7.86
RDA trial 5	0.808	0.607 to 0.912	0.45s	0.80	4.63
RDA trial 6	0.543	0.188 to 0.772	0.78s	0.55	7.95
RDA trial 7	0.753	0.509 to 0.885	0.73s	0.64	7.44
RDA – Tt	0.878	0.739 to 0.945	2.78s	0.83	4.07
RDA – It	0.891	0.765 to 0.951	2.48s	0.85	3.89
RDA – DS	0.068	-0.336 to 0.451	3.90%	0.12	54.49

Table 49.2 Bivariate correlations between within-subject differences derived from repeated measurements and several other characteristics (training experience, chronological age, body size, estimated body composition and fitness parameters) for the total sample (*n*=25).

Variables	RDA TT 2 - RDATT 1	RDA IT 2 – RDA IT 1
Training experience (y)	-0.240	0.029
Chronological age (y)	-0.208	-0.179
Predicted mature stature (%)	-0.246	-0.136
Stature (cm)	-0.226	-0.095
Body mass (kg)	0.203	-0.021
Thigh volume (L)	0.142	0.067
Fat mass (%)	0.201	0.147
Fat free mass (kg)	0.155	-0.096
Standing long jump (cm)	-0.307	0.357
Sit-ups (#)	-0.248	-0.222
RSA – TT (s)	0.294	0.324
RSA – IT (s)	0.347	0.351
RSA – DS (%)	-0.081	0.028

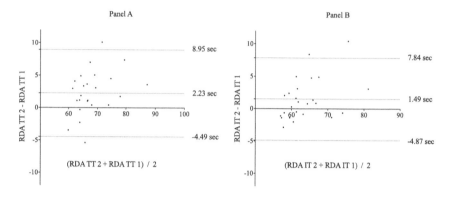

Figure 49.1 Bland-Altman plots between differences of RDA total time (panel A) and RDA ideal time (panel B) derived from session 2 and 1 (Y-axis) and the mean of the two sessions (X-axis considering limits of agreement at 95%).

49.4 DISCUSSION

The RDA protocol is a promising tool to combine physical fitness and soccer-specific control of the ball, but the current data suggest that the properties of the test may be influenced by experience in the sport and fitness level in other components such as lower limb and abdominal strength and RSA. A reliability coefficient of 0.88 for the mean of 7 sprints with young soccer players aged 11–14, using the same protocol has been reported (Figueiredo *et al.*, 2009). A similar reliability coefficient (0.83) was obtained with the repeated dribbling ability protocol in our study. Additional research is needed to determine the magnitude of learning effect and the content validity of the test to discriminate players by competitive level. However, based on a limited sample, the current study adds additional concerns about decrement scores in RSA and RDA. Future research needs to consider additional parameters (number of steps to complete the 34.2-m course from trials 1 to 7 in the RSA and RSA protocols; number of contact with the ball in the RDA protocol) and probably variation on the number of trials. It is believed that high trained late adolescent and young adult soccer players would need 10 or 12 trials to attain fatigue. This effort to test protocols with larger number of trials may be combined with different distances and resting time.

49.5 ACKNOWLEDGMENTS AND CONTRIBUTIONS

JPD was supervised by MJCS and VS. Data collected by JPD, JRP, RAF, FS, RRG, VS, JVS, VV. Analyses performed by RRG and MJCS. AS critically reviewed the chapter. All authors approved the final version.

49.6 REFERENCES

Bangsbo, J., 1994, *Fitness Training in Football: A Scientific Approach*, (Bagsvaerd: HO and Storm).

Bishop, D., Spencer, M., Duffield, R. and Lawrence, S., 2001, The validity of a repeated sprint ability test. *Journal of Science and Medicine in Sport,* **4**, pp. 19–29.

Bradley, P.S., Sheldon, W., Wooster, B., Olsen, P., Boanas, P. and Krustrup, P., 2009, High-intensity running in English FA Premier League soccer matches. *Journal of Sports Sciences,* **27**, pp. 159–168.

Council of Europe, 1988, *Eurofit: Handbook for the Eurofit tests of Physical Fitness*, (Rome: Council of Europe).

Figueiredo, A.J., Goncalves, C.E., Coelho-e-Silva. M.J. and Malina, R.M., 2009, Youth soccer players, 11–14 years: maturity, size, function, skill and goal orientation. *Annals of Human Biology,* **39**, pp. 60–73.

Huijgen, B.C., Elferink-Gemser, M.T., Post, W. and Visscher, C., 2010, Development of dribbling in talented youth soccer players aged 12–19 years: A longitudinal study. *Journal of Sports Sciences,* **99**, pp. 689–698.

Khamis, H.J. and Roche, A.F., 1994, Predicting adult stature without using skeletal age: the Khamis-Roche method. *Pediatrics,* **94**, pp. 504–507.

Mueller, W. and Martorell, R., 1988, Reliability and accuracy of measurement. In *Anthropometric Standardization Reference Manual*, edited by Lohman T., Roche A. and Martorell R., (Champaign, Illinois: Human Kinetics).

Slaughter, M.H., Lohman, T.G., Boileau, R.A., Horswill, C.A., Stillman, R.J., Van Loan, M.D. and Bemben, D.A., 1988, Skinfold equations for estimation of body fatness in children and youth. *Human Biology,* **60**, pp. 709–723.

CHAPTER NUMBER 50

ALLOMETRIC MODELLING OF PEAK POWER OUTPUT OBTAINED FROM A FORCE-VELOCITY PROTOCOL IN PREPUBERTAL BOYS

R. Baptista[1], A. Cupido-dos-Santos[1], J.P. Duarte[1], J.R. Pereira[1], R. Rebelo-Gonçalves[1], V. Severino[1], J. Valente-dos-Santos[1], I. Rego[1], M.J. Coelho-e-Silva[1], C.A. Fontes-Ribeiro[1], L. Capranica[2], and N. Armstrong[3]

[1]University of Coimbra, Portugal; [2]University of Rome Foro Italico, Italy; [3]University of Exeter, UK

50.1 INTRODUCTION

The majority of studies reporting peak power (PP) in children and youth have obtained their data from the Wingate anaerobic test (WAnT), although it may not be the best protocol for quantifying PP because of its reliance on a single braking force (usually set as 0.74 N.kg^{-1} of body mass). The WAnT was developed to optimize mean power over the 30 seconds test rather than PP. In cycle ergometry, power is a function of flywheel velocity (revs.min^{-1}) and braking force (Fb). Previous studies identified a quasi-linear relationship between force and velocity, at pedal rates between 50 and 150 revs.min^{-1}, and a parabolic Fb-power relationship (Vandwalle et al., 1987; Winter, 1991). These functions enable the determination of the optimal load for each individual. The force-velocity test (FVT) is a promising alternative with which to determine PP. The protocol is based on a set of maximal sprints (<10-s) performed against a range of contrasting braking forces. Additionally, the appropriate normalization of performance outputs for inter-individual variability in body size underpins the clarification of growth and maturation as independent and combined determinants of PP. A previous study used multiple linear regression analyses to estimate the interrelationship between chronological age, skeletal maturation, stature, leg length, body mass, fat free mass and lower-limb volume on short-term performance assessed with both repeated sprints and a WAnT (Carvalho et al., 2011). In this study with adolescent basketball players aged 14–16 years, skeletal maturation, body mass and leg length were primary predictors for the maximal short-term power outputs, while stature and body mass appeared in the model with the running test as dependent variable. Based on a similar set of total body and lower limb size descriptors and an indicator of biological maturation, the current study was designed to obtain allometric models of PP derived from the FVT.

50.2 METHODS

The sample is composed of 66 healthy boys aged 9.0–12.0 years. All participants were classified in stage 1 of pubic hair. In addition to stature, sitting height and body mass, anthropometry included variables needed to determine lower limb volume (Jones and Pearson, 1969), fat and fat-free masses (Slaughter et al., 1988). Age at peak height velocity (APHV) was determined (Mirwald et al., 2002). The FVT was performed using a Monark 814 E (Monark-Crescent AB, Varberg, Sweden) cycle ergometer. The protocol involved a series of 4–6 maximal exercise bouts against a variety of Fb (range: 0.29 to 1.10 $N.kg^{-1}$). The initial Fb was always set at 0.74 $N.kg^{-1}$ with subsequent forces above and below this intensity (Santos et al., 2002). FVT optimal load (FVT-OL), FVT optimal velocity (FVT-OV) and resultant FVT peak power (FVT-PP) were calculated (Winter, 1991). Simple allometric exponents were obtained and subsequently stepwise multiple linear regression on log-transformed variables was used to obtain proportional multiplicative allometric models (Nevill and Holder, 1994).

50.3 RESULTS

Mean and standard deviation of the present sample is 145.4±7.1 cm (133.1-164.5 cm) for stature, 41.4±10.9 kg (26.0-86.5 kg) for body mass, 32.8±5.8 kg (23.7-57.8 kg) for FFM, 8.32±1.57 L (6.50-14.90 L) for lower limb volume, and 330±73 (190-532) W for FVT-PP. Correlations between PP and size descriptors were 0.68 (95%CI: 0.52 to 0.79) for stature, 0.65 (95%CI: 0.48 to 0.77) for leg length, 0.65 (95%CI: 0.48 to 0.77) for body mass, 0.76 (95%CI: 0.63 to 0.84) for FFM and 0.66 (95%CI: 0.50 to 0.78) for lower limb volume.

Table 50.1 Summary of multiplicative allometric models combining one size descriptor (X_i) with chronological age (CA) and estimated APHV to explain variance on FVT-PP.

X_i	Model summary combining CA			Model summary combining APHV		
	R (95%CI)	Adj R^2	SEE	R (95%CI)	Adj R^2	SEE
Stature (cm)	0.69 (0.54 to 0.80)	0.46	0.16	0.67 (0.51 to 0.79)	0.43	0.17
Leg length (cm)	0.71 (0.57 to 0.82)	0.49	0.16	0.70 (0.55 to 0.81)	0.47	0.16
Body mass (cm)	0.67 (0.45 to 0.75)	0.44	0.16	0.63 (0.45 to 0.75)	0.37	0.17
FFM (kg)	0.77 (0.64 to 0.85)	0.57	0.14	0.77 (0.66 to 0.86)	0.59	0.14
LLV (L)	0.69 (0.54 to 0.80)	0.46	0.16	0.66 (0.50 to 0.78)	0.42	0.17

Log (FVT-PP) = k . Log (X_i) + a + b (CA or APHV) + Log ε

Significant allometric exponents were obtained to produce PP outputs independent from body size: 2.97 (stature), 1.85 (leg length), 0.61 (body mass), 1.01 (FFM), 0.83 (lower limb volume). Multiplicative allometric models combining one size descriptor with chronological age (CA) or APHV are presented in Table 50.1.

50.4 DISCUSSION

In contrast to the continued application of the ratio standard to partition body size effects from performance, the current study offers scaling exponents for size descriptors. The data suggest a quasi-isometry between FFM and FVT-PP amongst individuals, that is, proportions of FVT-PP to FFM are constant regardless of size. In contrast, scaling coefficients are substantial >1.0 for stature and leg length and substantially <1.0 for body mass and LLV. The size exponents derived from the simple allometric models confirmed the observations in the literature (Carvalho *et al.*, 2011) that the relationship between stature, body mass, leg length and lower limb volume dimensions and PP is not proportional.

Explained variance in FVT-PP among prepubertal boys in multiplicative allometric models ranged from 37–59% combining CA or APHV, and above mentioned size descriptors. The most relevant model emerged from FFM (57% with CA, and 59% with APHV). Much of the variation in scaling exponents obtained from different studies is likely to be explained by differences in sample size. Additional research is needed with more accurate indicators of biological maturation such as skeletal age. Agreement between maturity status derived from skeletal age and APHV is weak (Malina *et al.*, 2012). Finally, it is important to recognize the limitations of the application of the equation used to estimate lower limb volume. For example, a recent study obtained a correlation of 0.846 between estimates of thigh volume by dual energy x-ray absorptiometry and anthropometry in Portuguese school adolescents aged 10–14 years (Coelho-e-Silva *et al.*, 2012).

50.5 ACKNOWLEDGMENTS AND CONTRIBUTIONS

RB is a PhD student at the University of Coimbra (obtained the master degree supervised by ACS and CAFR and is being provisionally supervised by MJCS, ACS, LC. Data collected by RB, ACS and CAFR. This particular output was planned by MJCS and data analysed by RB and MJCS. ACS substantially contributed in the interpretation of data. NA critically reviewed the chapter. All authors approved the final version.

50.6 REFERENCES

Carvalho, H.M., Coelho-e-Silva, M.J., Gonçalves, C.E., Philippaerts, R.M., Castagna, C. and Malina, R.M., 2011, Age-related variation of anaerobic power after controlling for size and maturation in adolescent basketball players. *Annals of Human Biology*, **38**, pp. 721–727.

Coelho-e-Silva, M.J., Malina, R.M., Simões, F., Valente-dos-Santos, J., Martins, R.A.,Vaz-Ronque, E.R., Petroski, E.L., Minderico, C., Silva, A.M., Baptista, F. and Sardinha, L.B., 2013, Determination of thigh volume in youth with anthropometry and DXA. *European Journal of Sport Science*, doi: org/10.1080/17461391.2013.767945.

Jones, P.R., and Pearson, J., 1969, Anthropometric determination of leg fat and muscle plus bone volumes in young male and female adults. *Journal of Physiology*, **204**, pp. 63–66.

Malina, R.M., Coelho-e-Silva, M.J., Figueiredo, A.J., Carling, C. and Beunen, G.P., 2012, Interrelationships among invasive and non-invasive indicators of biological maturation in adolescent male soccer players. *Journal of Sports Sciences*, **30**, pp. 1705–1717.

Mirwald, R.L., Baxter-Jones, A.D.G., Bailey, D.A. and Beunen, G.P., 2002, An assessment of maturity from anthropometric measurements. *Medicine and Science in Sports and Exercise*, **34**, pp. 689–694.

Nevill, A. and Holder, R., 1994, Modelling maximum oxygen uptake - A case study in non-linear regression model formulation and comparison. *Journal of the Royal Statistic Society*, **43**, pp. 653–666.

Santos, A.M.C., Welsman, J.R., De Ste Croiz, M.B.A. and Armstrong, N., 2002, Age-and sex-related differences in optimal peak power. *Pediatric Exercise Sciences*, **14**, pp. 202–212.

Slaughter, M.H., Lohman, T.G., Boileau, R.A., Horswill, C.A., Stillman, R.J., Van Loan, M.D., Bemben, D.A., 1988, Skinfold equations for estimation of body fatness in children and youth. *Human Biology*, **60**, pp. 709–723.

Vandewalle, H., Peres, G. and Monod, H., 1987, Standard anaerobic exercise tests. *Sports Medicine,* **4**, pp. 268–289.

Winter, E.M., Brookes, F.P.C. and Hamley, E.J., 1989, Optimised loads for external power output during brief, maximal cycling. *Journal of Sports Sciences*, **7**, pp. 69–70.

IS GYMNASTICS EXPOSURE ASSOCIATED WITH SKELETAL BENEFITS IN THE FOREARM IN YOUNG CHILDREN?

S.A. Jackowski [1], M.C. Erlandson [1,2,3], R. Gruodyte-Raciene [1,4], S.A. Kontulainen[1], and A. Baxter-Jones[1]

[1]College of Kinesiology, University of Saskatchewan, Canada; [2]University Health Network, Osteoporosis and Women's Health, Canada; [3]Department of Medicine, University of Toronto, Canada; [4]Lithuanian Sports University, Lithuania

51.1 INTRODUCTION

The amount of bone gained during childhood and adolescence impacts greatly on lifetime skeletal health and it is well accepted that physical activity during growth increases bone acquisition. Gymnastics training results in unique high mechanical loading to the skeleton and therefore, provides an excellent model for assessing the effects of weight-bearing physical activity on bone development (Daly *et al.*, 1999). Young recreational gymnasts experience loads up to 3–10 times that of body weight on their feet and hands. Previous studies in young adolescent competitive female gymnasts have shown that they have 8–23% areal bone mineral density (aBMD, cm/g^2), at the total body, lumbar spine and hip (Laing *et al.*, 2002; Faulkner *et al.*, 2003; Erlandson *et al.*, 2011a). It is often presumed that higher the aBMD or BMC translates to greater bone strength but when estimating whole bone strength (resistance to fracture) it is important to assess bone size and geometry in addition to parameters charactering bone mass and areal density (Kontulainen *et al.*, 2007). Therefore, it is important to assess the geometrical indices of bone and not simply aBMD or BMC. Peripheral quantitative computed tomography (pQCT) is a novel technology that is able to measure bone cross sectional properties in three dimensions. It has been recently observed that early recreational and precompetitive gymnastic participation may confer 6–25% greater adjusted bone strength, as assessed by pQCT, at the distal radius compared to individuals not involved in gymnastic training (Erlandson *et al.*, 2011b). What remain unsubstantiated are the long term effects of early recreational gymnastics on the development of childhood bone strength. Therefore, the primary purpose of this study was to investigate whether gymnastics exposure was associated with estimated bone strength development derived from pQCT at the distal radius in young males and females.

51.2 METHODS

Participants were drawn from the University of Saskatchewan's Young Recreational Gymnast Study. This cohort consists of 178 children recruited into a mix-longitudinal study examining the influence of early life gymnastic participation on bone development (2006–2012; Erlandson *et al.*, 2011a). pQCT scan were implemented into the study in 2008 and by 2012, there were 3 years of pQCT data collected in children between 4 and 10 years of age. The gymnasts consisted of individuals who were participating in recreation and/or precompetitive gymnastics programmes at one of three competitive gymnastics clubs in Saskatoon. The non-gymnastic controls were individuals recruited from other local recreational sport programmes and camps (soccer, T-ball, basketball and karate). Participants were excluded from the current study if they had any condition that prevented them from performing exercise safely, had any condition known to affect bone development, or did not have a valid distal radius scan at two or more assessment occasions. This resulted in the inclusion of 126 participants (58 males, 68 females) consisting of 75 gymnasts (35 males, 40 females) and 51 non gymnasts (23 males, 28 females). Consent was obtained from all parents and/or guardians and verbal assent was obtained from all children. All procedures and protocols were approved by the Biomedical Research Ethics Board at the University of Saskatchewan.

Height was recorded without shoes to the nearest 0.1 cm using a wall mounted stadiometer. Weight was measured on a calibrated digital scale to the nearest 0.5 kg. Cross sectional slices of the left radius and tibia were measured by pQCT (XCT, Stratec Medizintechnik GmbH, Pforzheim, Germany). For this present study only data from the radius are presented. The radius was scanned at the distal and shaft sites represented by the 4% and 65% of the limb length proximal to the wrist, respectively. All scans were performed using a voxel size of 0.4mm at a speed of 20mm/s. All scans were analyzed using Stratec software, Version 6.0. Scans obtained from the distal radius and tibia 4% site were analyzed for total cross sectional bone area (ToA, mm2), bone density (ToD, mg/cm3), and bone content (ToC, mg/mm). All images at the 4% distal sites were analysed using contour mode 1, 280 mg/cm^3 to separate bone from surrounding soft tissue. Peel mode 2 with the inner threshold of 480 mg/cm^3 was used to separate trabecular bone. Additionally, at the distal radius bone strength index (BSI) was calculated (ToA x ToD^2) as a measure of estimate compressive strength. Images at the 65% radius site were analyzed using contour mode 1, 480mg/cm^3 to separate bone from the surrounding soft tissue. Separation Mode 4 with inner and outer thresholds of 480 mg/cm^3 was used to determine the cortical bone cross-sectional area (CoA, mm^2), density (CoD, mg/cm^3), content (CoC, mg/mm), and polar stress strain index (SSIp, mm^3). Forearm muscle area was measured and analyzed according to the manufacturer's recommendations, using Contour Mode 1 with a threshold of 40 mg/cm^3 and muscle filter C02 at the 65% sites.

Physical activity was assessed annually using the Netherlands Physical Activity Questionnaire (NPAQ). The NPAQ ranks individuals based on parental reports of their child's current activity preferences and everyday activity choices. The questionnaire response ranges from 7 (low level physical activity) to 35 (high level physical activity).

All variables were assessed for normality and violations were adjusted using logarithmic transformations. Multilevel random effects models were constructed to assess association in the development of pQCT estimated bone strength measures between individuals exposed and not exposed to gymnastics whilst controlling for age, radius length, weight, physical activity, muscle area, sex and hours of training. A total of 8 independent multilevel random effects models were constructed using MLwiN version 2.26 (Centre for Multilevel Modelling, University of Bristol, UK). Significance was accepted if the estimate mean coefficient was greater than twice the standard error of the estimates (SEE, ie. $p<0.05$).

51.3 RESULTS

Distal Radius (4% Site): Once age, radius length, weight, muscle area, physical activity, sex and hours of gymnastic training were accounted, it was observed that individuals exposed to recreational gymnastics had significantly greater ToA ($+18.0 \pm 7.5$ mm^2), and ToC ($+6.0 \pm 3.0$ g/cm) than individuals not exposed to gymnastics. ($p<0.05$). It was observed that weight, muscle area, and sex contributed to the prediction of ToA, and ToC, while physical activity and muscle area contributed to the prediction of ToD and only muscle area contributed to the prediction of BSI. Males were observed to have greater ToA ($+ 17.6 \pm 5.3$ mm^2), and ToC ($+5.6 \pm 1.9$ g/cm) regardless of their gymnastic exposure compared to females; **Proximal Radius (65% Site):** No significant differences between individuals who were exposed and not exposed to gymnastics were observed for any bone measure at the radial shaft ($p>0.05$); however, it was observed that weight, physical activity and muscle area contributed to the prediction of CoD ($p<0.05$). In contrast, only weight and muscle area significantly contributed to the prediction of CoC ($p<0.05$), while only muscle area contributed significantly to the prediction of CoA ($p<0.05$). For SSIp, radius length and muscle area significantly contributed to the prediction models ($p<0.05$).

51.4 DISCUSSION

Young children who were exposed to recreational level gymnastics were observed to develop significantly greater ToA and ToC at the distal radius than children not exposed to gymnastics, once confounders had been controlled. Gymnastics participation involves movements that dynamically load the upper and lower body. These unique movements may help to stimulate skeletal adaptation especially at regions, such as the distal radius, that do not typically undergo daily loading. These observations parallel previous findings that have documented skeletal benefits associated with gymnastics training (Laing *et al.,* 2002; Faulkner *et al.,* 2003; Erlandson *et al.,* 2011a; b) and further suggest that early life gymnastics participation may be advantageous to bone size and mass development. Additionally, it was observed that there were significant sex differences in the development of bone strength measures at the distal radius, with males having greater ToA and ToC. No sex differences, however, were observed at the radial shaft. These findings support previous literature that suggests the sex differences in bone strength development may be site specific (Ward *et al.,* 2005). In conclusion, there are site and sex specific differences in the development of forearm bone strength, but despite the differences, early life recreational gymnastic participation provides skeletal benefits at the distal radius. Thus, childhood gymnastics may be advantageous to forearm bone strength development.

51.5 REFERENCES

Daly R.M., Rich, P.A., Klein, R. and Bass, S., 1999, Effects of high-impact exercise on ultrasonic and biochemical indices of skeletal status: A prospective study in young male gymnasts. *Journal of Bone and Mineral Research,* **14**, pp. 1222–1230.

Erlandson, M.C., Kontulainen, S.A., Chilibeck, P.D., Arnold, C.M. and Baxter-Jones, A.D., 2011a, Bone mineral accrual in 4- to 10- year old precompetitive, recreational gymnasts : a 4-year longitudinal study. *Journal of Bone and Mineral Research,* **26**, pp. 1313–1320.

Erlandson, M.C., Kontulainen, S.A. and Baxter-Jones, A.D., 2011b, Precompetitive and recreational gymnasts have greater bone density, mass and estimated strength at the distal radius in young childhood. *Osteoporosis International,* **22**, pp. 75–84.

Faulkner, R.A., Forwood, M.R., Beck, T.J., Mafukidze, J.C., Russell, K. and Wallace, W., 2003, Strength indices of the proximal femur and shaft in prepubertal female gymnasts. *Medicine and Science in Sports and Exercise,* **35**, pp. 513–518.

Kontulainen, S.A., Hughes, J.M., Macdonald, H.M. and Johnston, J.D., 2007, The biomechanical basis of bone strength development during growth. *Medicine and Sport Science;* **51**, pp. 13–32.

Laing, E.M., Massoni, J.A., Nickols-Richardson, S.M., Modlesky, C.M., O'Connor, P.J. and Lewis, R.D., 2002, A prospective study of bone mass and body composition in female adolescent gymnasts. *Journal of Pediatrics,* **141**, pp. 211–216.

Ward, K.A., Roberts, S.A., Adams, J.E. and Mughal, M.Z., 2005, Bone geometry and density in the skeleton of pre-pubertal gymnasts and school children. *Bone;* **36**, pp. 1012–1018.

MATURITY OF CHILDREN AND ADOLESCENTS BELONGING TO WELL DEFINED ACTIVITY GROUPS: SEDENTARY, LEISURE, SPORTS

I. Fragoso[1], J.Teles[1], L. Massuça[1,2], J. Albuquerque[1], and C. Barrigas[1]

[1]Faculty of Human Kinetics, Technical University of Lisbon, Portugal; [2]Faculty of Physical Education and Sport, ULHT, Portugal

52.1 INTRODUCTION

Regular physical activity (PA) and sport participation are generally associated with both immediate and long-term health, as well as wellness benefits. During the last decades adults turned child routines into adult-like routines, changed children's free time into institutionalized time, turning children into small adults. Children stay away from their family all day long and, when they return home, they have to do their homework and play within the house (gameboy, playstation or watching television). In other words, children's free time has been significantly reduced and the time spent in sedentary activities increased drastically and radically. Although children demonstrate an extraordinary capacity for mobility during childhood, they have no time to express it (except during a short period when they are engaged in any organized activity).

The health benefits of PA are well documented (e.g., Fragoso *et al.*, 2007), and data show a weaker, but significant, association between PA and maturity status during childhood (Ekelund *et al.*, 2005) and a strong association during adolescence (Fragoso *et al.*, 2004). However, most of the studies focused on the benefits and disadvantages of young people's sport participation are based on the assumptions that different types of sport participation are associated with different levels of daily life energy expenditure and that chronological age can be a good indicator of biological and social characteristics of an adolescent population.

There is a lack of confirmation whether different groups of sport participation have different maturity status. Thus, this study aimed to investigate the association of well-defined PA groups (i.e., sedentary, leisure, sports) with biological maturity of children and adolescents.

52.2 METHODS

The objective and procedures of the study were explained to parents and only those children whose legal guardians had signed an informed consent were included in the sample. The sample was composed of 835 children and adolescents of both sexes, with ages between 11 and 16 years old, engaged in different sport participation groups. The independent variable, PA group, was divided into three categories: (i) Sedentary or non active (male, n=154; female, n=249), gathering children with a PA time lower than or equal to 60 min; (ii) Leisure PA (male, n=115; female, n=93), composed by children with a weekly PA time higher than 60 min, from which at least 75% accounting for leisure sport; and (iii) regular competitive Sports (male, n=168; female, n=56), with children that have a weekly time of PA higher than 60 min with at least 75% accounting for competitive sport.

The anthropometric measures were obtained according to the ISAK procedures (Marfell-Jones *et al.*, 2006) and included: stature, sitting height and weight. All anthropometric measures were taken by accredited Level 2 ISAK anthropometrists under the supervision of an ISAK Level 4 anthropometrist (Intra-observer TEM for stature: $R \geq 0.98$).

Maturity measures were: skeletal age (SA) obtained through radiographs of the left hand and wrist and physical maturity (PM) calculated by the formula: PM = PS/PAS, where PS is the child's present stature and PAS is the child's predicted adult stature (through SA or through Khamis and Roche, 1994). Radiography was performed in one session, and the maturity ratings were done by two examiners trained at the Faculty of Human Kinetics of Lisbon blinded to the chronological age of the subjects. Thirteen bones were rated by comparing the ossification stage of each bone according to the Tanner-Whitehouse III Method – TW3 method (Tanner *et al.*, 2001). PAS was also calculated according to the method reported by KR (Khamis and Roche, 1994), and current stature, current weight and mid-parent stature were used as predictor variables, i.e., PAS = $\beta0$ + $\beta1$stature + $\beta2$weight + $\beta3$mid-parent stature (where $\beta0$ is a constant, and $\beta1$, $\beta2$, $\beta3$ are coefficients). Finally, weight, standing height, sitting height and estimated leg length (stature minus sitting height), were used to predict maturity offset (time before or after peak height velocity – PHV). Age at PHV (APHV; years) was estimated from chronological age and maturity offset at each observation (Mirwald *et al.*, 2002).

Descriptive statistics were performed using the mean and standard deviation. Several analysis of covariance (univariate ANCOVA), were conducted to evaluate the association between the PA group and maturity, controlling by decimal age. Preliminary checks were conducted to ensure that there was no violation of the ANCOVA assumptions. The statistical analyses were performed with the software IBM SPSS v.21 and the level of significance was set at 5%.

52.3 RESULTS

For APHV, skeletal age and maturity offset variables, no significant differences were found, after controlling by decimal age, for both boys and girls. Relative to percentage of child's predicted adult stature variables (PPAS; TW3 and KR methods), and after controlling for decimal age, no significant differences were found in boys, but significant differences were attained in girls (PPAS: TW3, low effect; KR, low effect). Multiple comparisons showed that sedentary girls have significant higher PPAS than: (i) sports girls (TW3 method; p = 0.042), and (ii) leisure girls (KR method; p = 0.023) (see Table 52.1).

Table 52.1 Summary statistics and ANCOVA results when evaluating the effect of Activity group on maturity variables, after controlling for the effect of decimal age, for boys and girls

Activity group	Boys					Girls				
	Descriptive			ANCOVA		Descriptive			ANCOVA	
	N	Mean	SD	Mean	SE	N	Mean	SD	Mean	SE
APHV (years)										
Sedentary	154	13.87	0.66	13.87	0.05	249	12.46	0.70	12.45	0.03
Leisure	115	13.80	0.67	13.81	0.06	93	12.45	0.71	12.54	0.05
Sports	166	13.79	0.64	13.78	0.05	56	12.60	0.61	12.48	0.06
	F(2,433) = 1.022, p = 0.361 (n.s.)					F(2,394) = 1.378, p = 0.253 (n.s.)				
Skeletal age (years)										
Sedentary	154	13.28	2.56	13.35	0.11	247	14.06	2.21	14.03	0.08
Leisure	115	13.17	2.53	13.28	0.12	93	13.52	2.48	13.85	0.12
Sports	166	13.37	2.40	13.23	0.10	56	14.10	2.27	13.68	0.16
	F(2,431) = 0.352, p = 0.703 (n.s.)					F(2,392) = 2.395, p = 0.093 (n.s.)				
PPAS (TW3 method) (%)										
Sedentary	154	90.33	6.90	90.54	0.23	233	96.14	4.29	96.07	0.17
Leisure	115	90.02	6.76	90.35	0.26	93	94.70	4.97	95.35	0.26
Sports	166	90.68	6.57	90.26	0.22	56	95.89	4.22	95.14	0.34
	F(2,431) = 0.392, p = 0.676 (n.s.)					F(2,378) = 4.669, p = 0.010, η_p^2 = 0.024				
PPAS (KR method) (%)										
Sedentary	154	90.16	6.82	90.36	0.22	249	95.51	4.33	95.46	0.15
Leisure	115	89.85	6.23	90.16	0.25	93	94.06	4.98	94.69	0.25
Sports	168	90.56	6.25	90.16	0.21	56	95.54	4.45	94.70	0.32
	F(2,433) = 0.271, p = 0.763 (n.s.)					F(2,394) = 4.918, p = 0.008, , η_p^2 = 0.024				
Maturity offset +10 (Mirwald et al., 2002)										
Sedentary	154	9.64	1.71	9.70	0.05	249	11.27	1.39	11.26	0.03
Leisure	115	9.67	1.67	9.76	0.06	93	10.94	1.58	11.17	0.05
Sports	168	9.90	1.71	9.80	0.05	56	11.54	1.56	11.23	0.06
	F(2,433) = 1.022, p = 0.361 (n.s.)					F(2,394) = 1.378, p = 0.253 (n.s.)				

52.4 CONCLUSION

This study aimed to investigate the association of well-defined PA groups (sedentary, leisure, sports) on biological maturity of children and adolescents. No significant effects of activity groups were observed (for both boys and girls) in age at peak height velocity, skeletal age and maturity offset variables. However, sedentary girls, showed a significantly higher percentage of child's predicted adult stature than: sports (TW3 method), and leisure (KR method) girls. These findings are in accordance with the literature (Cumming et al., 2012; Hunter Smart et al., 2012; Sherar et al., 2010), and confirm: (i) that less active girls are advanced in maturity status, and (ii) that there is an inverse association between biological maturity and PA in well defined PA groups. Moreover, the different effect of PA groups in boys and girls, emphasize the study of sex-related variance.

52.5 REFERENCES

Cumming, S.P., Sherar, L.B., Pindus, D.M., Coelho-e-Silva, M.J., Malina, R.M. and Jardine, P.R., 2012, A biocultural model of maturity-associated variance in adolescent physical activity. *International Review of Sport and Exercise Psychology*, **5**, pp. 23–43.

Ekelund, U., Neovius, M., Linné, Y., Brage, S., Wareham, N.J. and Rossner, S., 2005, Associations between physical activity and fat mass in adolescents: the Stockholm weight development study. *American Journal of Clinical Nutrition*, **81**, pp. 355–360.

Fragoso, I., Fortes, M., Vieira, F. and Canto e Castro, L., 2004, Different maturational levels during adolescence: A methodological problem. In *Kinanthropometry VIII*, London, edited by Reilly, T. and Marfell-Jones, M., (London: Routledge. Taylor & Francis Group), pp. 68–81.

Fragoso, I., Vieira, F., Barrigas, C., Baptista, F., Teixeira, P., Santa-Clara, H., Mil-Homens, P. and Sardinha L., 2007, Influence of Maturation on Morphology, Food Ingestion and Motor Performance Variability of Lisbon Children Aged Between 7 to 8 Years. In *Kinanthropometry X. Proceedings of the 10th Conference of the International Society for the Advancement of Kinanthropometry (ISAK)*, London, edited by Marfell-Jones, M. and Olds, T., (London: Routledge. Taylor & Francis Group), pp. 9–24.

Hunter Smart, J.E., Cumming, S.P., Sherar, L.B., Standage, M., Neville, H. and Malina, R.M., 2012, Maturity associated variance in physical activity and health-related quality of life in adolescent females. A mediated effects model. *Journal of Physical Activity and Health*, **9**, pp. 86–95

Khamis H.J. and Roche A.F., 1994, Predicting adult height without using skeletal age: the khamis-roche method. *Pediatrics*, **94**, pp. 504–507.

Marfell-Jones, M., Olds, T., Stewart, A. and Lindsay Carter, J.E., 2006, *International Standards for Anthropometric Assessment*, (Potchestroom: ISAK).

Mirwald, R.L., Baxter-Jones, A.D.G., Bailey, D.A. and Beuner, G.P., 2002, An assessment of maturity from anthropometric measurements. *Medicine and Science in Sports and Exercise*, **34**, pp. 689–694.

Sherar, L.B., Cumming, S.P., Eisenmann, J.C., Baxter-Jones, A.D.G. and Malina, R.M., 2010, Adolescent biological maturity and physical activity: biology meets behavior. *Pediatric Exercise Science*, **22**, pp. 332–349.

Tanner, J.M., Healy, M.J.R., Goldstein, H. and Cameron, C., 2001, *Assessment of Skeletal Maturity and Prediction of Adult Height (TW3 Method)*, (London: W.B. Saunders).

This research was supported by *Fundação para a Ciência e a Tecnologia* [PTDC/DES/113156/2009].